SETON HALL UNIVERSITY

S0-BJH-689

DATE DUE

JAN 2 2 2001		4445 782	
GAYLORD			PRINTED IN U.S.A.

THE BLOODBORNE PATHOGENS STANDARD

THE BLOODBORNE PATHOGENS STANDARD

A Pragmatic Approach

Jon T. O'Neal, M.D., M.P.H.

SETON HALL UNIVERSITY
WALSH LIBRARY
SO. ORANGE, N.J.

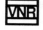 VAN NOSTRAND REINHOLD
I(T)P A Division of International Thomson Publishing Inc.

New York • Albany • Bonn • Boston • Detroit • London • Madrid • Melbourne
Mexico City • Paris • San Francisco • Singapore • Tokyo • Toronto

Copyright © 1996 by Van Nostrand Reinhold

I(T)P® A division of International Thomson Publishing, Inc.
The ITP logo is a trademark under license

RA
642
.B56
O54
1996

Printed in the United States of America
For more information, contact:

Van Nostrand Reinhold
115 Fifth Avenue
New York, NY 10003

Chapman & Hall GmbH
Pappelallee 3
69469 Weinheim
Germany

Chapman & Hall
2-6 Boundary Row
London
SE1 8HN
United Kingdom

International Thomson Publishing Asia
221 Henderson Road #05-10
Henderson Building
Singapore 0315

Thomas Nelson Australia
102 Dodds Street
South Melbourne, 3205
Victoria, Australia

International Thomson Publishing Japan
Hirakawacho Kyowa Building, 3F
2-2-1 Hirakawacho
Chiyoda-ku, 102 Tokyo
Japan

Nelson Canada
1120 Birchmount Road
Scarborough, Ontario
Canada M1K 5G4

International Thomson Editores
Campos Eliseos 385, Piso 7
Col. Polanco
11560 Mexico D.F. Mexico

All rights reserved. No part of this work covered by the copyright hereon may be reproduced or used in any form or by any means—graphic, electronic, or mechanical, including photocopying, recording, taping, or information storage and retrieval systems—without the written permission of the publisher.

1 2 3 4 5 6 7 8 9 10   BKR   01 00 99 98 97 96

Library of Congress Cataloging-in-Publication Data

O'Neal, Jon T.
    The bloodborne pathogens standard : a pragmatic approach / Jon T. O'Neal.
        p.   cm.
    Includes bibliographical references and index.
    ISBN 0-442-01779-0 (hardcover)
    1. Bloodborne infections—Prevention—Standards—United States.
2. Occupational diseases—Prevention—Standards—United States.
I. Title.
    [DNLM: 1. Infection Control—standards—United States. 2. Blood-Borne Pathogens.
3. Occupational Exposure—prevention & control—United States. 4. Disease Transmission,
Patient-to-Professional—prevention & control—United States. 5. HIV Infections—transmission.
6. Hepatitis B—transmission. WX 167 O58 1995]
RA642.B56O54   1995
614.4—dc20   95-19093
                                                                                        CIP

For the nurse in the emergency room who taught me during the first months of my internship, whom I later saw as an inpatient with hepatitis on the medicine floor.

Contents

Preface

During the summer of 1991, I was an occupational medicine resident who rotated through the Occupational Safety and Health Administration's (OSHA) Occupational Medicine Department at the Department of Labor in Washington, D.C. Quite by chance I was there during the last 2 months of the final preparation of the Bloodborne Pathogens Standard (BBPS, or the Standard), and I was tasked to write the first draft of the medical portion of the summary and explanation section. Not only did I get to review the history of the Standard, but I was also an active participant in its formation. I contributed very little to the Standard and the work group, but I gained a great deal of insight into the politics of medicine and compromise.

Understanding how and why the Bloodborne Pathogens Standard became a reality made me truly appreciate and respect the Standard, its intent, and the people who worked on it for over 5 years. This book is biased toward the Standard, not only because I was personally (though minimally) involved with it, but because I believe in it and support its goal of preventing occupational illness.

The information presented in the first part of this book is my interpretation of and comments on an important U.S. government regulation. I have used a pragmatic, simplified approach intended to help others understand and appreciate a complicated document and the actions it requires of employers and employees. The simplification process obscures fine details, and it is attention to detail that makes fine lawyers, or at least wealthy ones. My comments on this book should not be regarded as a substitute for the Standard itself, the regulatory text of which is included as Appendix A. In all cases of practical (or legal) interpretation:

> Refer to the Regulatory Text of the Standard.

If the regulatory text doesn't help, refer to the summary and explanation section of the Standard (170 pages of microscopic *Federal Register* print), which gives background information and reasoning for the regulatory text (a mere 7 1/2 pages of microscopic *Federal Register* print). Because of space constraints, and the fact that almost no one reads it, the summary and explanation section is not included in this book. Anyone charged with knowing the Standard in depth should have a complete copy of the 29 CFR Part 1910.1030 Occupational Exposure to Bloodborne Pathogens, Final Rule, as published in the *Federal Register* on Friday, December 6, 1991, which can be requested from your OSHA regional office. Note that it is the text of the 7 1/2 pages of regulatory text that is binding, not the information presented in the summary and explanation section, and certainly not my comments or the simplified explanations presented here. If you're still confused about a specific issue, call the regional or national OSHA office for clarification. If OSHA can't help, you'll have to wait for the courts to define and interpret the meaning and intent of the Standard.

Because I am a physician, I am most attuned to medical issues; therefore, I apologize for my bias toward occupational issues relating to nurses, doctors, and hospital employees. This book (like the Standard) was also written for dentists and dental personnel; nursing home, hospice, lab, research, funeral home, law enforcement, fire/rescue, and correctional facility personnel; and all others who may incur occupational exposure to bloodborne pathogens.

Readers already acquainted with the BBPS may find parts of Chapters 1–17 old news. Advanced readers, however, will benefit from the appendixes, which include not only a reformatted, and thus readable, BBPS regulatory text, but the OSHA BBPS compliance guide, the Centers for Disease Control's Universal Precautions, and other HBV and HIV resources that never seem to be available when you need them. A word of caution, however: Some of the appendixes, especially Appendix G (dated January 1990), relating to postexposure treatment, may provide recommendations and medication doses that are no longer considered treatment of choice. Readers are advised to check with qualified physicians for current recommendations before considering medical treatment related to HIV. On the other hand, most of Appendix I (dated 1987) provides recommendations for the prevention of HIV transmission in health care settings that are as appropriate today as the day they were published. At worst, the appendixes offer an easily accessible one-stop shopping guide and a historical perspective on the Standard.

For some nonmedical personnel, reading this book may be technically difficult; for others, it may seem trite and elementary. Nevertheless, both firefighters and infectious disease subspecialists should be able to learn something valuable from reading it.

Acknowledgments

W ith special thanks to Angela, Elise, Susan, Karen, Claudia, Ruth, and later Melissa, who guided me through the maze that is OSHA; Dr. Kantrowitz and the Polaroid Medical Department, who taught me about practical applications of government regulations; Phoebe, who provided insightful comments on the draft manuscript; and George, who put me up, put up with me, and laughed at my jokes.

THE BLOODBORNE
PATHOGENS
STANDARD

Chapter 1

Introduction

In the arts of life man invents nothing; but in the arts of death he outdoes Nature herself, and produces by chemistry and machinery all the slaughter of plague, pestilence, and famine.

—George Bernard Shaw

Between 200 and 300 health care workers die each year in the United States as a result of occupationally acquired hepatitis. About 2,100 per year develop symptoms of acute hepatitis. Most of these infections could be prevented by two actions—preventing exposure to hepatitis virus and preventing disease if exposure occurs. The Occupational Safety and Health Administration's Bloodborne Pathogens Standard, when condensed to its most important elements, deals with these same two actions:

Preventing exposure and preventing disease if exposure occurs.

The Bloodborne Pathogens Standard prevents exposure by mandating the use of Universal Precautions, an approach to infection control that assumes all blood is infectious (see Appendix B). Although the guidelines for Universal Precautions were published in 1988, they were only recommendations, and they were intended for health care settings, not for all workplace settings. The Standard made those recommendations into enforceable (i.e., fineable) requirements that apply to all workplaces where exposure to blood or other potentially infectious materials may occur.

The Standard prevents disease after exposure by requiring employers to provide hepatitis B vaccination free of charge (i.e., at the employer's expense) to employees. Though long recommended for workers exposed to hepatitis, the complete series of three shots is expensive (around $100 for the series), and many health care workers were hesitant to take the series because of both cost and concerns about possible infectiousness.

The now mandatory use of Universal Precautions also prevents exposure to other bloodborne pathogens, including the human immunodeficiency virus (HIV), the virus that causes acquired immunodeficiency syndrome (AIDS). Unfortunately, there is no vaccine or medication that prevents the development of AIDS after exposure or infection.[1] During the first 10 years of the AIDS epidemic, fewer than 100 cases of occupationally acquired HIV infections and fewer than 20 deaths due to AIDS were documented in health care workers. This is not to belittle concerns about occupationally acquired HIV infection; it is a real risk, it's just not as important in numbers as occupational hepatitis B virus (HBV) infection.

When compared to hepatitis, the risk of acquiring HIV infection on the job is minimal.[2] The fear of acquiring AIDS on the job is great. The increasing real risk of HIV infection outside the workplace created an AIDS hysteria that led to creation of the Bloodborne Pathogens Standard, which helps prevent hepatitis B infection in the workplace.

OSHA estimates that the Standard will prevent approximately 8,500 cases of hepatitis B infection and 190 deaths per year in workers.[3] Quite simply, and above all other considerations, the pragmatic reason for the Bloodborne Pathogens Standard is to prevent hepatitis B infections and deaths in workers.

---

1. Some medications may delay the development of symptoms, or treat certain infections, but none are thought to prevent the eventual development of AIDS after HIV infection.

2. Except, possibly, in sex workers, one of the few occupations OSHA doesn't regulate.

3. OSHA estimates that compliance with the Standard will prevent 8,383–8,858 occupational and nonoccupational cases of HBV infection per year, of which 2,096–2,215 would have resulted in acute symptoms and 187–197 in death. Moreover, OSHA estimates that the Standard will prevent 253–578 employees from becoming HBV carriers, thereby stemming the spread of this disease to others.

Chapter 2

OSHA: An Overview

An Act to assure safe and healthful working conditions for working men and women. . . .

—OSHAct opening statement

THE BIRTH OF THE OSHACT[1]

Throughout the 1960s, a body of medical and scientific evidence accumulated to show that diseases such as lung cancer, asbestosis, black lung disease, and brown lung disease were associated with occupational exposures and were killing many American workers. Better mortality statistics were making these "invisible" occupational killers much more visible. During the same decade, the incidence of industrial accidents increased 29%, possibly due to increased accident rates in the war-related industries supporting the Vietnam War. In the late 1960s, the National Safety Council estimated that more than 14,000 workers were killed and 2 million workers were injured and disabled on the job each year. There was clear evidence that both illnesses and injuries were increasing in the U.S. working population.

---

1. This introductory history is taken from Nicholas Ashford's and Charles Caldart's book *Technology, Law, and the Working Environment.* New York: Van Nostrand Reinhold, 1991.

In 1968, President Johnson submitted a bill to Congress that would have created a comprehensive occupational health and safety program. Because of intense industry opposition, the bill never reached the House or Senate floor. In November 1968, 78 miners were killed in a mine explosion in Farmington, West Virginia. A few weeks later, an oil rig off the southern California coast exploded, covering miles of beach with black sludge. These two incidents received extensive media coverage and heightened public concern over occupational and environmental safety issues, setting the political stage for congressional action.

In 1969, striking workers shut down West Virginia's mines and marched on the state capitol to demand workers' compensation for black lung disease. The threat of a national expansion of the strike forced Congress to pass the Coal Mine Health and Safety Act of 1969 and gave impetus to the demands for comprehensive occupational safety and health legislation. Finally, in 1970, during the Nixon administration, and after considerable debate and compromise, the 91st Congress passed the Occupational Safety and Health Act of 1970 (OSHAct), which was signed into law on December 29, 1970.

THE OSHACT

The OSHAct created OSHA, placing it within the Department of Labor, and the National Institute for Occupational Safety and Health (NIOSH), placing it within the Department of Health, Education and Welfare (now Health and Human Services). NIOSH does research and makes recommendations to OSHA, which develops and enforces standards. NIOSH makes health-based recommendations to OSHA, which makes labor-based standards, but both agencies are charged with ensuring safe and healthy working conditions for workers.

Since the actual rulemaking and enforcement powers (i.e., inspections and monetary fines) are delegated to OSHA, this agency is more well known. NIOSH actually does great work, but OSHA is not obligated to follow its recommendations. Before a final standard is created, OSHA receives input from many different sources, such as NIOSH, the Centers for Disease Control (CDC, also within the Department of Health and Human Services), employees, employers, unions, and other executive branch departments and interested parties.

Coverage of the OSHAct extends to all employers and their employees in the 50 states, the District of Columbia, Puerto Rico, and all other territories under federal government jurisdiction. "Employer" is defined as any person engaged in a business affecting commerce who has employees, but does not include the United States or political subdivision of a state, which means that federal and state government employees are not covered.[2] Nor are self-employed persons and family farm employers covered under the Act.[3]

OSHA, in addition to developing standards, has the authority to require recordkeeping, employee education, and workplace inspections, as well as issue citations and penalties. Each of these areas, except standards development, will be covered in later chapters specifically as they relate to the Bloodborne Pathogens Standard (BBPS).

STANDARDS DEVELOPMENT

OSHA can begin the process of developing standards either on its own initiative, or in response to petitions from other groups, such as the Department of Health and Human Services, NIOSH, employer or labor representatives, or any other interested person—i.e., anyone who may be affected by a workplace hazard. If OSHA is looking for background information, it may publish an Advance Notice of Proposed Rulemaking (ANPR) in the *Federal Register,* a government publication that notifies the general public of proposed and final regulations and standards. An ANPR is published to solicit information that can be used in drafting a proposal. If OSHA has enough initial information and decides to develop a standard, it publishes its intentions in the *Federal Register* as a Notice of Proposed Rulemaking (NPR).

The Notice of Proposed Rulemaking includes the terms of the new rule and states a specific time, usually 60 days or more from the date of publication, during which the public may respond in written form.[4] Information received in response to an NPR is catalogued and stored in the docket department for review and use in making the final standard. Interested persons or groups who submit arguments and pertinent information may request a public hearing, in which case OSHA may

---

2. Actually, the Act requires these agencies to comply with standards consistent with those OSHA issues for private sector employers, but government agencies are not liable for fines.

3. Farmers have some of the highest rates of injury and death of any occupation but, unfortunately, are not covered.

4. The OSHAct states that the NPR should give interested persons 30 days after publication to submit written data or comments, but they usually allow more time than the Act states. In turnaround play, OSHA usually takes more time to publish the final standard than the Act stipulates. A currently pending OSHA legislative reform act provides greater time limits for standard development.

schedule a public hearing, announcing the time and place for it in the *Federal Register*. After the close of the comment period and public hearing, OSHA must publish—again, in the *Federal Register*—the full, final text of the standard, the date it becomes effective, an explanation of the standard, and the reasons for implementing it.

The standards development process was designed to allow any and all interested parties to have a say in the standard. OSHA must therefore weigh all information it receives, not just NIOSH input, in making the final standard. Business, employer, employee, union, and health comments are rarely the same, and it's left up to OSHA to determine the scientific, political, and economic impact of a standard. It is not an easy job, and in the end, it seems no one is ever completely happy.

The vast majority of businesses, employers, and employees around the country are not aware of or involved with the standards development process and probably have never seen a copy of the *Federal Register*. The first they hear about an OSHA standard is a week or so after it's been published, giving them only a few weeks to comply with a standard they know nothing about. But the process was designed to solicit the active participation of interested parties, and it works reasonably well.[5]

INSPECTIONS

OSHA is given authority to enforce its standards by conducting workplace inspections. The OSHA inspector, called a "compliance officer," is authorized to enter, without delay and at reasonable times, any place where work is performed by an employee. Unlike standards development, inspections are conducted *without* advance notice. The inspection process is covered in Chapter 15, which also goes into more detail about compliance issues.

Inspections related to bloodborne pathogens were, however, conducted by OSHA even before the Standard came into effect. This was possible because OSHA has the authority to inspect and fine based on the General Duty Clause of the OSHAct, which states: "Each employer shall furnish to each of his employees employment and a place of employment which are free from recognized hazards

---

[5]In recent years, the greatest barrier to standards development has been not the employers, employees, or unions, but the executive branch. President Reagan, during his first month in office, issued an executive order giving the Office of Management and Budget (OMB) power to do economic analysis of the implementation costs of federal regulations. During some cases in the Reagan years, OMB delayed standards for several years. Until 1980, OSHA had been averaging two to three health regulations per year. Not one standard was issued during the first 2 1/2 years of the Reagan administration.

that are causing or are likely to cause death or serious physical harm to his employees."

After Universal Precautions became the standard of good preventive practice in many hospitals, and since HBV and HIV were recognized hazards, OSHA compliance officers were fining employers for gross abuses of Universal Precautions recommendations. However, because the protective procedures were merely recommendations, OSHA was still on shaky ground in cases where fines were legally challenged by employers. Following the issuance of the Standard, OSHA could cite the provisions of the Standard instead of relying on the somewhat vague theory of the General Duty Clause.

> The codification of Universal Precautions is the first of the two triumphs of the Bloodborne Pathogens Standard.

Chapter 3

Hepatitis B

Groups as diverse as the AMA, who stated "the loss of health care workers to hepatitis B virus infection overshadows the risk of AIDS and is almost entirely preventable," to ACTUP, who "encourages OSHA to continue to educate workers of their excessive risk of contracting hepatitis B as opposed to their extremely small risk of contracting HIV or AIDS through workplace exposure," concur that occupationally acquired hepatitis B infection affects a far greater number of workers than does occupationally acquired HIV infection.

—Summary and explanation section of the Standard

HEPATITIS VIRUSES

Hepatitis is an inflammation of the liver caused by drugs, chemicals, alcohol, or infectious agents. The most common cause of hepatitis is viral infection. There are several important types of viral hepatitis.[1]

Hepatitis A (HAV, formerly called "infectious hepatitis") is spread through fecal contamination. Although outbreaks of infection in health care workers have been reported, it is not considered a significant occupational risk. Most hepatitis A infections are minor, and patients have subclinical or unrecognized symptoms.

Hepatitis B (HBV, formerly called "serum hepatitis") is spread through sexual

---

1. See Appendix F for a more thorough discussion of hepatitis.

contact and bloodborne transmission. The Standard, quite simply, was created to deal with occupational hepatitis B infection.

> Hepatitis B is the most significant infectious occupational risk in the United States.

Non-A, non-B hepatitis is caused by viruses other than hepatitis A and B. The CDC estimates that about 3,400 non-A, non-B hepatitis infections occurred in health care workers during 1988. Approximately 20–40% of all bloodborne hepatitis infections are caused by non-A, non-B viruses. Some specific types have recently been identified:

Hepatitis C Virus (HCV) has recently been shown to be responsible for a large proportion of the non-A, non-B bloodborne hepatitis infections. HCV can be occupationally transmitted. A test to detect antibodies to HCV was licensed in 1990 and is now used in screening blood donations, but it is still too soon to judge how significant HCV infection is in the workplace. Though there is no HCV prophylactic vaccination, the precautions set forth in the Standard can be expected to greatly decrease the number of occupational HCV infections.

Hepatitis D Virus (HDV) causes infection only in the presence of active HBV infection.

Hepatitis E, which is spread through fecal-oral routes, is not a significant concern in the United States.

HBV infection is the major infectious bloodborne occupational hazard to health care workers. The CDC estimates that approximately 8,700 health care workers are occupationally infected with HBV each year in the United States. Of these, 2,100 will have acute hepatitis; about 400 will be hospitalized; and 200 health care workers will die each year from effects of acute and chronic HBV infection. Asymptomatic HBV-infected health care workers can spread the infection to family members, and, rarely, to their patients.

> The procedures set forth in the Standard[2] can prevent almost all HBV and most other hepatitis infections in occupational settings.

---

[2] Including HBV vaccination, engineering controls, work practice controls, and personal protective equipment.

BIOLOGY

HBV invades and replicates inside liver cells. Like most viruses, HBV uses host cell mechanisms to reproduce itself, instead of allowing the host cell to perform normal cellular functions. The virus disrupts and may kill the host cell, eventually destroying the whole organ.

HBV has an inner core that contains DNA and an outer shell of lipoprotein. This outer shell lipoprotein, called "hepatitis B surface antigen" (HbsAg), is produced in great quantities by liver cells commandeered by HBV to replicate itself. The presence of HbsAg in blood indicates that the person is currently infected with HBV and is potentially infectious. There is a relatively simple laboratory blood test for HbsAg, and anyone with a positive HbsAg test is considered to be actively infected and infectious.

About 6 months after an initial HBV infection, the host produces detectable levels of antibody to hepatitis B surface antigen (anti-HbsAg, which is referred to as Anti-HBs). The presence of Anti-HBs indicates that the person has been exposed to HBV, has developed protective antibodies, and is immune.[3] There is a laboratory blood test for Anti-HBs, and a positive test indicates immunity and noninfectiousness. Sometimes a person infected with HBV does not develop protective antibodies and may become what is called an "HBV carrier."

> HbsAg = Infected/Infectious
> Anti-HBs = Immune/Noninfectious

There are a whole slew of other HBV antigens and antibodies[4] that are used for tracking stages of HBV infection and immune response, as well as identifying chronic carrier states. To simplify: If, after the 6th month of HBV infection, someone tests HbsAg-positive and Anti-HBs-negative, he or she is most likely a chronic HBV carrier. Chronic carriers are usually infectious and asymptomatic.

DISEASE OUTCOMES

Infection with HBV in a susceptible person can produce either of two outcomes—self-limited acute infection or chronic infection.

---

3. Or has had a response from HBV vaccination, or a prophylactic injection of preformed HBV Immune Globulin, HBIG.

4. Including e, c, IgM. See Appendix F, Table F1, for clarification.

Self-limited acute HBV infection is the most frequent response in healthy adults. About one-third of individuals acutely infected with HBV have no symptoms; one-third have a relatively mild clinical course of a flulike illness, which is usually not diagnosed as hepatitis; and one-third have a severe clinical course. Those with severe infection usually have jaundice, dark urine, extreme fatigue, anorexia, nausea, abdominal pain, and sometimes joint pain, rash, and fever. Fulminant hepatitis, the most severe form, is about 85% fatal and occurs in about one in 1,000 of all HBV infections. The CDC estimates that about 0.125% of HBV infections in health care workers result in death from acute fulminant hepatitis (or about 11 deaths per year.)

Chronic HBV infection occurs in about 6–10% of newly infected adults. Chronic carriers cannot clear the virus from their liver cells. They are infectious and continue to produce HBsAg for many years, usually for life. Unfortunately, because of developing immune system differences, over 70% of children infected at birth become chronic carriers. HBV carriers are at high risk of developing chronic hepatitis, cirrhosis of the liver, and liver cancer. About 25% of chronic carriers develop chronic active hepatitis, often leading to end-stage cirrhosis after 5–10 years. The CDC estimates that about 1.7% of HBV infections in health care workers result in death from cirrhosis (or about 148 deaths per year).

Integration of HBV DNA into liver cells may result in malignant transformation and the development of liver cancer (primary hepatocellular carcinoma). Liver cancer usually only develops in HBV carriers after a latency period of 20–60 years. Liver cancer deaths from occupational exposure thus usually occur late in a career or after retirement. The CDC estimates that about 0.4% of HBV infections in health care workers result in death from liver cancer (or about 35 deaths per year). These mortality estimates from occupational HBV exposure show that only about 11 health care workers die from HBV infection during the first year of infection. The vast majority die years after HBV infection.[5]

Morbidity (illness/suffering) estimates from HBV infection must also be included. Many more people infected with HBV suffer and survive HBV infection than die from it. The amount of time lost and pain suffered due to the annual estimated 2,100 symptomatic occupational health care worker HBV infections is significant and difficult to measure.

---

5. The estimated 148 deaths due to cirrhosis occur 5–10 years postexposure, and the 35 deaths from liver cancer occur more than 20 years postexposure.

MODES OF TRANSMISSION

HBV is spread occupationally through the following routes: direct injection (parenteral), eye or mouth contamination (mucous membranes), sexual, and from mother to newborn (perinatal transmission). Though sexual and perinatal transmissions are not normally considered occupational routes, secondary HBV transmission from an occupationally infected worker can lead to HBV infection of a sexual partner or child.

HBV transmission is quite efficient: 1 ml of infected blood may contain as many as 100 million infectious doses of the virus. Studies have shown that 7–30% of susceptible health care workers with needlestick injuries from HBsAg-positive patients become infected. Transfer of HBV-contaminated blood, via inanimate objects or environmental surfaces has also been shown to cause infection.

Fewer than 20% of HBV-infected health care workers report direct needlestick injuries from a known infected patient. Preexisting cuts, sores, or dermatitis on the hands or other parts of the skin may provide a route of entry for HBV. Although gloving may not stop direct puncture injuries, it can provide a barrier between infected blood and an open sore or cut area, denying HBV access to the worker. Experimental studies have shown that HBV is transmitted through blood placed in animals' eyes and mouths. Therefore, splashes of blood into eyes and mouths must be considered potentially serious exposures.

Nonsexual family contacts of HBV carriers are also at risk of infection. Studies have shown that 40–60% of household contacts of carriers show signs of infection. Because perinatal HBV transmission is extremely efficient (infected mothers pass the infection to between 70–90% of their newborns), pregnant workers must be doubly concerned about acquiring HBV through occupational infection.

EPIDEMIOLOGY[6]

HBV infection does not occur uniformly in the United States. There are significant differences in HBV prevalence in geographic regions and among ethnic and racial populations. The prevalence of HBV antibodies in the general population is 3–4% for whites, 13–14% for African-Americans, and greater than 50% for some foreign-born Asians.

Outbreaks of clinical hepatitis have been reported in health care workers for

---

6. Epidemiology is the study of infectious patterns in populations—i.e., the study of epidemics.

many years. It was not until the development of HBV antigen and antibody tests (markers) that the true risk to workers was well defined, and it was shown that HBV was the type of hepatitis occurring more commonly in health care workers. Some of the early studies of occupational infection showed that dentists were more likely than attorneys to have had clinical hepatitis. During the decade after these markers were developed, studies were performed that showed the prevalence of HBV infection in various health care settings. Two general conclusions were drawn from these studies:

- Workers exposed to blood had a prevalence of HBV markers several times that of nonexposed workers and the general population; and
- The prevalence of HBV markers was related to the degree of blood exposure and frequency of needle exposure, and not to patient contact per se.[7]

Before the development of HBV markers, the only way to tell if workers were infected was if they got sick, which is only the tip of the exposure iceberg. With HBV markers, it became possible to determine which workers were infected and had no symptoms and which were infectious carriers. Studies showed that most infected health care workers were unaware that they had been exposed to or infected with HBV; other studies found that approximately 1% of hospitalized patients were HBV carriers, and most of these were asymptomatic, with no evidence of infection documented in their hospital charts.

Health care workers may take extraordinary precautions when working with a known carrier, but they may be unaware that they are likely to treat five unknown carriers for each carrier they recognize. This is a key point in understanding the rationale for Universal Precautions.

> The vast majority of patients who are HBV-infectious are unrecognized at the time of treatment.

Exposure to blood through needlesticks and cuts with sharp instruments are efficient modes of HBV transmission, but reported injuries do not account for the majority of infections in health care workers. Some workers get cuts and needlesticks or large blood exposures so often that they neglect to report them; others become infected when the blood of an unknown carrier gets into preexisting

---

7. Workers in hospital labs, who have relatively little patient contact, had a high HBV marker prevalence.

cuts or is rubbed into eyes. Workers' compensation boards usually deny coverage to infected workers who do not report discrete needlesticks or injuries from a known HBV carrier. Unfortunately, the vast majority of occupational HBV transmissions are undocumented. It's a goal of the Standard to prevent these undocumented occupational infections.

TRANSMISSION FROM HEALTH CARE WORKERS TO PATIENTS

More than 20 clusters of patients infected with HBV through transmission from health care workers have been reported. It is assumed that many instances of this type of transmission involving only one or a few patients go unrecognized. Most of the documented transmissions involved oral surgeons, dentists, gynecologists, or surgeons, where significant blood exposure, trauma, and use of sharp instruments occur. Some of these clusters involved transmission from health care workers to 20–55 patients, with deaths and secondary transmission to family members of patients. Several common factors have contributed to these transmissions:

- The health care workers were chronic carriers who were unaware they were infected.
- Transmission usually occurred during traumatic procedures.
- Dental personnel did not routinely wear gloves.
- Dentists and surgeons often had a medical problem, such as dermatitis.
- Gynecologists used their index finger to feel for tips of suture needles.

Guidelines for HBV- and HIV-infected healthcare workers were published by the CDC in 1991, too late to be included in the Standard. These guidelines, Recommendations for Preventing Transmission of Human Immunodeficiency Virus and Hepatitis B Virus to Patients during Exposure-Prone Invasive Procedures, are included as Appendix E.

TRANSMISSION VIA THE ENVIRONMENT

Transmission of HBV from contaminated environmental surfaces has been documented, especially in hemodialysis units, where HBV-contaminated blood from the surface of the dialysis machines may make contact with the hands of health care workers. In addition, use of unsterilized acupuncture needles has been indicated in outbreaks of HBV infections.

> HBV can survive for at least 1 week dried at room temperature on environmental surfaces.

Because of this long survival time, it is extremely important to use disinfection and sterilization techniques to prevent the spread of HBV. Sterilization or disinfection procedures, sterilizing agents, and high-level disinfectants will kill HBV if used as directed. If used properly, diluted solutions (1:10 or 1:100) of household bleach (sodium hypochlorite) are effective and inexpensive, although they may be corrosive to some materials.

HBV VACCINE

Gloving and other protective devices cannot completely prevent puncture injuries from needles and other sharp instruments; therefore,

> HBV vaccination is the most important part of any HBV control program.

A safe and effective HBV vaccine derived from human plasma was licensed in the United States in 1982. Unfortunately, because it was derived from the blood of persons previously infected with HBV, many of whom were homosexuals or IV drug abusers, many people feared vaccination would cause hepatitis. After HIV was identified in 1983, there was great concern about HIV transmission through HBV vaccination. Even though the procedures used to manufacture the HBV vaccine inactivated HIV, the vaccine did not contain HIV DNA, and those receiving the HBV vaccine did not develop antibodies to HIV, there was still an underlying fear that HBV vaccination might spread HIV.[8]

---

8. This first, serum-derived HBV vaccine is no longer available in the United States.

In 1987, a second HBV vaccine, produced in yeast cells by a gene recombinant technique, was licensed. This vaccine contains no human blood and there is no possibility it could be infected with HIV. Recombinant HBV vaccine is given intramuscularly in the deltoid, in three doses over a 6-month period. When given according to directions, the vaccine induces protective antibody responses in 85–97% of healthy adults. Protection against illness and the carrier states lasts at least 9 years (the period of the prelicensing follow-up studies) and probably longer. Unfortunately, this vaccination series costs around $100, and employers have often been hesitant to pay for it.

Prevaccination screening with HBV markers raises a number of complex issues. This screening may be cost-effective if there is a high likelihood of prior HBV infection. In most cases, however, prevaccination screening is not cost-effective, and there is little harm in vaccinating those who may have already been exposed to HBV and developed protective antibodies on their own. The Immunization Practices Advisory Committee (ACIP) of the U.S. Public Health Service has published an algorithm to help determine the usefulness of prevaccination screening (see Appendix F, Table F5).

Postvaccination screening with HBV markers is also a thorny issue. Unless recipients received the vaccination series inappropriately in the buttock, are over age 50, or are infected with HIV, this screening is usually not indicated. On an individual basis, postvaccination testing may be indicated to find out if a person responded to vaccination in the course of postexposure prophylaxis. In most cases, however, postvaccination screening, for a particular population, is neither helpful nor indicated.

The medical community accepts that HBV vaccination is safe and prevents HBV infection. OSHA estimates that over a 45-year working lifetime, HBV vaccination will prevent between 5,000 and 6,000 deaths.

Requiring employers to provide employees with HBV vaccination[9] is the second of the two triumphs of the Standard.

POSTEXPOSURE PROPHYLAXIS

Preexposure vaccination is the most effective method of preventing HBV infection. However, some unvaccinated workers may have exposure incidents. Luck-

9. At no cost to the employees.

ily, postexposure prophylaxis for HBV is available. The ACIP recommendations specify that if the source individual is known to be HBV-infectious (i.e., HBsAg-positive), the exposed individual should be given hepatitis B immuneglobulin (HBIG), and the HBV vaccination series should be started. HBV vaccination is recommended for any unvaccinated health care worker who has an exposure incident.

Chapter 4

HIV and AIDS

*A pestilence isn't a thing made to man's measure; therefore we tell ourselves
that pestilence is a mere bogey of the mind, a bad dream that will pass away. But
it doesn't always pass away, and from one bad dream to another, it is men who
pass away. . . .*

—*Albert Camus*
The Plague

On December 12, 1977, Dr. Grethe Rask died of *Pneumocystis carinii* pneumonia.[1] A Danish physician, she had practiced in Zaire in the early 1970s,
performing surgery with minimal equipment and protection; sterile gloves were
rarely available and were used till they were worn out, needles were used and
reused, surgeons often just stuck their bare hands into the patient's blood. She
returned to Denmark after being plagued by 3 years of diarrhea, weight loss, and
fatigue, only to find that the best medical specialists back home had no idea what
was going on. Dr. Rask's longtime female companion, a nurse, was with her
when she died.[2]

This, the first documented case of AIDS mortality in the Western world,

1. Randy Shilts, *And the Band Played On: Politics, People, and the AIDS Epidemic.* (New York:
St. Martin's Press), 1987.

2. This information is important because it implies that Dr. Rask, while in Africa, was not infected
through male-to-female sexual transmission. Female-to-female HIV sexual transmission is quite
rare without other risk factors, such as sharing IV drug needles.

occurred in a surgeon. A female surgeon. A female surgeon probably not infected through sexual activity. Her death was the result of an occupational infection.

There have been 42 confirmed cases, and 91 more possible reported cases, of occupational HIV transmission in the United States since the start of the AIDS epidemic.[3] Although the number of occupationally related AIDS deaths is unknown at this time, it is probably less than 50. The assumption, unfortunately, is that all HIV-infected people will eventually die of HIV-related complications.[4] The combination of newness and virulence makes HIV infection much more frightening to most people than HBV infection.

THE HUMAN IMMUNODEFICIENCY VIRUS

The first cases of what was to become known as acquired immunodeficiency syndrome (AIDS) were reported in the United States in June 1981. Two unusual illnesses, *Pneumocystis carinii* pneumonia and Kaposi's sarcoma (a rare cancer of blood vessels), had been reported in young homosexual men. By early 1982, 159 AIDS cases had been identified in the United States and two foreign countries. By late 1982, cases of AIDS had been reported in IV drug users, blood transfusion recipients, hemophiliacs, and Haitians. The actual virus that caused AIDS was identified in 1983 and 1984, first by a French scientist, Dr. Luc Montagnier, and later by an American, Dr. Robert Gallo.

A simple test to detect HIV infection was developed incredibly quickly and was approved for use in early 1985. The discovery, isolation, replication, and development of a detection test for this virus was an astounding medical accomplishment. In a sense, it was a medical miracle, except that it did not directly save lives. However, the test for the presence of antibodies to HIV did save lives, indirectly, because it prevented countless unknown transmissions of HIV through blood transfusions.

The CDC estimates that 1–1.5 million people in the United States are infected with HIV. This is of great importance to health care workers who may treat patients who are unaware that they are infected. There are increasing numbers of HIV-infected persons in the United States, and the number of occupational HIV infections

---

3. A confirmed case must have a documented HIV-negative status, followed by a conversion to HIV-positive after the exposure. Possible reported cases have unknown preexposure status. Centers for Disease Control, *HIV/AIDS Surveillance Report,* cases reported through December 1994. Vol. 6, No. 2.

4. This differs from HBV infection, where the vast majority of those infected not only do not die, but do not have symptoms requiring hospitalization.

is likely to grow as the number of infected individuals requiring health care and other services increases. The growing number of individuals with AIDS, the large number of unidentified HIV infections, and the numerous reports of occupational infection all indicate that health care workers, as well as police, firefighters, and others, will be at increasing risk for occupationally acquired HIV infection in the future.

THE BIOLOGY OF HIV

HIV is a retrovirus—it goes backward. Its genetic material is ribonucleic acid (RNA) rather than deoxyribonucleic acid (DNA). Instead of the normal host DNA producing host RNA that produces normal cellular material, the retrovirus uses its own RNA to produce virus DNA. The reason HIV is so frightening is that some of this virus DNA may become integrated into human genetic material.

Because viruses lack the necessary machinery to reproduce, they must borrow cellular material from host cells, in order to reproduce. HIV replicates inside two specific types of human cells involved in the immune response—macrophages and T4 lymphocytes. These cells normally function to help fight off infections. HIV replicates and destroys these cells, gradually depleting the number of cells until the host individual is unable to fight off infections. People with AIDS die because their immune system is so damaged they become succeptible to infections.

THE HIV ANTIBODY TEST

Infection with HIV is identified by testing the blood for the presence of HIV antibodies. The HIV test does not measure the presence of virus in the blood.

> The HIV test is an indirect test that measures antibody, not virus.

When exposed to viruses or bacterias (called "antigens"), the body's immune system produces proteins (called "antibodies") that help destroy the antigens upon reexposure. For HIV and HBV, it may take anywhere from 6 weeks to 6 months after an exposure to develop detectable levels of antibodies. During this time, even though the virus may replicate and be present in extremely high concentrations in the blood, the blood tests antibody-negative. In actuality, during this initial stage of virus replication (called "viremia"), when the body has yet to produce a strong antibody response, the blood is teaming with newly produced HIV and is probably quite infectious, even though it tests antibody-negative.[5]

By the time the antibodies are detectable, the level of virus in the blood has decreased significantly, sometimes to the point where it cannot even be found on routine virus testing.[6] This phase, where HIV virus but not HIV antibodies are present in the blood, is the so-called "window phase" of infection. Because blood may be most infectious during this window phase, when it tests HIV antibody-negative, health care workers cannot rely on testing patients for their HIV status (direct HIV virus tests, called "antigen tests," are not yet accurate enough to be widely used). For this reason, it must be assumed that all blood is possibly infectious. It may seem strange to consider blood that tests positive as safer than blood that tests negative. Therefore, to be safe, we must assume that all blood is infectious, and we must take precautions for all the human blood in the *universe*. This extreme-sounding statement can be used to help remember the importance of *Universal Precautions* for blood and body fluids.

HIV TRANSMISSION

HIV is not transmitted by casual contact. Successful transmission of HIV requires direct contact into the host's blood system. The virus, whether in blood, semen, vaginal secretions, or breast milk, must have direct contact with the exposed person's blood or white blood cells.

In the United States, the primary route of nonoccupational transmission is through homosexual rectal intercourse, where trauma to the rectal mucosa (which is only one to a few cells thick) easily allows for microtears and rectal bleeding. HIV, which is present in semen (probably due to the presence of white blood cells in semen) thus has a direct route of entry into the receptive partner's blood system.

---

5. Levels of virus have also been shown to be elevated during the later stages of HIV infection, when actual AIDS symptoms are present.

6. It is speculated that the HIV virus becomes integrated into the genetic material, possibly in cells located in lymph nodes, and lies there dormant until the virus expresses itself and starts replicating again. Recently, however, it has been shown that even though the virus may not be found in blood samples, it may be "sequestered" in lymph nodes, continuing to be active and reproduce there.

HIV transmission throughout the world occurs predominantly through hetero-sexual contact. Male-to-female transmission is probably most effective because virus in semen has a direct route of entry into the highly vascular female genital tract area. Female-to-male transmission requires virus present in vaginal secretions to enter directly into microtears in the penis (less likely), or through areas already infected and inflamed by another sexually transmitted disease (more likely). Entrance through weeping or open penile and vaginal lesions is probably the primary route of HIV transmission in the world. The process of inflammation is associated with a localized accumulation of white blood cells (WBCs), and HIV needs these WBCs to reproduce. Thus, transmission is most likely when HIV is exposed to areas with a high concentration of WBCs and nonintact skin.

As for occupational transmission, which accounts for a minuscule percentage of the total HIV transmission, HIV also must have direct access to a worker's blood. Direct injection of HIV into the bloodstream is an extremely efficient route of transmission. Thus, the majority of occupational infections occur through needlesticks, which inject infected blood directly into subcutaneous tissue or muscles. WBCs accumulate around this injured area to help fight off foreign-body infection, but, unfortunately, the WBCs may become infected with HIV. Transmis-sion through sharing of IV needles or by hemophiliac use of blood products are even more efficient routes, because infected blood and virus is introduced directly into the host's blood system, giving excellent viral access to WBCs.

Intact skin provides an effective barrier to HIV infection; no blood-to–intact skin infections have been documented.

- **Blood-to-blood contact is most efficient.**
- **Blood to nonintact skin, or infected body fluid to blood, is efficient.**
- **Infected body fluid to nonintact skin is less efficient.**
- **Blood or infected body fluid to intact skin is not efficient.**

OCCUPATIONAL CASE HISTORIES

The case histories of occupational HIV transmission date from 1985, the year the first blood test for HIV infection became available. Possible cases of conversion before 1985 are not well documented because no such test was available, and the only infection marker would have been symptom development, which usually occurs a few years after initial infection. Just as the development of hepatitis markers allowed tracking of HBV infection in the 1970s, the development of HIV markers allowed tracking of HIV infection in the late 1980s. A synopsis of a few of the first occupationally transmitted HIV infection case reports (see Appendix H, Table H2) follows:

- While obtaining blood in a vacuum collection tube from an AIDS patient, a hospital health care worker sustained an accidental self-inflicted injection of several milliliters of blood.
- A previously healthy 33-year-old Navy hospital corpsman punctured his fingertip while disposing a needle used to draw blood from a patient later diagnosed with AIDS.
- A phlebotomist reported that blood splattered on her face and in her mouth when the top of a vacuum blood collection tube flew off while she was collecting blood from an HIV-positive patient. She was wearing gloves and glasses. She reported that no blood got in her eyes and that she had no open wounds, but she did have facial acne.
- A 24-year-old student nurse pricked the fleshy part of her index finger with a needle used to draw blood from an AIDS patient.
- A clinical laboratory worker sustained a cut that penetrated through a glove and the skin when a vial of HIV-infected blood broke in the worker's hand.
- A nurse received a puncture wound from a colonic biopsy needle visibly contaminated with the blood and feces of an AIDS patient.
- A 37-year-old intensive care nurse in Italy had her hands, eyes, and mouth heavily splashed with blood from an HIV-infected hemophiliac. She also developed non-A, non-B hepatitis.
- A health care worker applied pressure to an HIV-infected patient's arterial catheter insertion site to stop bleeding. She had chapped hands and was not wearing gloves. A small amount of blood may have remained on her index finger for 20 minutes before she washed her hands.
- More needlesticks, needlesticks, needlesticks. (The majority of occupational infections have occurred through needlesticks. This list actually understates this fact, in order to emphasize the other important routes of documented transmissions. OSHA considered all these routes when formulating the Standard and its preventive requirements.)

WORKERS WITH AIDS

The vast majority of HIV-infected workers or those with AIDS acquired the virus through nonoccupational transmission. And most continue to work. In fact, the Americans with Disabilities Act (ADA) specifically prevents the firing of a worker on the basis of his or her HIV status. There has been only one set of documented cases of HIV transmission from health care worker to patients in the United States, and it occurred in a dentist. (The specifics of the Acer case will be discussed more fully in Chapter 5.)

> There has not been a single documented case of physician-to-patient HIV transmission in the United States.

By law, the Standard does not apply to worker-to-nonworker transmissions, since this would not comprise an occupational exposure. Thus, the Standard does not apply to possible—though highly improbable—worker-to-patient exposures.

The Creation of the Bloodborne Pathogens Standard

I blame every one of you bastards.

—Kimberly Bergalis, referring to physicians

THE EARLY YEARS

Before the 1970s, and thus pre-OSHA, thousands of people died as a result of occupationally acquired hepatitis B infection. Like tuberculosis before antibiotics, hepatitis was considered an occupational hazard of health care workers. Because there was no treatment for infection, deaths from hepatitis were, unfortunately, tolerated, and many deaths occurred so many years after exposure that they were not causally associated with the original occupational exposure. A short synopsis of the major milestones relating to the creation of the Standard follows:

1970s: The risk to workers became better defined when studies showed that dentists were more likely than attorneys to have clinical hepatitis. Tests for HBV antibodies and other serologic markers became available and allowed, for the first time, the evaluation of nonclinical hepatitis infection. Studies showed that dentists and physicians were four to 10 times more likely to have prior HBV infection than first-time blood donors.

Dozens of subsequent studies showed that workers exposed to blood on the job had a prevalence of HBV infection several times that of non-exposed workers and the general population.

1981: The first cases of what would become known as AIDS were reported to the CDC.

1982: A plasma-derived vaccine against hepatitis B became available. When given pre-exposure, it prevented the vast majority of postexposure infections. The vaccine was derived from donated blood, and the presence of HBV antibodies implied that the plasma donors had been previously infected with HBV. Unfortunately, many people refused vaccination because they feared it would cause hepatitis.

1983: OSHA issued a set of guidelines designed to reduce the risk of occupational exposure to hepatitis B virus. These voluntary guidelines, sent to health care industry employers, made recommendations on work practices and the use of hepatitis B vaccine. That same year, the virus thought to casuse AIDS was discovered in France.

1984: The AIDS virus was officially identified. Initially called HTLV-III in the United States and LAV in France, it is now called HIV.

1985: The HIV antibody test became available. As with the introduction of HBV antibody testing a decade earlier, it allowed the evaluation of early and nonclinical cases of HIV infection. Asymptomatic HIV infection could now be identified. The film star Rock Hudson died of AIDS, bringing AIDS into the public consciousness. The first cases of occupational HIV infection were reported.

1986: Four unions[1] petitioned OSHA during the month of September to take action to reduce the risk to employees from exposure to certain infectious agents. A genetically engineered hepatitis B vaccine became available.

1987: On October 22, over a year after being petitioned, OSHA denied the petition for an emergency temporary standard and determined that the appropriate course of action was to initiate rulemaking and the collection of information. A week later the Departments of Labor and Health and Human Services published a Joint Advisory Notice dealing with protection against occupational HBV and HIV exposure and sent information to over half a million employers and employee representatives.

1987: In November, an Advance Notice of Proposed Rulemaking (ANPR) was published in the *Federal Register,* requesting information relevant to reducing occupational exposure to HBV and HIV. OSHA received an

---

1. The American Federation of State, County and Municipal Employees petitioned OSHA on September 19, 1986, requesting an emergency temporary standard. The Service Employees International Union, the National Union of Hospital and Healthcare Employees, and the Drug, Hospital and Healthcare Union petitioned OSHA on September 22, 1986, to promulgate a standard.

overwhelming response to the ANPR, and these public comments were analyzed and used in the preparation of the first draft of the Standard.

The major advances made in the 1970s relating to HBV were paralleled by advances made relating to HIV in the 1980s. Unfortunately, a protective HIV vaccine has not yet been discovered, and the parallels between HBV and HIV stop here. Prevention of HIV infection rests solely with education and avoidance of exposure.

THE FIRST DRAFT

In May 1989, a year and a half after the publication of the Advance Notice of Proposed Rulemaking, OSHA published the Notice of Proposed Rulemaking (NPRM) in the *Federal Register*. The NPRM, basically a first draft of the standard, resulted from the analysis of over 350 comments filed by employers, unions, health professionals, trade representatives, professional associations, manufacturers, and federal, state, and local governments, among others. There were 25 reported cases of apparent HIV infection through occupational exposure by then, and the CDC had reported 88,000 cases of AIDS and estimated that 1–1.5 million people were infected with HIV in the United States.

The CDC also estimated that 1.4 million people had received HBV vaccination at that time. Although over 85% of them were health care workers, only 30–40% of high-risk health care workers had been vaccinated. Early efforts to immunize health care workers were hampered by the fear that the plasma-derived vaccine might be infected with HIV. However, the newer yeast-derived HBV vaccine contained no human plasma and therefore could not possibly transmit HIV.[2]

A series of public hearings were held in Washington, D.C., Chicago, New York City, Miami, and San Francisco between September 1989 and January 1990. OSHA presented 10 expert witnesses; and over 400 persons, representing a wide range of interested parties, participated in the hearings. May 21, 1990, was set as the deadline for the submission of comments and exhibits. OSHA received over 4,000 dockets relating to the Standard, by far the largest number of comments and exhibits ever received in the history of OSHA standard making.[3] The final Bloodborne

---

2. There are no known cases of HIV transmission through either the plasma or yeast-derived HBV vaccination.

3. This record was broken in 1994, when OSHA received over 10,000 dockets relating to a proposed Indoor Air Quality Standard. Most of these comments, however, were related to environmental tobacco smoke in the workplace.

Pathogens Standard was based on consideration of the entire record of the proceedings, including materials in the proposal, the record of the hearings, and all written comments and exhibits received.

THE FINAL CUT

The Bloodborne Pathogens Standard working group at OSHA completed the final draft of the Standard during the summer of 1991. The major roadblock to many OSHA standards has been the OMB, Office of Management and Budget, an executive branch agency that evaluates the financial feasibility of regulations passed by the federal government. It was widely suspected that OMB would stall the Standard for months, or years, pending requests for further cost analysis. OSHA estimated that compliance costs would run approximately $813 million a year.[4] OMB was bound to look carefully and skeptically at any regulation that would cost nearly a billion dollars a year. At the same time, the health care industry could not be expected to be enthusiastic either, even though most of the cost would be passed on to medical consumers and third-party payers. Certainly, it would not help contain the skyrocketing costs of medical care.

The forces in OSHA and OMB might have stalled the Standard for years, or cost-effectively neutered it, had it not been for a young girl from Florida and a senator from North Carolina. Kimberly Bergalis claimed to have been infected with HIV by her dentist, Dr. David J. Acer, who had recently died of AIDS. Scientists were now able to identify different strains of HIV, and they were relatively certain that the virus that infected Bergalis was identical to Acer's virus. Bergalis not only blamed her dentist, she indicted the entire dental and medical profession.

Senator Jesse Helms of North Carolina jumped on the bandwagon. At that time, there was not one single documented case of a patient who had died of AIDS acquired from any type of doctor. Pushing a thinly disguised anti-gay agenda,

---

4. Personal protective equipment accounted for the largest amount of estimated compliance costs ($327 million per year). Training ($134 million), vaccine and postexposure follow-up ($107 million), and housekeeping ($102 million) were the other significant annual cost components.

5. The Helms amendment dealing with deliberate transmission of the AIDS virus read: "Whoever, being a registered physician, dentist, nurse, or other health care provider, knowing that he is infected with the Human Immunodeficiency Virus, intentionally provides medical or dental treatment to another person, without prior notification to such person of such infection, shall be fined no more than $10,000, or imprisoned not less than ten years, or both." *Congressional Record-Senate*, July 11, 1991.

Senator Helms introduced legislation that would require jail time for practicing doctors who tested positive for HIV antibodies, the vast majority of whom were homosexual.[5]

Soon thereafter, Kimberly Bergalis died of AIDS. Several other patients of Dr. Acer's, including a grandmother in her 60s, were identified as having been infected by the dentist. The CDC has no official or scientific explanation for how these isolated infections might have occurred. One rumor had it that Dr. Acer had stated that "When AIDS starts affecting grandmothers and young people, then you'll see something done." Thus, there is a question whether Acer purposely injected his blood into these patients.[6,7]

The Helms rhetoric, combined with Bergalis's emotional appeals, was so intense, and general concern was so strong about HIV infection and health care, that Congress had to act to reassure the electorate. Wisely, the Senate defeated the Helms amendment; and within a week, passed the Mitchell, Kennedy, Dole, and Hatch amendment, which adopted guidelines for preventing the transmission of HIV and HBV from health care professionals to patients during exposure-prone procedures (see Appendix E).

Aware that OMB and OSHA were stalling the Standard, Congress threatened to adopt, as law, the proposed standard as written in the Notice of Proposed Rulemaking. Players from OSHA, OMB, and Congress met during the summer of 1991 and came to a compromise solution: The OSHA Standard must be finalized within a few months, receive its blessing from OMB, and be published in the *Federal Register* by the end of the year. All players made minor compromises and the final rule was published on December 6, 1991—over 5 years after the request for an emergency temporary standard, but sooner than many had anticipated, considering the constrictive legislative pressure exerted by the Bush administration.

The public fear of contracting AIDS from health care workers forced the completion of a regulation to protect health care workers from getting HBV from the public.

---

6. R. Lang, Did Dr. Acer murder his patients? *Oral Health* 1993; 83(9): 3.

7. This may not be such a far-out idea. Some AIDS patients, or PWAs (People With AIDS), develop psychiatric or thought problems in advanced stages of infection. PWAs may also have helpless anger about the perceived—and real—inaction of the government and scientists because of sexual orientation prejudice. Another theory questions whether Bergalis was infected through her own sexual activity, not by exposure from Dr. Acer.

Chapter 6

Paragraph (a):
Scope and Application

I can also tell you that on a daily basis, some of us would be chagrined to admit to you that even though we consider ourselves to be firefighters, that most of our calls are emergency medical calls.

—Statement to OSHA from Eric Lamar,
firefighter and emergency medical technician

The Standard applies to all occupational exposure to blood or other potentially infectious materials.

O SHA believes that:

- A single exposure incident may result in infection and subsequent illness and death.
- There is no population that is risk-free for HBV or HIV infectivity.

Therefore, any employee who has occupational exposure to any population's blood or other potentially infectious material (OPIM) has the potential for infection and is included within the scope of the Standard. The risk of occupational blood-borne pathogen infection is most thoroughly documented in health care workers employed by hospitals; however, the risk is not confined only to hospitals but is present whenever blood/OPIM is present.

Coverage by the Standard is not based solely on job classifications; it is based on an employee's occupational exposure. There are, for example, psychiatrists who limit their practice to outpatient group settings. They would not have reasonably anticipated occupational exposure and would not be covered by the Standard. On the other hand, an ocean lifeguard could be reasonably anticipated to have exposure to blood while rescuing a swimmer bleeding from coral cuts; similarly, an equipment repair person who works once a week on transfusion machines would also have occupational exposure. Both of these employees would be covered.

By relating coverage to occupational exposure, OSHA hopes to protect all at-risk employees regardless of their job title or place of employment. OSHA is careful, and correct, to base coverage on occupational exposure and not on generalized job classifications. The regulatory text therefore does not list jobs or job classifications. The compliance guide (Appendix C), in reverse logic, lists the following jobs in which the employees are not automatically covered unless they have occupational exposure:

Physicians, physician's assistants, nurses, nurse practitioners, and other health care employees in clinics and physicians' offices

Employees of clinical and diagnostic laboratories

Housekeepers in health care facilities

Personnel in hospital laundries or commercial laundries that service health care or public safety institutions

Tissue bank personnel

Employees in blood banks and plasma centers who collect, transport, and test blood

Freestanding clinic employees (e.g., hemodialysis clinics, urgent care clinics, health maintenance organization (HMO) clinics, and family planning clinics)

Employees in clinics in industrial, educational, and correctional facilities (e.g., those who collect blood, and clean and dress wounds)

Employees assigned to provide emergency first aid

Dentists, dental hygienists, dental assistants, and dental laboratory technicians

Staff of institutions for the developmentally disabled

Hospice employees

Home health care workers

Staff of nursing homes and long-term care facilities

Employees of funeral homes and mortuaries

HIV and HBV research laboratory and production facility workers

Employees who hande regulated waste

Medical equipment service and repair personnel

Emergency medical technicians, paramedics, and other emergency medical service providers

Firefighters, law enforcement personnel, and correctional officers (employees in the private sector, the federal government, or a state or local government in a state that has an OSHA-approved state plan)

OSHA received comments from employers or employees in each of these occupations. Employers often argued for exemption from the Standard ("Hey, it's expensive, a lot of work, and we've never had anyone get sick"); individual workers and unions most often pressed for inclusion of their occupation. Because of OSHA's philosophical stance that all exposures are possibly infectious and no population is risk-free, all it took was one worker testifying or commenting that he or she had been exposed or knew someone who had been infected and the occupation went on record as having potential risk.

Though no specific occupations are listed in the regulatory text, there are 10 pages in the summary and explanation section stating reasons for including specific occupational exposures in various jobs. The publication of reasons why employees, such as dental equipment repair personnel, should be covered by the Standard decreases the chances that employers will successfully sue OSHA. Once published in the *Federal Register,* the comments become an official part of the Standard's legislative history and can be cited in legal battles. A documented case or story of exposure to blood/OPIM in an occupation makes the exposure a recognized hazard, and the General Duty Clause states that employers must provide a place of employment that is free from recognized hazards.

The Bloodborne Standard Docket file contains numerous statements from dentists and dental associations arguing that they should not be covered. The comment period had closed before the controversy surrounding Dr. Acer and Kimberly Bergalis exploded. Even though the Bergalis case did not deal with occupational exposure, it inspired widespread fear about HIV transmission. Just 2 years after the close of the comment period in 1990, it would have been difficult to find any dentist or dental association that would publicly state that dental personnel should be excluded from coverage.

A phlebotomist drawing blood, a firefighter resuscitating a victim, a police officer struggling with a bleeding criminal, and a virologist transferring HIV cultures all have occupational exposure. The Standard is worded to protect an employee drawing blood, an employee resuscitating a victim, an employee struggling with a bleeding criminal, and an employee transferring HIV cultures.

QUESTIONS

1. *Do I have to cover a part-time housekeeping worker in my dental clinic?*

Yes. Part-time or temporary employees and per diem health care workers are covered by the Standard. Individuals who perform housekeeping duties in patient care and laboratory areas have occupational exposure when they perform tasks such as cleaning blood spills or encounter contaminated equipment or sharps.

2. *Are first-aiders in my company covered by the Standard?*

Yes and No. If employees are trained in first aid and designated by the employer as responsible for providing medical assistance as part of their job duties, they are covered by the Standard. If the first-aiders are paid or receive special compensation, it is assumed to be a special job duty and most likely would be covered. If employees organize on their own or individually and function more as "Good Samaritans" at the work-place, they probably would not be covered.

The high cost of HBV vaccination for first-aiders in major companies resulted initially in these programs being suspended by management. OSHA, realizing that there was greater risk to ill or injured employees who did not have access to first-aiders than there was risk for first-aiders of acquiring infection from coworkers, quickly changed the enforcement procedures. Policy violations relating to first-aiders are now considered *de minimis*, and citations will not be issued if first aiders are not offered HBV vaccination, though employers still must follow the other require-ments of the Standard (see Appendix D). OSHA, in a parallel action to some states' liberalizing marijuana laws, decriminalized the act of em-ployers not paying for HBV vaccination. That is, the law still stands, it's just not fiscally enforced for this section.

3. *Since construction and maritime workers are exempt from other OSHA standards, are they exempt from the Standard?*

No. Employees in the construction and maritime industries who have occupational exposure to blood/OPIM are covered by the Standard.

4. *I work at a military dental clinic and my boss claims that the government doesn't have to follow OSHA standards. Is she right?*

The OSHAct defines "employer" as a person engaged in business who has an employee and specifically excludes the United States as an employer. Thus, OSHA standards do not apply to federal agencies and the Department of Defense (DOD), and OSHA cannot fine these agen-cies. However, DOD agencies have regulations that require compliance with OSHA standards, and DOD medical and dental facilities therefore follow Universal Precautions and the requirements of the Standard. If the OSHA reform act currently in Congress is passed, it may have a provision to include federal agencies, in which case OSHA may in the future be able to fine DOD facilities for noncompliance.

Chapter 7

Paragraph (b):
Definitions

Fe fi fo fum!
I smell blood and/or OPIM;
Be he alive or be he dead,
I'll grind his bones and protect my head.

—*Anonymous fractured orthopedic nursery rhyme*

Paragraph (b) defines specific terms as they relate to the interpretation, implementation, and enforcement of the Standard. These definitions must be understood to adequately comprehend the Standard. Simplified interpretations of selected definitions follow:

Blood Human blood, human blood components,[1] and products made from human blood.[2]

Bloodborne pathogens Disease-causing organisms carried in blood.

>   **HBV** and **HIV** are discussed because they are the most important pathogens and present the greatest risk to workers, but the following other diseases[3] are also included in the summary and explanation section:

---

1. Plasma, platelets, and the gooey fluids from wounds (exudates).

2. Including Factor VIII, a clotting substance required by hemophiliacs that was contaminated with HIV in the early 1980s.

3. Precautions designed to minimize transmission of HBV and HIV would be effective in minimizing occupational transmission of all these infections.

Hepatitis C   Recently discovered virus responsible for a large percentage of hepatitis cases not caused by hepatitis B or A.

Malaria   Parasitic infection of blood cells, transmitted by mosquitos, causing fever, chills, anemia, and sometimes death.

Syphilis   Usually a sexually transmitted disease caused by spirochetes, though transmission from mother to fetus and through blood has occurred.

Babesiosis   Disease similar to malaria, infecting blood cells and carried by ticks.

Brucellosis   Illness causing fevers, associated with livestock or ingestion of unpasteurized dairy products.

Leptospirosis   Spirochete infection characterized by fever and rash, typically acquired through contact with animal urine.

Arboviral infections   Arthropod-borne (transmitted by insects, usually mosquitos and ticks) virus infections, including Colorado tick fever.

Relapsing fever   Disease transmitted by lice or ticks causing recurring episodes of fever separated by periods of relative well-being.

Creutzfeld-Jakob disease   Rare degenerative viral disease of the brain.

Human T-lymphotropic virus type 1   Human retrovirus infection associated with a cancer of the blood known as T-cell leukemia/lymphoma.

Viral hemorrhagic fever   Severe viral illness that often causes hemorrhage and death; not common in the United States.

Contaminated   Presence of blood or other potentially infectious materials (OPIM).

Decontamination   Removal, inactivation, or destruction of bloodborne pathogens.

Engineering Controls   Things that isolate or remove blood/OPIM (sharps disposal containers, self-sheathing needles).

Exposure Incident   Eye, mouth, mucous membrane (lip, nose, anus), or non-intact skin, including under-the-skin (parenteral) contact with blood/OPIM. Non-intact skin includes skin with dermatitis, hangnails, cuts, abrasions, chafing, etc.

Note: An exposure is not necessarily always an exposure incident. Blood dripping on intact skin, or nonbloody urine contacting skin with cuts or sores would be defined as an exposure, not an exposure incident and would not require follow-up medical care or postexposure evaluation. However, the occurrence of an exposure implies potential for an exposure incident. Reporting of employee exposures to medical personnel, who would be better able to differentiate between exposures and exposure incidents and evaluate the need for procedural changes to avoid future exposure, is recommended.

Licensed health care professional   Person who is licensed to independently, or under supervision, perform duties such as vaccination or medical evaluation. Assumed to include doctors, nurses, and physician's assistants.

HBV   Hepatitis B virus.

HIV   Human immunodeficiency virus.

Occupational exposure   Contact or *potential contact*[5] of blood/OPIM with eye, mucous membrane, nonintact skin, including under-the-skin contact, occurring as a result of performance of work duties.

Other potentially infectious materials (OPIM)   Body fluids[6] other than blood, and tissues, organs, or cells that may contain bloodborne pathogens. The Standard lists the following body fluids as OPIM:

> Semen
> Vaginal secretions
> Saliva in dental procedures
> Any body fluid visibly contaminated with blood
> Any unidentified body fluid
> Special fluids[7]
> > Cerebrospinal (brain/spinal cord)
> > Synovial (joint)
> > Pleural (chest)
> > Pericardial (heart)
> > Peritoneal (abdominal)
> > Amniotic (pregnant uterus)

Also considered OPIM are:

> Tissue or organs from living or dead humans
> HIV- or HBV-containing cells, cultures, mediums, or solutions
> Blood, organs, or tissues from experimental animals infected with HIV or HBV

---

5. Potential contact is called "reasonably anticipated contact" in the Standard. Alas, "reasonably anticipated" is not well defined. The compliance manual says "reasonably anticipated" includes the potential for as well as actual exposure—i.e., a nurse who has never had actual contact with blood while starting IV lines has the potential for contact and therefore has occupational exposure to blood/OPIM.

6. Sweat, tears, and urine that are not visibly contaminated with blood are not OPIM.

7. If you see body fluid coming from some place you don't recognize, or can't pronounce, consider it OPIM.

Parenteral   Piercing into or under skin or mucous membranes, as occurs with needlesticks, human bites,[8] cuts, and abrasions.

Personal Protective Equipment (PPE)   Special equipment or clothing[9] worn to protect against a hazard.

PPE =

Masks	Respirators
Gloves	Goggles
Gowns	Protective clothing
Face shields	

Regulated waste   Liquid or dried blood/OPIM or items contaminated with or capable of releasing liquid or dried blood/OPIM.

Source individual   A person (living or dead) whose blood/OPIM is the source of occupational exposure.[10]

Universal Precautions   An approach to controlling infections that assumes all blood/OPIM is infectious (see Appendix B). Because the most infectious blood may test antibody-negative, and blood that tests antibody-positive may not be infectious, antibody testing is basically useless for emergency preventive measures and it must be assumed that all blood is infectious.[11]

Work practice controls   Processes or procedures that reduce the likelihood of exposure by altering the performance of a task (like prohibiting the recapping of needles).

---

8. Human bites that break the skin may occur in violent situations encountered by police or by prison, emergency room, and psychiatric ward personnel.

9. General work clothes, such as uniforms, pants, shirts, or blouses not intended to provide protection from bloodborne hazards, are not considered to be PPE.

10. An **exposed employee** is a person who has contact with a source individual's blood/OPIM.

11. After HIV antibodies are produced during initial infection, HIV itself (an antigen) may not be detectable. HIV may become detectable in higher concentrations in the blood of people in the later stages of AIDS. In early infection, the HIV antibody test may show a false negative; and in later stages, a false positive. Quite simply, antibody testing is confusing and often inaccurate. Thus, to be safe, we must not rely on antibody testing; we must assume that *all* blood is infectious.

QUESTIONS

1. *Do I have to use Universal Precautions when collecting routine urine samples?*

No. The definition of OPIM does not include urine, but it does include any fluid that is visibly contaminated with blood. Thus, the use of protective procedures or equipment is not required when obtaining routine urine samples, but it would be required if the urine appeared pink (visibly contaminated with blood.)

2. *Are "Good Samaritan" acts performed by employees covered by the Standard?*

No. "Good Samaritan" acts while assisting a fellow employee and which result in exposure to blood/OPIM are not covered by the Standard, although OSHA encourages employers to offer medical follow-up and evaluation. These acts are not considered to be reasonably anticipated; however, if first-aid or emergency response is listed in a job description, or the employee gets some type of compensation for being a first-aider, the rules of the Standard apply.

3. *Does the presence of stool /feces on something cause contamination?*

No, not as long as the stool is not visibly contaminated with blood. If, however, blood is visible on the stool, it would be considered contaminated by the Standard's definition.

4. *I heard that saliva has been shown to contain HIV. Why isn't saliva listed as OPIM?*

HIV has been isolated from most body fluids from People With AIDS (PWAs), but the concentrations are so low in urine, sweat, tears, or saliva that the risk of HIV transmission is thought to be minimal or nonexistent. There have been no documented cases of HIV transmission attributed to these fluids, and the Standard does not consider them to be OPIM, unless they are visibly contaminated with blood.

Saliva in dental procedures, however, is considered to be OPIM. Occupationally acquired infection with HBV in dental workers has been documented, and two possible cases of occupationally acquired HIV infection involving dentists have been reported. During dental procedures, the contamination of saliva with blood is predictable, trauma to health care workers' hands is common, and blood spattering may occur.

5. *Who is considered a licensed health care professional?*

The legal scope of practice for health care professionals, including doctors and registered nurses, is regulated by each state. In some states, nurse practitioners may prescribe and administer vaccinations independently, as well as perform other requirements of the Standard. Other health care workers may perform certain procedures, such as administration of vaccines, only under the supervision of another licensed health care professional. The regulating body for your state can provide information about the scope of practice for licensed health care professionals.

6. *Is breast milk considered to be OPIM?*

Breast milk is not included in the Standard's definition of OPIM. Therefore, contact with breast milk, unless it is visibly, or expected to be, contaminated with blood, does not constitute occupational exposure. This determination was based on the CDC's findings that human breast milk has not been implicated in the transmission of HIV or HBV to workers; however, it has been implicated in perinatal transmission of HIV, and the hepatitis surface antigen has been found in the milk of mothers infected with HBV. For this reason, gloves should be worn by health care workers in situations where exposures to breast milk might be frequent—for example, in milk banking.

7. *I saw an ad that said the prostitutes working at the legal houses in Nevada are tested for HIV every 2 weeks, and they'll show you the card to prove it.*

You can look at the card, but that's all I'd look at. Since it takes up to 6 weeks to develop detectable levels of HIV or HBV antibodies in blood tests, and the virus concentration in the blood may be highest before any antibodies are detected, a card proving HIV negativity 2 weeks earlier in a sexually active person is worthless and may even make business contact with the oldest occupation more dangerous, since the client may assume noninfectiousness and fail to use PPE—i.e., a condom.

Chapter 8

Paragraph (c):
Exposure Control

The sole end for which mankind are warranted, individually or collectively, in interfering with the liberty of action of any of their number is self-protection.

—*John Stuart Mill*

T he goal of the Standard is to reduce the risk of infection by decreasing or eliminating occupational exposure to bloodborne pathogens and by providing HBV vaccination and postexposure medical follow-up. The goal of this section is to identify employees who have a risk of infection in their jobs. Paragraph (c) is a key section because it requires the employer to identify the employees who fall under the provisions of the standard.

> Exposure Control = Infection Control

Paragraph (c) was initially called Infection Control in the proposed standard. OSHA changed the title to Exposure Control because "infection control" is typically used in health care settings to mean prevention of transmission of disease from employee to patient, whereas the Standard aims to prevent transmission of disease from patient to employee. Unfortunately, "exposure control" does not translate easily into non–health care settings and may confuse those of us who understand the concept of controlling infections better than the concept of controlling exposures. A major part of the Standard deals with HBV vaccination, which helps prevent postexposure infection, and this implies an exposure-control failure. This paragraph is better understood as Infection Control, subdivided into Infection Control Plan and Risk of Infection Determination (we're concerned about exposure because people who are exposed are at risk of infection).

EXPOSURE CONTROL PLAN

The first part of this section states that employers who have employees with occupational exposure must establish a written **exposure control plan (ECP)** that contains, at least, the following:

- Exposure determination
- Implementation plans
- Procedures for evaluating exposure incidents

The exposure control plan also must:

- Be accessible to employees
- Be reviewed and updated at least annually (or whenever new occupational exposes are possible)
- Be made available to OSHA personnel upon their request

Note that the first thing an OSHA inspector will ask to see, even before the coffee machine, is the ECP. The BBPS compliance guidelines state simply: "The compliance officer shall review the facility's written exposure control plan."

EXPOSURE DETERMINATION

The second part of paragraph (c) states that employers must prepare an **exposure determination.** This exposure determination is supposed to identify job classifications where occupational exposure may occur. Instead of requiring identification of each specific task or procedure that may incur an occupational exposure (as originally recommended in the proposed standard), the final Standard allows identification of broader categories of jobs where infection may occur. Employees who perform these jobs have exposure; thus, they are at risk of infection and must be protected.

Exposure Determination = Identifying Jobs with Risk of Infection
---

The exposure determination is required to contain:

- A list of jobs in which *all* employees have occupational exposure
- A list of jobs in which *some* employees have occupational exposure

The all-employees-with-occupational-exposure list may include jobs such as nurse, doctor, or phlebotomist. Listing of specific risky tasks and procedures (called "activities") is not required. However, the some-employees-with-occupational-exposure list also requires another list of activities that, when performed by employees, result in occupational exposure. Thus, if some employees in a job have occupational exposure, the specific risky activities must be defined in order to identify which employees require protection. If an employee in one of these jobs is not required to perform the risky activity, he or she is not covered by the Standard.

For example, the summary and explanation section includes the job of funeral director. Some, but not all, employees classified as funeral directors perform embalming or other tasks with potential blood/OPIM contact, while the duties of other funeral directors are limited to arranging and conducting services, and they have no occupational exposure. The job of funeral director thus must be on the some-employees-with-occupational-exposure list, and the activities that place some, but not all, funeral directors at risk must be described.

OSHA does allow the grouping of risky activities, so tasks such as starting or stopping IVs, drawing blood, and inserting arterial catheters may be grouped into the broad category of "vascular access procedures," and tasks such as washing, cleaning, and disposing of contaminated needles, knives, or razors may be classified as "handling of contaminated sharps."

On the lighter side, there is no requirement to list jobs in which employees do not have occupational exposure.

The last sentence of this paragraph is particularly important. It states that:

Exposure determination shall be made without regard to the use of personal protective equipment (PPE).

There is valid reasoning for this requirement, since several conditions must be met for PPE to effectively protect employees: The employee must be trained to use the PPE properly; it must be used each time the task is performed; it must fit properly; and it must be free of flaws. If any of these conditions are not met, PPE use is less effective and a worker may be at increased risk of exposure. To be safe, OSHA therefore does not allow the consideration of PPE use when identifying jobs with risk of infection.

QUESTIONS

1. *Can I keep our exposure control plan on a computer?*

In the compliance guidelines, OSHA states that the location of the ECP may be adapted to the circumstances of a particular workplace provided the employee can access a copy at the workplace and during the work shift. If the plan is maintained solely on a computer, employees must be trained to operate the computer. A hard copy of the ECP must be made available to an employee within 15 working days of the employee's request.

2. *I work in the laundry room of a large hospital. Do I have to get a hepatitis vaccination?*

That depends. If your job in the laundry room does not require you to handle contaminated laundry (e.g., if all you do is to fold and store cleaned laundry), you would not be reasonably anticipated to have occupational exposure to bloodborne pathogens, so your employer would not be obligated to offer HBV vaccination to you. However, if you occasionally loaded dirty laundry into the washing machine, you could reasonably anticipate occupational exposure, and you would fall into the exposure determination list for jobs in which some employees have occupational exposure. The loading of contaminated laundry would therefore make all provisions of the Standard apply to you. You cannot be forced to take HBV vaccination, but you must be offered it (and I would certainly recommend having the vaccination series).

3. *If we get an OSHA BBPS inspection, what will the compliance officer look for?*

The compliance guidelines state that the content of the ECP will be reviewed for at least the following elements:

- Exposure determination lists
- Schedule and method of implementation of the Standard
- Procedures for evaluating circumstances surrounding exposure incidents
- Location of the plan

Of course, the compliance officer will look for the coffee pot after finding the ECP.

4. *Do I have to make a list of employees who have no occupational exposure?*

No. You are not required to make an exposure determination on employees such as receptionists, bookkeepers, or office managers who do not have occupational exposure. The exposure determination need only be made for employees who have occupational exposure.

Chapter 9

Paragraph (d): Methods of Compliance

Beware of all enterprises that require new clothes.

—Henry David Thoreau

P aragraph (d) contains the true meat of the Standard. It outlines the procedures that must be followed in order to achieve the goal of reducing risk of exposure and infection. One dictionary definition of compliance is "a yielding to a demand." Thus, paragraph (d) could be appropriately called Ways of Yielding to Demands.

UNIVERSAL PRECAUTIONS

Appendix B contains the complete CDC guidelines for universal blood and body fluid precautions. "Universal Precautions" is simply defined as an approach to controlling infections that assumes all blood/OPIM is infectious. I have never been able to find a copy of Universal Precautions in a medical library; somehow, it always gets borrowed. So Appendix B is one of the most important parts of this book. Read it. There will be no CliffNotes to Universal Precautions presented here. Just read it.

The first sentence of paragraph (d) is the single most important one in the whole Standard:

> Universal Precautions shall be observed to prevent contact with blood or other potentially infectious material.

Prior to the Standard, Universal Precautions were mere recommendations. Now they are requirements, *enforceable* requirements. This is the first of the two most important end results of the BBPS (the other being that employers must provide HBV vaccination for at-risk employees).

The second sentence of the paragraph says that if you can't tell what type of body fluid it is, consider it potentially infectious.

ENGINEERING AND WORK PRACTICE CONTROLS

Engineering controls (EC) are methods used to reduce workplace exposure by either removing the hazard or isolating the employee from exposure. Ideally, the problem is *engineered* away. Seat belts and airbags are engineering controls used to remove hazards of driving. Needleless IV lines, negative-pressure isolation rooms, and sharps disposal containers are all medical engineering controls. Engineering controls are the most effective means of reducing exposure because they deal with the source of the hazard and they decrease exposure without reliance on the actions of employees.

Work practice controls (WPC) are methods used to reduce exposure by changing human behavior. Ideally, the work practices that cause exposures are modified. For those of you who don't know it, human behavior is hard to change. Hand washing, wearing gloves, not recapping needles, and using a mouth guard for CPR are all work practice controls. Work practice controls also act on the source of the hazard, but because they are based on the actions of employees, they are fallible. Thus, work practice controls are usually less effective than engineering controls. These types of controls often work together; a sharps container (EC) is not effective unless a worker puts the sharp in the container instead of on the bed (WPC).

The Standard states that engineering and work practice controls should be used to eliminate or minimize employee exposure, but if risk still exists once these controls are in place, **personal protective equipment (PPE)** should also be used. PPE consists of clothing, devices, or things that are used or worn personally by the worker (gloves, masks, shields, etc.). Use of PPE is the least desirable method of decreasing exposure because its use assumes the continuation of the risky work practices. The reality is that risky work practices must be performed (CPR, surgery, etc.), and PPE offers at least some added protection. Although considered least effective, the use of PPE is what is noticed most by workers.

Engineering controls must be reevaluated on a regular schedule to ensure that they work. The term "regular schedule," intentionally vague, is used here because OSHA believes that the reevaluation (examination, maintenance, replacement) should be individualized to each particular engineering control—i.e., sharps boxes should not be changed every year; some of them may need changing every few hours. Engineering controls should be checked, as needed, to ensure their effectiveness.

The Standard requires employers to:

- Provide readily accessible hand-washing facilities[1]
- Ensure that employees wash their hands promptly[2] after removing gloves or other PPE
- Ensure that employees wash their hands/skin with soap and water, or flush mucous membranes with water, promptly following contact with blood/OPIM
- Provide appropriate containers[3] for sharps and also for blood/OPIM specimens

Employees must *not:*

- Bend, recap, remove, or break contaminated needles or sharps[4]
- Eat, drink, smoke, apply cosmetics or lip balm, or handle contact lenses in areas with a reasonable likelihood of exposure

---

1. If this is not feasible, as in an ambulance, antiseptic hand cleanser and clean towels or towelettes must be provided.

2. "Promptly = immediately or as soon as feasible" and is added as legalese to clarify that workers are not required to wash their hands immediately after removal of all PPE. It might be dangerous to a patient if workers were required to wash their hands after removing blood-covered goggles blocking their view during emergency surgery. Throughout the Standard, things that are to be done quickly are stated to be done "immediately" or "as soon as feasible."

3. Appropriate sharps containers are puncture-resistant, labeled or color-coded, and leakproof on sides and bottoms (see Chapter 12). Appropriate blood/OPIM specimen containers must prevent leakage during collection, handling, processing, storage, transport, or shipping and be labeled or color-coded when leaving the facility (no labeling/color-coding is required inside a facility if Universal Precautions is used for handling of all specimens). If outside contamination of a container occurs, is must be placed within a second container that meets the same requirements.

4. Contaminated needles or sharps may be recapped or removed if the employer can demonstrate that no alternative is feasible or that the action is required by a specific medical procedure. Such recapping or removal must then be accomplished through the use of a mechanical device or one-handed process.

- Keep food or drink in refrigerators, freezers, shelves, cabinets, or on countertops or benchtops where blood/OPIM is present
- Perform mouth pipetting or suctioning of blood/OPIM

In addition, equipment that may be contaminated with blood/OPIM must be examined before servicing or shipping and be decontaminated, if possible. Parts that remain contaminated must be labeled as contaminated (see Chapter 12), and the employer must inform appropriate employees, servicing representatives, and manufactures so that precautions are taken.

PERSONAL PROTECTIVE EQUIPMENT

The most important part of the Standard, as it relates to everyday job performance, is the requirement that employers provide appropriate personal protective equipment, *at no cost to the employee.* "Appropriate" PPE is defined as PPE that does not permit blood/OPIM to pass through or reach clothes, undergarments, skin, eyes, mouth, or other mucous membranes under normal conditions.

PPE includes, but is not limited, to:

Gloves
Gowns
Laboratory coats
Face shields/masks
Eye protection
Mouthpieces
Resuscitation bags
Pocket masks or other ventilation devices

Employers must:

Ensure that employees use appropriate PPE
Ensure that PPE is easily accessible and in appropriate sizes[5]
Clean, launder, and dispose of PPE[6]
Repair and replace PPE[6]

---

5. Employees who are allergic to normally used gloves must be provided with hypoallergenic gloves, glove liners, powderless gloves, or similar alternatives.

6. At no cost to the employee.

PPE that is penetrated by blood/OPIM must be removed promptly (i.e., immediately or as soon as feasible), and it must be removed prior to leaving the work area. Used PPE must be placed in a designated area or container.

An employee may, under rare and extraordinary circumstances, decline to use PPE when, in the employee's professional judgment, use of PPE would prevent the delivery of care or would pose a hazard to the safety of the employee. For example, obtaining and properly donning gloves, a mask, gown, and a face shield before defibrillating a bleeding patient may place the patient's life at risk. The employee has the option, in this or similar serious scenarios, not to wear PPE. When a judgment not to wear appropriate PPE has been made, the circumstances surrounding the incident must be investigated and documented so that similar incidents are prevented.

Gloves must be worn if hand contact with blood/OPIM is reasonably anticipated (as when drawing blood or performing other vascular access procedures); when hands may contact mucous membranes or nonintact skin; and when handling or touching contaminated items or surfaces. Disposable gloves intended for single use must be replaced promptly[7] when contaminated, torn, or punctured, or when they fail to provide a protective barrier. They may not be washed or decontaminated for reuse. Utility gloves intended for multiuse may be reused if the integrity of the glove is not compromised, but they must be discarded if cracked, peeled, torn, or punctured, or if they show signs of deterioration.

The Standard has one important exception to required glove use. Experienced phlebotomists at volunteer blood centers may opt not to use gloves, as long as they have no cuts, scratches, or skin breaks, and the employee believes that hand contamination will not occur. If hand contamination may occur (the example given is when drawing blood on an uncooperative patient—highly unlikely in a volunteer blood center!) or if the employee is being trained in phlebotomy, gloves must be used. The employer must periodically reevaluate this policy, make gloves available to all who wish to use them, and not discourage the use of gloves for phlebotomy. This exception is strictly limited to phlebotomy performed in volunteer blood centers and does not apply to phlebotomy conducted in other settings, such as hospitals, or to plasma collection and private medical or dental offices.

It's an illogical policy that came about as a result of politics. During the final evaluation by OMB (the Office of Management and Budget, the agency that evaluates the fiscal implications of legislation), blood bank representatives lobbied hard to exempt phlebotomists from glove wearing. Their argument was that blood

---

7. "Promptly" in this sentence is defined as *as soon as practical* when contaminated and *as soon as feasible* if torn or punctured. OSHA legalese here does not state "Change PPE as soon as possible" because there may be procedures, such as surgery, where it may be possible to change gloves but not practical to interrupt the procedure.

donations were down because of unfounded fears of contracting AIDS from donating blood. They contended that if phlebotomists started wearing gloves, they would scare away some of the prospective blood donors, and blood supplies would decrease. This imminent medical catastrophe resulted in a compromise at the OMB level; OSHA, to get the Standard passed quickly, reluctantly consented to this exemption. Unfortunately, it leaves phlebotomists at increased risk of infection, and donors who may be used to having blood drawn by someone without gloves now think something terrible is happening in hospitals when they have blood drawn by gloved phlebotomists.

Masks, eye protection, and face shields must be worn whenever splashes, spray, spatters, or droplets of blood/OPIM may be generated and eye, nose, or mouth contamination may be reasonably anticipated. Gowns, aprons, and other protective body clothing must be worn in occupational exposure situations. Surgical caps or hoods and/or shoe covers or boots must be worn in instances when gross contamination can be reasonably anticipated (as in deliveries or surgeries).

HOUSEKEEPING

The employer is responsible for maintaining, cleaning, and sanitizing the workplace. Employers are required to prepare a written schedule for cleaning and decontamination to ensure that routine and appropriate cleaning is performed. Employees can use the schedule to determine when the cleaning should be done and what method should be used. The Standard makes no reference to specific appropriate disinfectants or exact cleaning procedures. It states that specifying particular disinfectants and procedures might limit their use and discourage the development of new products and procedures. The defining sentence of this section is:

> All equipment and environmental and working surfaces shall be cleaned and decontaminated after contact with blood or other potentially infectious materials.

"Environmental surfaces" refers to floors, walls, ceilings, etc., that may become contaminated but are not normally considered working surfaces.

In general, contaminated **work surfaces** and **protective coverings** used to cover equipment and environmental surfaces must be decontaminated:

- After the completion of procedures
- Promptly when they are overtly contaminated (as in a spill)
- At the end of the work shift if they may have become contaminated since the last cleaning

Receptacles intended for reuse that have a reasonable likelihood of becoming contaminated (such as bins, pails, and cans) must be inspected and decontaminated on a regularly scheduled basis. They must be cleaned and decontaminated promptly when visibly contaminated.

Broken glassware that may be contaminated must be cleaned up using mechanical means (such as a brush and dustpan, tongs, or forceps) and must not be picked up directly with the hands. Contaminated reusable sharps must not be stored or processed in a manner that requires employees to reach by hand into containers to obtain them.

The Standard is quite specific regarding containment and discarding of **regulated waste** and **contaminated sharps.** In general, contaminated sharps and regulated waste must be promptly placed in a container that is:

- Closable
- Puncture-resistant
- Leakproof
- Labeled or color-coded in accordance with paragraph (g)
- Closed prior to removal

If the first container leaks or becomes contaminated on the outside, it must be placed in a secondary container that meets the same requirements.

Containers for contaminated sharps must be easily accessible to employees and located as close as feasible to the area where the sharps are used; they must be kept upright, be replaced routinely, and not be allowed to overfill. Reusable containers must not be manually opened, emptied, or cleaned in any manner that would expose employees to risk of injury.

OSHA defers to the Environmental Protection Agency (EPA) and state regulations by requiring that disposal of regulated waste be in accordance with applicable regulations of the United States and its territories.

Contaminated laundry must be:

- Handled as little as possible and with minimum agitation
- Handled by employees wearing protective gloves and appropriate PPE

- Bagged or containerized at the location of use but not sorted or rinsed there
- Placed and transported in labeled or color-coded bags or containers[8]
- Placed in leakproof bags or containers if wet

Questions

1. *Do we have to double-bag blood-soaked linens?*

No, not unless the outside of the bag or container is contaminated, or the wet linens are likely to soak through the first bag. OSHA did not intend to imply that all regulated waste needs to be double-bagged, but it wanted to ensure that waste was placed in a second bag or container if the first one had been splashed with blood or handled by an employee wearing bloody gloves, or if the bag was leaking blood/OPIM—all cases when contact with the outside of the contaminated bag presents a hazard.

2. *I just can't feel veins well if I wear gloves when drawing blood. I heard that I don't have to wear gloves if I don't want to, but one of my coworkers said I had to. What's the story?*

There was considerable concern during the formulation of the Standard that requiring gloves for drawing blood would make it difficult to feel veins and would decrease manual dexterity, possibly resulting in an increased risk of needlestick or missing the stick. Most of the comments received by OSHA agreed that once the worker got used to it, drawing blood while using gloves was no more difficult than when not using them, as long as the gloves fit well. The only exception to this rule applies to experienced phlebotomists working in volunteer blood donation centers who have no sores or nonintact areas of skin. All other employees performing vascular access procedures (including routine blood drawing) must wear gloves.

Since gloves may not prevent needlesticks, think about what happens if you get a needlestick while wearing a glove. Recent studies have shown

---

8. If a facility uses Universal Precautions in the handling of all soiled laundry, methods of labeling or color-coding other than that outlined in paragraph (g) are sufficient so long as all employees in the facility recognize the containers as requiring Universal Precautions. If the laundry is shipped off-site to a facility that does not utilize Universal Precautions for all laundry, then bags or containers must comply with labeling and color-coding as required in paragraph (g).

that a glove provides a "squeegee" effect when a needle passes through it. As much as 50% of the blood on the outside of a needle or suture is wiped off when it penetrates the glove. It makes sense to wear gloves in procedures where needlesticks may occur because they could decrease the amount of exposed blood by a factor of one-half! Your coworker is right.

3. *Why can't I wash my lab coat at home? The laundry takes weeks, and always I end up with someone else's coat.*

OSHA believes that if an item is to function as PPE, it is the employer's responsibility to provide that item, clean it, repair it, replace it, and dispose of it. If employers permit home laundering of PPE, they cannot be sure that proper handling or laundering procedures are being followed. OSHA recognizes no distinction between dealing with contaminated institutional linens and the procedures for cleaning and laundering PPE. If a lab coat is used to prevent an employee's uniform from becoming contaminated with blood/OPIM, then the lab coat is PPE and is the responsibility of the employer.

4. *I'm a plastic surgeon in Hollywood. Washing my hands after removing my gloves is ludicrous, and it slows down my production line timing.*

Paragraph (d)(2)(v) of the Standard states that the employer shall ensure that employees wash their hands immediately or as soon as feasible after removal of gloves or other PPE. Most likely you, as a plastic surgeon, are an employee *and* employer; therefore, you are responsible for ensuring post–glove removal hand washing. The CDC's guideline for Hand-washing and Hospital Environmental Control, 1985[9] states:

. . . handwashing is indicated, even when gloves are used, after situations during which microbial contamination of the hands is likely to occur, especially those involving contact with mucous membranes, blood and body fluids, and secretions or excretions, and after touching inanimate sources that are likely to be contaminated, such as urine-measuring devices.

OSHA believes that hand washing after removal of gloves or other PPE is consistent with these CDC guidelines and is appropriate for preventing occupational exposure. Interestingly, OSHA has no jurisdiction over patient protection and cannot require that gloves be changed between

---

9. J. S. Garner and M. S. Farero, Guideline for handwashing and hospital environmental control, 1985. *Am Journal Inf Control* 1986; 14(3):110–29

patient contacts; however, this is certainly good infection control practice and helps to eliminate patient-to-patient transmission of disease.

5. *Head Nurse Ratchit has just issued an edict stating that we can't drink at our nurses' stations. Does she mean all alcohol?*

No, she means all beverages. The Standard prohibits the consumption of food and drink in areas where work involving exposure or potential exposure to blood/OPIM occurs, or where the potential for contamination of work surfaces exists. In addition to possible contamination of the food and drink itself, the food and beverage containers may also become contaminated, resulting in unsuspected contamination of the hands or mucous membranes. This prohibition against eating and drinking in work areas is consistent with other OSHA standards and is good industrial hygiene practice.

6. *Do I have to wear PPE when performing dental treatment on children?*

Yes. Children, like adults, may be infected with HBV, HIV, or other bloodborne pathogens without exhibiting overt symptoms of disease. Therefore, exposure to blood/OPIM of children also presents a risk of occupational infection. OSHA had testimony from many dentists who treated children while using PPE without frightening the children. Dentists and dental personnel are not required to wear PPE when first meeting the child, which is the appropriate time to explain the procedures and to demonstrate and explain the PPE to be used.

7. *How do I clean up a blood spill?*

Carefully. First, clean up or wipe up the initial blood spill while wearing appropriate PPE. Do not use your hands to pick up broken glass or sharps that may cause cuts or punctures. The wiped-up blood and towel or linen are considered contaminated waste and must be disposed of appropriately. A solution of bleach (sodium hypochlorite) diluted 1:10 with water is acceptable for the disinfection of environmental surfaces and site decontamination following the initial cleanup. Unfortunately, bleach may harm some surfaces after extended use.

Chapter 10

Paragraph (e): HIV and HBV Research Laboratories and Production Facilities[1]

Shun those studies in which the work that results dies with the worker.

—Leonardo da Vinci

Paragraph (e) sets additional requirements that must be followed by research laboratories and production facilities involved in the culture, production, and concentration of HIV/HBV. It does not apply to clinical or diagnostic laboratories that analyze blood, tissues, or organs. Requirements stated elsewhere in the Standard, such as the prohibition of mouth pipetting or recapping needles, are not repeated in this chapter, but they still apply.

RESEARCH LABORATORY AND PRODUCTION FACILITY RISKS

People working in laboratories have contracted infections throughout the history of microbiology. HIV/HBV laboratories are no exception. Of the first 19 cases of health care workers reported to CDC who became HIV-infected through occupa-

---

1. If you are not associated with an HIV/HBV research/production facility, you will probably want to skip over Chapter 10 and go directly to Chapter 11.

tional exposure, two worked in laboratories. The first of these infections occurred in an employee who worked with concentrated HIV. Although no specific exposure incident was identified, it was concluded that infection most likely occurred through undetected skin contact with concentrated virus. The other lab worker handled large volumes of concentrated HIV and recalled having cut his finger with a blunt steel needle while cleaning some contaminated equipment.

OSHA defines a **research laboratory** as a facility producing or using small quantities of highly concentrated HIV or HBV, and **production facilities** as places that produce large quantities of highly concentrated HIV/HBV. Facilities that use unconcentrated blood as the only source of HIV/HBV do not have to follow the requirements of paragraph (e).

It makes sense that when the concentration of virus is increased by growing the virus in cell culture (or through simple concentration procedures), the risk to workers increases also. The increased risk associated with working in research/production facilities warrants additional protective measures.

ADDITIONAL PROTECTIVE MEASURES

Paragraph (e) of the Standard restates the need for standard microbiological practices, including the requirement that regulated waste be incinerated or decontaminated by methods known to destroy bloodborne pathogens (such as autoclaving). It also requires these special practices:

- Closing lab doors when working with HIV/HBV
- Placing materials to be decontaminated into appropriate and identifiable containers and removing them from the work area[2]
- Limiting access to the work area to authorized persons
- Posting the universal biohazard symbol on doors when OPIM or infected animals are present
- Conducting work involving OPIM in biological safety cabinets or other physical-containment devices
- Using appropriate PPE in the work area and animal rooms[3]
- Wearing gloves when handling infected animals or when hand contact with OPIM is unavoidable

---

2. "Appropriate and identifiable containers" are durable, leakproof, and labeled or color-coded. They must be closed before removing them from the work area.

3. Protective clothing is not to be worn outside the work area and must be decontaminated before being laundered.

- Decontaminating or incinerating all contaminated waste from work areas or animal rooms before disposal[4]
- Protecting vacuum lines with liquid disinfectant traps and high-efficiency particulate air (HEPA) filters, and checking and maintaining them routinely
- Using hypodermic needles and syringes only for parenteral injection and aspiration of fluid from animals or diaphragm bottles[5]
- Having properly trained personnel immediately contain and clean up all spills
- Immediately reporting exposure incidents to the lab director or other responsible person
- Preparing a biosafety manual that will be periodically reviewed and updated[6]
- Using certified containment equipment[7] when working with potentially infectious materials that might spill, splash, or become aerosolized
- Certifying biological safety cabinets when installed or moved, and at least annually

Research laboratories must contain facilities for hand and eye washing that are readily available in the work area. They must also have available an autoclave for decontamination of regulated waste.

Production facilities must have:

- Work areas separated from open areas in the building in order to decrease traffic flow into the area
- Two sets of doors to pass through to enter the work area from an access area[8]
- Work areas with water-resistant and easily cleanable doors, walls, floors, and ceilings

---

4. By a method, such as autoclaving, that is known to effectively destroy bloodborne pathogens.

5. Workers are advised to use extreme caution when handling needles and syringes; not to bend, shear, or recap needles following use; and to place used sharps promptly into appropriate containers.

6. At least annually, or more often if necessary. Personnel must be advised of potential hazards and be required to read about and follow the practices and procedures.

7. Such as certified biological safety cabinets, or other protective devices such as respirators, centrifuge safety cups, sealed centrifuge rotors, containment caging for animals, and protective clothing.

8. Other methods of physical separation, such as double-doored clothes changing rooms or airlocks, may be used.

- Readily available facilities for hand and eye washing in each work area[9]
- Self-closing access doors into the work or containment area
- A readily available[10] autoclave
- A ducted exhaust-air ventilation system that draws air into the work area and discharges it to the outside without recirculation[11]

SPECIAL TRAINING REQUIREMENTS

Although additional training requirements for employees in HIV/HBV research/production facilities are stated in paragraph (g), they are presented here for consistency. Remember that these training requirements are *additional,* and employers must also fulfill all the other training requirements set forth in Chapter 12.

Employers in research/production facilities must:

- Ensure that employees are proficient in standard microbiological practices and techniques before being allowed to work with HIV/HBV
- Ensure that employees have prior experience in handling pathogens and tissue cultures before working with HIV/HBV
- Provide training to employees who have no prior experience in handling human pathogens
- Not allow the initial work activities of inexperienced workers to include the handling of pathogens
- Not allow employees to work with infectious agents until they demonstrate handling technique proficiency

QUESTIONS

1. *There is a whole paragraph of the Standard devoted to research and production facilities. Why isn't there a paragraph on dental facilities?*

---

9. The sink for hand washing must be foot-, elbow-, or automatically operated and located near the work area exit.

10. Within or as near as possible to the work area.

11. This ventilation system should create a negative air pressure, drawing air into the work area from the entry area, and the exhaust air must be dispersed away from occupied areas and air intakes. The proper airflow direction in the work area must be verified.

Even though HBV transmission to and from dental workers has been documented quite frequently, at the time of the first draft (Advance Notice of Proposed Rulemaking), there had been no reported cases of HIV transmission to or from dentists. There had, however, been two documented cases of HIV transmission in laboratory workers. Furthermore, the high concentration of virus found in these facilities increases the risk of infection. On the other hand, it could be that this paragraph is here because the chair of the OSHA Bloodborne Pathogens working group was a virologist, not a dentist.

2. *You seemed to gloss over this paragraph without giving much detail. Why?*

The requirements in paragraph (e) were derived primarily from the CDC/NIH recommendations found in their guidelines on Biosafety in Microbiological and Biomedical Laboratories, first published in 1984 and revised in 1988. It is assumed that laboratory employers and employees are familiar with these recommendations, though only the provisions that relate to the health and safety of employees are included in the Standard. If you are not already familiar with these recommendations, you should become familiar with them.

Briefly, these biosafety guidelines classify infectious agents and laboratory activities into four classes, denoted as biosafety levels (BSL) 1 through 4. In 1988, the CDC also published an Agent Summary Statement for Human Immunodeficiency Virus, which outlines biosafety levels for activities involving HIV. This summary classifies activities performed in clinical laboratories as BSL 2 and activities performed in facilities with concentrated HIV as BSL 3. The special training requirements outlined in Chapter 12 are based on the recommendations of an expert team brought together by the National Institutes of Health (NIH).

There apparently has been little dissension about this section from the research and production community, who are well aware of the extra risk they have in their workplace. It is beyond the scope of this book to go into depth about the specific requirements of this paragraph.

Chapter 11

Paragraph (f):
HBV Vaccination and Postexposure Follow-up

Vaccination is the medical sacrament corresponding to baptism.

—*Samuel Butler*

EMPLOYER RESPONSIBILITIES

Paragraph (f), the medical section of the Standard, is broken down into two parts: **preexposure** (HBV vaccination[1]), and **postexposure** (medical evaluation and follow-up). It begins by charging the employer with the responsibility to provide employees with pre- and postexposure medical evaluation. This is consistent with the OSHAct's General Duty Clause, which places the burden for employee health issues directly on employers.

---

1. "HBV vaccination" refers to the HBV vaccine and vaccination series. OSHA formally states "HBV vaccine and vaccination series" throughout the Standard. If they stated, "The employer must provide HBV vaccine," employers might only give one shot of the vaccine, instead of the complete series of three shots. The term "HBV vaccination" always means the complete set of three HBV shots.

The second most important sentence in the Standard follows:

> The employer must make free HBV vaccination available
> to all employees who have occupational exposure.

"Free" means at no cost to the employee. It's certainly not free to the employer, who must pay for it! "Make available" means that the employer must actually provide the vaccination. The first draft stated that employers must "provide" HBV vaccination and postexposure evaluation. The wording of the final Standard was changed from "provide" to "make available" in order to emphasize that employee participation in these programs is optional. The employer must make the programs available, but the employee has the choice to participate or not (however, participation is highly recommended). Unfortunately, these are the types of fine details that are lost when we try to simplify the language of the Standard.

The employer also must provide postexposure evaluation and follow-up to all employees who have had an exposure incident. In regard to both HBV vaccination and postexposure evaluation, the employer must:

- Pay the bills[2]
- Make vaccinations and evaluations convenient for employees[3]
- Ensure that they are performed by licensed physicians or health care professions[4]
- Ensure that they are provided according to current U.S. Public Health Service (USPHS) recommendations

---

2. Make available at no cost to the employee.

3. Make available to the employee at a reasonable time and place. OSHA worried that employers might discourage participation by making these programs difficult to participate in, so they added this important requirement. Unfortunately, "reasonable time and place" is not defined. It is assumed to mean during normal working hours for the employee and at the workplace, if possible (which may not always be feasible.) If these programs are not convenient for the worker, OSHA feared they may not be done.

4. Vaccinations and evaluations must be performed by or under the supervision of a licensed physician or licensed health care professional. Other OSHA standards require physician participation, but it was thought that many of these requirements (like vaccination) could be performed by appropriately licensed nurses or nurse practitioners.

■ Ensure that laboratory tests are performed by an accredited laboratory[5]

Since HBV vaccination has only been around since 1982, it is still unclear whether booster doses will be needed. If, in the future, routine HBV booster doses are recommended by the USPHS, these booster doses must be made available under the same above requirements.

The Standard does not specify medical treatment but defers to other agencies. OSHA recognizes the dynamic nature of medical knowledge relating to bloodborne pathogens and notes that USPHS recommendations current at the time the Standard is published may differ from those current at the actual time of vaccination or evaluation. OSHA thus appropriately defers specific details of medical practice to the USPHS.

HEPATITIS B VACCINATION

General information on HBV vaccination can be found in Chapter 3 and specific information in Appendix F. Only OSHA requirements will be presented here.

HBV vaccination must be made available to employees within 10 working days of initial assignment to jobs with occupational exposure.

Before the vaccination series is started, however, employees must receive the training required in paragraph (g). OSHA believes that it is necessary to accomplish this training before the employee makes a decision regarding acceptance of the HBV vaccine. HBV vaccination does *not* have to be provided if:

■ The employee has previously received the complete HBV vaccination series
■ Antibody testing shows that the employee is already HBV-immune
■ The vaccine is contraindicated for medical reasons

---

5. OSHA defines "accredited laboratory" as one that has participated in a recognized quality assurance program and has received accreditation from a national accrediting body or its state equivalent.

There is debate about the usefulness of HBV vaccination prescreening programs, which may identify workers who are immune to HBV because of previous infection or workers who have had an inadequate response to prior HBV vaccination. Prevaccination screening is usually only cost-effective if the cost of the vaccine is high and many in the population have been infected and are already immune (and therefore need not be revaccinated).[6] There is minimal danger in revaccinating those already immune through prior infection,[7] so it is usually easiest just to vaccinate everyone who has not yet been vaccinated. Because of the above concerns about prescreening programs, OSHA states that employers may not make participation in prescreening program a prerequisite for receiving HBV vaccination. Employees have the right to decline prevaccination testing and yet still receive HBV vaccination.

If an employee initially declines HBV vaccination, but later decides to accept vaccination, the employer still must provide the vaccination series at no cost to the employee.[8] This provision ensures that employees who are initially reluctant to accept vaccination have an opportunity to receive vaccination later if they change their mind (i.e., figure out that the benefits of vaccination far outweigh the risks). Remember, there was significant unfounded concern about HIV contamination of the early HBV vaccine, as well as some concern that employers might try to discourage vaccination to save money.

Employers are required to have employees who decline HBV vaccination sign the following declination statement:

> I understand that due to my occupational exposure to blood or other potentially infectious materials I may be at risk of acquiring hepatitis B virus (HBV) infection. I have been given the opportunity to be vaccinated with hepatitis B vaccine, at no charge to myself. However, I decline hepatitis B vaccination at this time. I understand that by declining this vaccine, I continue to be at risk of acquiring hepatitis B, a serious disease. If in the future I continue to have occupational exposure to blood or other potentially infectious materials and I want to be vaccinated with hepatitis B vaccine, I can receive the vaccination series at no charge to me.

OSHA thinks that employers will benefit from signed declinations because the

---

6. If the vaccination series costs $100 and screening costs $25, more than one-quarter of the population must be immune before prevaccination screening is cost-effective, i.e., the employer would spend $100 to identify the one person out of four ($4 \times \$25$) who is already immune and does not need revaccination, just to save that $100 cost of one revaccination series.

7. As with any vaccination, there is always some risk of an allergic reaction. Luckily, allergic reactions to HBV vaccination are relatively rare.

8. As long as the employee still has occupational exposure and is working for the same employer.

statements make it easy to identify employees who have not been vaccinated, so that the employers can then improve the vaccination acceptance rate. This rationale seems dubious, at best, as I doubt many employers will analyze declination statements in order to improve vaccination rates. More likely, the signed declination statements just make it easier for compliance officers to enforce the requirements of the Standard. As will be explained later in this chapter, all employees with occupational exposure must have documented evidence that they either have had complete HBV vaccination, are immune, that vaccination is contraindicated, or that they declined vaccination. This is what I call "the HBV vaccination paper chase."

POSTEXPOSURE EVALUATION AND FOLLOW-UP

Once an exposure incident has been reported, the employer must *immediately* provide the exposed employee a *confidential* medical evaluation and follow-up. The adjective "immediately" emphasizes the importance of prompt medical evaluation and prophylaxis.[9] "Confidential" is used to underscore the importance of maintaining strict confidentiality throughout these evaluations.

The postexposure medical evaluation and follow-up must include:

- Documentation of the route and circumstances of the exposure
- Identification of the source individual
- Testing of blood for HBV and HIV status
- Postexposure prophylaxis, as recommended by the USPHS
- Counseling
- Evaluation of reported illnesses

Again, all postexposure medical evaluation and follow-up must be provided by the employer at no cost to the employer.

The route and circumstances of exposure must be documented in order to allow employers to receive feedback about the circumstances of employee exposures. Ideally, this information will be used to prevent future similar exposures. Review of this documentation may show that PPE is not being used because it is uncomfortable. In this case, the employer should make an effort to provide more comfortable, and thus usable, PPE.

The source individual must be identified, if feasible, and this information must be documented, unless prohibited by state or local law. It is the responsibility of

---

9. Some HBV prophylaxis must be done within the first few days after exposure, and HIV prophylaxis may need to be done within the first few hours after exposure.

the employer to establish the identification of the source individual, or to establish that identification is infeasible or prohibited by law. Exposure incidents involving unmarked sharps may make identification impossible, and it would be in the employer's best interest to document the infeasibility or impossibility of identification.

If available, the source individual's blood must be tested for HBV/HIV status promptly and after consent is obtained. If consent is not obtained, the employer must document this. Some states do not require consent from the source individual for postexposure testing. The words "if available" apply to blood samples that have already been drawn from source individuals for other tests. Postexposure blood drawing specifically for HBV/HIV status should not be done without the source individual's consent. Drawing blood without consent would be considered bodily assault and could be reason for legal action. The Standard also specifically states that if the source individual is already known to be HBV/HIV-infected, testing for HBV/HIV status need not be repeated.

Results of the source individual's testing must be provided to the exposed employee. The exposed employee must also be informed about confidentiality laws concerning the source individual, in order to protect the source's privacy rights.

The exposed employee's blood must be collected promptly after consent is obtained.[10] Exposed employees have the right to decline postexposure HBV/HIV testing; however, they would lose legal standing if they declined this baseline testing and were later to claim that they were infected by the exposure. OSHA gives the exposed employee an option to have baseline blood collected promptly, but not to give consent for HIV testing for up to 90 days.[11] This provision was added to give the employee time to think and to learn more about HIV testing instead of immediately demanding a decision. The employer is responsible for preserving this sample for at least 90 days, so that if at a later date the exposed employee so decides, the preserved sample can be tested for HIV status. This 90-day holding provision

---

10. The one important addition I made to the Standard was the specific inclusion of this statement requiring consent of the employee before postexposure testing. In an oversight, the OSHA working group had left out the employee consent statement, though they were careful to have it in for the source individual. I pointed out that consent must be specifically stated here for employees also, or the procedures could be interpreted as absolutely requiring testing of employees. For better or worse, the exposed employee has the legal right to decline this testing.

11. I disagreed with this holding provision and recommended that it be deleted, but I was overruled. The employer should be required to adequately educate employees promptly after an exposure incident. If I were skeptical of having blood drawn in the first place, I'd certainly be skeptical of having it held for later testing. The thousands of employees who are HIV-positive or at risk of being HIV-positive from nonoccupational exposure would most likely decline testing so that they would not be identified as being baseline positive. In my practice as a physician, I would have a difficult time explaining to you that I wanted to draw blood for a test, then hold it without testing until you became informed enough to have the sample tested.

includes the 12-week postexposure period when acute HIV illness may develop and the employee's HIV antibody status would most likely convert to positive if he or she was infected.

Although it is not specifically stated in the Standard, the employer does not have the right to know the results of either the source individual's or exposed employee's testing. It's a little confusing because what is stated is that the employer shall make the results of the source individual's testing available to the exposed employee. The employer must pay for the tests and provide the results to the exposed employee, but the employer has no right to be informed of the actual results. A problem arises when the employer, as in a doctor's office, is also the health care professional working with the exposed employee. OSHA says only that matters of consent and confidentiality are extremely important in this setting, but it gives no specific guidance, even though this creates a major confidentiality conflict in occupational medicine when the employer acts as the health care provider for employees.

INFORMATION PROVIDED TO THE HEALTH CARE PROFESSIONAL

The employer must make sure the health care professional (HCP) working with the HBV vaccination program and postexposure evaluations has a copy of the Standard. The employer must also ensure that the HCP performing the postexposure evaluations is provided with:

- A description of the exposed employee's duties relating to the exposure
- Documentation of the circumstances of the exposure
- The source individual's blood test results
- All relevant medical records[12]

It is the employer's responsibility to maintain employee HBV vaccination records.

Again, the employer does not have a specific right to know the results of the source individual's blood testing. The employer is merely responsible for ensuring the evaluating HCP is provided with the results of the testing. The employer also has no right to know information contained in medical records, which must be kept confidential.

------

12. "Relevant medical records" are those that are needed for the appropriate postexposure treatment of the employee and include HBV vaccination status.

THE HEALTH CARE PROFESSIONAL'S WRITTEN OPINION

The HCP working with the HBV vaccination program or performing the postexposure evaluation must produce what OSHA calls a "written opinion." The employer does have the right to know what is contained in a written opinion and may even keep a copy. The employer must provide the employee with a copy of the written opinion within 15 days of the completion of an evaluation. Note that there are two distinct types of written opinions—one for HBV vaccination evaluation, and one for postexposure evaluation. The purpose of the written opinion is to ensure that the employer has knowledge and documentation of the employee's HBV vaccination and postexposure evaluation status.

The HBV vaccination written opinion is limited to whether HBV vaccination is indicated for an employee, and if the employee has received vaccination. Appropriate written opinions may be as simple as:

HBV vaccination indicated for this employee; vaccination received.
HBV vaccination indicated for this employee; vaccination not received.
HBV vaccination not indicated for this employee; vaccination not received.

The postexposure evaluation written opinion is limited to stating that the employee has been informed of the evaluation results and has been told about any medical conditions that may result from the exposure. Appropriate written opinions may be as simple as:

This employee has been informed of postexposure evaluation results and has been told about any medical conditions that may result from the exposure.

OSHA specifically states that both types of written opinions should contain no other findings or diagnoses.

MEDICAL RECORDKEEPING

Medical recordkeeping is discussed in paragraph (h), but is mentioned here so that employers, physicians, and other HCPs are made aware that there are medical recordkeeping requirements elsewhere in the Standard. See Chapter 13 for further information. All medical records must be kept confidential.

QUESTIONS

1. *My boss said that if I have a needlestick I should get it evaluated through our employee health plan, which has a $100 deductible charge. Should I have to pay if it happened on the job?*

No. The employer must pay all costs relating to HBV vaccination and postexposure evaluation. If your health plan is completely employee noncontributory (e.g., no premium charge, deductible, copayment, or other form of payment required by the employee), then your boss could use the health plan to cover the expenses, as long as those expenses are covered in the plan. It is the employer's responsibility to pay for all the costs involved in pre- and postexposure evaluations.

2. *I have some employees who, for religious reasons, have declined HBV vaccination. They're even refusing to sign the required HBV vaccination declination form. What should I do?*

You cannot force employees to sign the declination. Don't get nasty about it, but I'd recommend fully annotating the circumstances, reasons, and names of the employees who refuse to sign the declination. Otherwise, if OSHA inspects your office, you could be fined for not having complete HBV vaccination information on your employees. Ideally, you should have either a declination statement or a written opinion on HBV vaccination from a health care provider for each of your employees with occupational exposure.

3. *Is it true that they make the hepatitis vaccine from the blood of homosexuals and drug users—the same groups most likely to have AIDS?*

No. The first hepatitis B vaccine was derived from the plasma of people who had already been infected with HBV, and many of these donors were IV drug abusers, homosexuals, or both. This first HBV vaccine is no longer being produced in the United States. The vaccine now in use is produced by a recombinant gene technique, contains no human blood, and therefore has no possibility of being HIV-infectious.

4. *We had some first-aiders in our company until the OSHA regulation came along. The company discontinued the program because they did not want to give employees hepatitis vaccinations. Does OSHA know about this?*

Yes. About a year after the Standard was released, OSHA issued a policy letter stating that failure to give vaccine in cases like this would be considered a *de minimis* violation and would result in no fine to the employer; however, the rest of the provisions in the Standard would apply (yearly training, etc.). If an exposure incident did occur for a first-aider, the employer would have to provide free postexposure HBV vaccination (which has shown to decrease risk of developing hepatitis but is not as helpful as vaccination before exposure) and free medical evaluation and follow-up (see Appendix D).

5. *Our city closed down the children's summer camp last year because the hepatitis vaccination required for the camp counselors was too expensive. This is unnecessary government intervention, and OSHA should be ashamed. Why is vaccination needed if all they do is put Band-Aids on the kids?*

The cost of the three-part HBV vaccination is about $100, and it's good for at least 9 years, maybe for life. OSHA requires that employees who may be reasonably anticipated to have occupational exposure to blood be offered HBV vaccination. Camp counselors who perform first-aid duties may be reasonably anticipated to have contact with blood. The OSHA policy letter mentioned in the previous question states that failure to offer (i.e., pay for) HBV vaccination preexposure to employees who render first aid only as volunteer duty will be considered a *de minimis* violation and carry no penalties, as long as the rest of the requirements of the Standard are met (see Appendix D). Camp nurses and doctors, who would be reasonably expected to have blood contact, must be offered the vaccine preexposure.

6. *I don't hear much about AIDS anymore. Is there an HIV vaccine?*

There is no HIV vaccine at this time, and it may be years until a safe one is developed, if ever. Hundreds of thousands of Americans have died and will continue to die of AIDS through nonoccupational exposure (fewer than 100 cases have been documented as occupationally related). If an HIV vaccine does become available, employers would undoubtedly have to provide it free to employees, just like HBV vaccination.

7. *I just had a needlestick from a patient with AIDS. Should I take AZT?*

OSHA does not make specific medical treatment recommendations; it defers these decisions to the Public Health Service (see Appendix G, but keep in mind that these recommendations may be outdated by the time this text appears). Medical knowledge in this area changes too rapidly and has too many unknowns for specific recommendations to be made in the Standard. The use of AZT in postexposure prophylaxis is controversial; it has many proponents and opponents. This is a decision you must discuss personally with your health care professional, who should be a fully qualified physician with experience in the treatment of HBV/HIV.

8. *I'm an oral surgery resident and had the complete HBV vaccination series a few years ago. Following a needlestick, I had a baseline hepatitis panel drawn. It showed HBsAg but no anti-HBs. The source individual was not infectious for HBV. I took another complete HBV vaccination series and a few months later was found to still have HBsAg but no anti-HBs. The employee health physician then made the diagnosis that I'm an HBV chronic carrier. He told my residency director, who said I could no longer perform invasive procedures, and thus could not finish my residency. Can they do this?*

Probably. Health care personnel who are chronic HBV carriers should not perform invasive procedures, per USPHS recommendations (see Appendix E). However, the medical results of your postexposure evaluation should not have been made known to your employer without your consent. The employer has the right to a copy of the postexposure written opinion, which is limited to stating that you have been informed of the results of the evaluation and any medical conditions that may result from the exposure. All other medical information is confidential.

Unfortunately, you are potentially infectious yourself, regardless of the needlestick, and may cause harm to your patients. You could probably sue the employee health physician for breach of confidentiality, but it would be a difficult case because the physician appears to be acting in the best interests of the employer and the general public health. Employee health physicians, though often employees of the employers, still have an obligation to protect the doctor-patient privacy privilege.

9. *I'm a male orthopedic surgeon at risk for HIV infection because of my sexual orientation. I've never been tested for HIV because I'm afraid of what the results would be and their implications for my career. I just had another exposure incident, and this time my favorite nurse saw it. I don't know what to do.*

First off, you're not at risk because of your sexual orientation, you're at risk because of your sexual activities. Second, it is irresponsible of you not to be aware of your HIV status, especially since you're in the health care field. You have a moral obligation to know your HIV status and act in the best interests of your patients.

All I can say is that you've got some tough decisions. You have a legal right to decline postexposure testing. Nothing in the Standard says you have to report an exposure incident, but other OSHA standards require the reporting of occupational injuries, and this could be considered one. If the nurse reports the incident, you can still decline evaluation, but you'll have a hard time explaining why you didn't want to get tested. The Standard does not address issues dealing with your infectiousness, because it is designed to protect employees, not patients. You must make these decisions yourself.

10. *OSHA does not address the appropriateness of returning an employee to work after an exposure incident. Shouldn't someone make a determination about an employee being possibly infectious to other workers before returning him or her to work?*

It is standard practice for an occupational physician to make a return-to-duty determination each time an employee is evaluated. This determination is done for two reasons—first, to ensure that the employee won't be harmed when returned; and second, to ensure that other employees won't be harmed by the employee being returned. During my short tenure with OSHA, I drafted a specific return-to-duty requirement for the postexposure evaluation paragraph, but it was deleted in the final draft, presumably because no one had commented on it during the notice of proposed rulemaking or during testimony. Unfortunately, no one formally trained in occupational medicine was included in OSHA's BBPS working group, so this important basic concept was ignored. For example, an HCP does have an obligation, if postexposure evaluation found that an employee was a chronic HBV carrier, to ensure that returning the employee to duty would not present a risk to other workers.

Chapter 12

Paragraph (g): Communication of Hazards

The scars of others should teach us caution.

—Saint Jerome

Paragraph (g) requires employers to tell employees about the hazards of blood-borne pathogens through the use of labels, signs, information, and training. The intent is to ensure that employees receive adequate warning and education to eliminate or minimize hazardous exposure.

LABELS AND SIGNS

The text of the 1970 OSHAct states that any standard made by OSHA must require labels or other appropriate forms of warning to make employees aware of occupational hazards. This part of the Standard thus is a direct requirement of the OSHAct. Labels and signs may be more important for bloodborne pathogens than other exposures because infectious material may not always be recognizable as blood/OPIM.

Warning labels must:

- Be affixed to regulated waste containers, refrigerators or freezers containing blood/OPIM, and containers used to store or transport blood/OPIM
- Include the word "biohazard" and the biohazard symbol
- Be fluorescent orange or orange-red with lettering and symbol in contrasting colors

- Be affixed on or close to the container by a method that prevents loss or unintentional removal

An example of an appropriately colored biohazard label can be found on the front cover of this book.

There are four exemptions to the biohazard labeling requirement:

- Red bags or containers may be substituted for labels.[1]
- Containers of blood or blood products that are labeled for release for transfusion or clinical use do not require biohazard labeling.
- Individual containers for blood/OPIM that are placed in a labeled container for storage or transport do not require labeling.[2]
- Regulated waste that has been decontaminated does not require labeling or color-coding.

In addition, contaminated equipment must be biohazard-labeled, and the parts of the equipment that remain contaminated must also be identified on the label. This ensures that employees who repair or service the equipment will be warned to take appropriate precautions.

Signs are required at the entrance to work areas in HIV/HBV research or production facilities. Like the labels, signs must be fluorescent orange or orange-red with contrasting lettering and symbols.

These signs must bear:

- The word "biohazard" and the biohazard symbol
- The name of the infectious agent
- Special requirements for entering the area
- The name and telephone number of the laboratory director or other responsible person

INFORMATION AND TRAINING

This section requires the employer to train all employees who have occupational exposure about the hazards associated with bloodborne pathogens and the pro-

---

1. As long as employees are trained about and informed of the meaning of red bags.

2. A phlebotomist drawing blood would not need to label individual blood tubes but must place them in a labeled container for storage and transportation.

tective measures to be taken to minimize their risk of exposure. Effective training is the critical preventive element in any exposure control plan.

> Employers must ensure that all employees with occupational exposure participate in a bloodborne pathogens training program.

The training program must be provided:

- At no cost to the employee
- During working hours
- At the time of initial assignment to tasks with occupational exposure
- At least annually
- In vocabulary and content appropriate to the employee's education level, literacy, and language

Annual training must be provided to employees within 1 year of their previous training. Additional training is required when new or modified tasks affect an employee's occupational exposure. This additional training may be limited to information about the new exposures, but the employee must have received and continue to receive the complete annual bloodborne pathogens training program.

There are 14 separate requirements listed for the training program. Unfortunately, there is no easy way to deal with them, except to just list them. At a minimum, the bloodborne pathogens training program must explain the following elements:

1. The regulatory text, a copy of which must be accessible to employees
2. The epidemiology and symptoms of bloodborne diseases
3. The modes of transmission of bloodborne pathogens
4. The exposure control plan and how to obtain a copy
5. Ways to recognize tasks or activities that may involve exposure to blood/OPIM
6. The use and limitations of methods that prevent or reduce exposure, including engineering controls, work practices, and PPE
7. The types and proper use of PPE[3]
8. The appropriate selection of PPE

---

3. PPE information should include types, proper use, location, removal, handling, decontamination, and disposal.

9. The hepatitis B vaccination, and that it will be provided free of charge[4]
10. The appropriate actions to take and persons to contact in an emergency involving blood/OPIM
11. The procedures to follow after an exposure incident
12. The postexposure evaluation and follow-up that an employer must provide after an exposure incident
13. The required labels, color-coding, or signs

Finally, the training program must offer:

14. An opportunity for interactive questions and answers with the person conducting the training session

The person conducting the training session must be knowledgeable in the preceding subject matters as they relate to the specific workplace. This means that employers cannot simply buy a general videotape on bloodborne pathogens and have employees watch it without having someone trained and knowledgeable present to answer questions.

Specific additional requirements for HBV/HIV research and production facilities are presented in this paragraph in the Standard, but they are discussed in this book in Chapter 10.

QUESTIONS

1. *Do I have to label every blood tube I draw on a patient? And what do I do about patients who I know have hepatitis or AIDS?*

Containers, such as phlebotomy blood tubes, that are easily identifiable by trained employees as containing blood/OPIM do not need to be labeled. Blood drawn from a source individual known to be HBV/HIV-infected does not need to be labeled differently from blood from an unknown or known negative source. Thus, a source individual's rights to confidentiality and privacy are preserved. Remember that Universal Precautions treats all blood/OPIM as possibly infectious, so there is no need to specifically identify known infectious blood. OSHA does require,

---

4. HBV vaccination information should include information on efficacy, safety, method of administration, the benefits of vaccination, and the fact that it will be offered free of charge to the employee.

however, that the outermost containers used to store, transport, ship, or dispose blood/OPIM bear a warning label signaling that appropriate precautions must be used.

2. *We send our infectious waste to an outside private contractor and have to label the transportation container with the DOT (Department of Transportation) infectious substances label. Do we have to also label the container with the DOL (Department of Labor) biohazard label?*

No. OSHA will accept the DOT label ("infectious substances") when it is required in lieu of the OSHA biohazard label on outer containers of regulated waste or containers of other materials that contain blood/OPIM. Labeling in accordance with the OSHA Bloodborne Pathogens Standard is required for such containers where DOT regulations do not apply. The Standard requires labeling when containers are functioning as collection receptacles within facilities generating contaminated waste. These containers would be exempt from the DOT labeling requirement because they are not being transported between facilities.

3. *If blood is so dangerous, why aren't there biohazard labels on blood for transfusion?*

Blood and blood products do not need to bear a biohazard label as long as they bear an identifying label, specified by the FDA (Food and Drug Administration), indicating that they have been screened for HBV/HIV antibodies and released for transfusion or other clinical use. Actually, even screened blood may still be infectious with HCV (hepatitis C virus) or even HIV if the blood was donated from someone in the "window phase" of infection, before detectable levels of antibodies had developed. It would be quite frightening, however, to watch blood from a bag labeled "Biohazard" being transfused into your body.

4. *My company just paid $749 for a videotape about bloodborne pathogens. Will this videotape be adequate for training?*

Self-study modules, videotapes, and interactive computer programs may all be used as part of the training program. However, the Standard specifically requires that there be an opportunity for interactive questions and answers with the person conducting the training session. Training employees solely by means of a videotape, without allowing an opportunity for a discussion period, would be a violation of the Standard. Videotaped programs may thus be useful as an aid in training, but they must be supplemented with site-specific information, and a qualified person must be accessible for questions.

Many of the requirements of the Standard are performance-oriented. Compliance officers, if they inspect your facility, will determine on a case-by-case basis whether the training you have provided is effective and adequate. They will accomplish their evaluation by observing work practices and interviewing employees to determine if the training has been presented in a manner appropriate to the employee's education, literacy level, and language.

5. *There are no physicians associated with the dental clinic where I've worked for the past 6 years. Whom should we employ for the required training?*

A qualified trainer does not have to be a physician. The trainer must be knowledgeable in the contents of the Standard, the site-specific hazards, and the exposure control plan. A dentist or a nurse in a dental office should certainly be able to train employees, provided she or he gains familiarity with the Standard and understands the topics required for the training program. A wide variety of health care professionals, as well as non–health care professionals such as industrial hygienists, epidemiologists, or professional trainers, may also be considered competent if they can demonstrate evidence of specialized training in bloodborne pathogens.

6. *I'm a mortician who shares an office with the dental clinic next door, but I don't know anything about the epidemiology, symptoms, and modes of transmission of bloodborne pathogens. How do I explain this to my employees?*

That's why Chapters 3 and 4 of this book were included—to offer a simple and practical understanding of the two most important occupationally transmitted bloodborne pathogens. You might also check with the dental clinic to see if it has a qualified trainer who would be willing to learn about your specific workplace and exposures and then do the required training for your employees.

7. *Paying for all these labels is too expensive. Can I just scan one into my computer and print out labels on my printer?*

Only if you have a color scanner and a fluorescent color printer. The Standard specifically states that the labels must be fluorescent orange or orange-red. The intent is to make sure that the labels are easily seen and thus provide a clear visual warning of the potential hazard. Using a nonfluorescent colored or black-and-white label would be a violation.

8. *We have 308 employees at our hospital who have occupational exposure. The annual training takes an hour, and we have to allow everyone half an hour to get to the auditorium, then back to work. That's 462 hours a year, at approximately $25 an hour (not including the doctors, who think they're worth $250 or more an hour), which amounts to about $12,000 annually just in lost productivity. How can we reduce these costs?*

Sorry, but you can't. OSHA estimates that implementation of the Standard will cost employers almost $813 million a year, of which about $134 million represents training costs, and $107 million goes for vaccine and postexposure follow-up. Note that the annual training costs are higher than the cost of the vaccine and medical evaluation. The largest expense is for compliance costs, estimated to be around $327 million per year. But the savings in life, suffering, productivity, legal fees, future infection, etc., are still greater. Besides, the total annual expenditure wouldn't even cover the cost of a B-2 bomber.

Chapter 13

Paragraph (h): Recordkeeping

How to save the old that's worth saving, whether in landscape, houses, manners, institutions, or human types, is one of our greatest problems, and the one that we bother least about.

—John Galsworthy

The OSHAact created the requirement for employers to keep necessary and appropriate records relating to the causes and prevention of occupational accidents and illnesses. OSHA believes that recordkeeping is necessary to ensure that employees receive appropriate information on the effective prevention and treatment of illnesses and injuries involving bloodborne pathogens. Thus, employers are required to maintain medical and training records for employees covered by the Standard—that is, for all employees with occupational exposure.

MEDICAL RECORDS

The maintenance of medical records is necessary to ensure the proper evaluation of employees' immune status and for proper medical management following an exposure incident. Interestingly, OSHA received little comment or testimony relating to this provision during the formation of the Standard, probably due, in part, to the common understanding that the maintenance of medical records is an important part of any occupational health program.

The medical record must include:

- The employee's name and Social Security number
- Information on HBV vaccination status
- Dates of all HBV vaccinations
- Medical records relative to HBV vaccination[1]
- All postexposure evaluation results, testing, and procedures
- The health care professional's written opinion (or opinions[2])
- Information provided to the health care professional after an exposure incident[3]

The employer must ensure that employee medical records are kept confidential and not disclosed to anyone within or outside the workplace without the employee's written consent.[4]

> The employer must maintain employee medical records for at least the duration of employment plus 30 years.

TRAINING RECORDS

The employer is also required to maintain bloodborne pathogens training records, which must include:

- Dates of training sessions
- Contents or summary of the training sessions

---

1. Relevant medical records may include information on completion of HBV vaccination, contraindication for vaccination, or results of HBV antibody testing.

2. A written opinion is required for HBV vaccination (unless the employee declines vaccination), and another is required for postexposure medical evaluation.

3. A description of the exposed employee's duties as they relate to the exposure, documentation of the circumstances of exposure, and results of the source individual's blood testing, if available.

4. An exemption is given here to allow OSHA representatives to examine employee medical records, as required, for evaluation of compliance. Of course, these representatives are required to maintain the confidentiality of the records.

- Names and qualifications of trainers
- Names and job titles of persons attending the training session

> Training records must be maintained for 3 years from the date of training.

These training records are not considered confidential and may be maintained in any file. OSHA does not require employers to maintain an individual training file for each employee, although employers may choose to keep the training records in each employee's personnel file. Employers can keep the training records wherever they want, as long as they exist and are maintained. OSHA believes that keeping the records for 3 years will be helpful in allowing the employer, the employee, and OSHA (the so-called OSHA Trinity) to evaluate the effectiveness and adequacy of the training program.

AVAILABILITY

Medical and training records must be made available to OSHA representatives upon request. Training records may be made available for examination and copying to employees and employee representatives. Medical records may be made available for examination and copying to the employee or anyone having written consent of the employee.

TRANSFER OF RECORDS

If an employer ceases to do business and there is no successor employer to keep the records for the required time, the employer must notify NIOSH at least 3 months prior to the disposal of the records and then transfer the records to NIOSH (if they so request). Records are kept at NIOSH because they have a vested interest in maintaining records of occupational injuries and illnesses (besides, someone's got to keep them).

QUESTIONS

1. *I'm worried about other employees having access to my medical record. What does the Standard say about this?*

Nonmedical employees of a company should not have access to the confidential medical records required by the Standard. In fact, the employer should not have access to the medical record—unless, of course, the employer is the designated health care provider for the employee. The Standard places responsibility for recordkeeping directly on the employer, but it does not require the employer to maintain possession of the records. It's probably best not to have the employer maintain possession of the medical records. If the employer already maintains a confidential medical record on employees, however, an additional medical record is not required, and the information relevant to bloodborne pathogens may be kept in this record. On the other hand, if the existing record is not confidential, a new medical recordkeeping system and/or record must be created.

2. *Why must records be kept for 30 years after the end of employment?*

Keeping medical records for 30 years past the time of employment is necessary because some complications of occupational exposure, such as hepatocellular carcinoma, which can occur as a result of HBV infection, can develop 20–30 years after initial infection. Employees who become HBV carriers or develop chronic hepatitis are often ill and infected for the rest of their lives. In addition, initial symptoms of HIV infection may not occur until 10 or more years after infection (though most people infected with HIV develop symptoms within 10 years). This time period is consistent with other OSHA standards requiring the retention of occupational medical records—specifically records related to asbestos exposure, where signs and symptoms of malignant mesothelioma normally don't develop until at least 20 years after exposure. Finally, OSHA believes that this requirement is not unduly burdensome for the health care industry, which is known for its long-term recordkeeping.

3. *Will an OSHA inspector review the training records?*

Yes. Reviewing training records is one of the first things an OSHA compliance officer does when inspecting a workplace.

Chapter 14

Paragraph (i):
Effective Dates

Time is the nurse and breeder of all good.

—*Shakespeare*
The Two Gentlemen of Verona

> All paragraphs of the Standard are in effect *now*.

The Standard had an initial effective date of March 6, 1992, with a phase-in of different paragraphs over 5 months. All paragraphs of the Standard have been in effect since July 6, 1992.

Chapter 15

Compliance

Roses have thorns, and silver fountains mud;
Clouds and eclipses stain both moon and sun,
And loathsome canker lives in sweetest bud.
All men make faults.

—Shakespeare

OSHA enforces the requirements of the Standard through inspections by compliance officers. With few exceptions, OSHA compliance officers have little or no medical background, except that some are trained industrial hygienists. The BBPS has been somewhat of a change for compliance officers, who, historically, have inspected industrial businesses. Only recently, with the institution of the Hazard Communications Standard (HAZCOM), has OSHA become involved with health care facilities. By the time you read this text, however, many of the compliance officers will be experienced at inspecting health care facilities, so expect them to know what they're doing.

INSPECTIONS

OSHA conducts both "programmed" and "unprogrammed" inspections. **Programmed inspections** are randomly chosen from a list of businesses and worksites in the area. **Unprogrammed inspections** result when OSHA visits a workplace because of an imminent danger situation, a fatality or catastrophe investigation, or because they received a complaint. Because OSHA has so few compliance officers (fewer than 2,000 for the whole country) and because fatality and complaint investigations receive the highest priority, very few inspections are programmed. In some states, the chances of having a routine programmed OSHA inspection at a worksite are less than 1% per year.

OSHA has issued a compliance guide that sets, explains, and clarifies inspection procedures for their compliance officers. The compliance guide is in the public domain and is therefore open for public scrutiny and use. Appendix C is the text of the March 6, 1992, OSHA compliance guide for the Bloodborne Pathogens Standard. You now have your own copy, and if you are in charge of the bloodborne pathogens program for your workplace, I suggest you read it.

States that run their own OSHA programs develop their own compliance programs. Unfortunately, the state-run OSHA program in North Carolina became so ineffective that businesses tried to recruit new industry to the state by advertising the fact that they had little or no possibility of getting inspected by OSHA if they moved there. The September 1991 catastrophic fire in a chicken processing plant in Hamlet, North Carolina, that had locked its escape doors to prevent employees from stealing chickens, resulting in the deaths of 25 employees, most certainly would not have occurred if the facility had had an OSHA inspection.

An inspection begins when the compliance officer arrives at the worksite. In most instances, the officer arrives unannounced, unless the visit is scheduled due to a catastrophe or fatality investigation. In fact, it is a violation of law to announce a programmed inspection, and compliance officers are trained not to give out this information. The compliance officer will display official credentials and ask to see an employer representative. OSHA does not collect penalties at the time of inspection. Anyone who tries to collect money at an inspection is not an OSHA compliance officer.

The compliance officer will hold an opening conference and explain why the facility was selected for inspection before beginning the inspection tour and examining work areas for compliance with OSHA standards. The officer may inspect the workplace for all OSHA standards, not just the Bloodborne Pathogens Standard. An inspection related to complaints about Hazard Communications in a dental clinic may also include checking for compliance with the Bloodborne Pathogens Standard. The compliance officer consults with employees during the inspection, usually stopping to question workers in private about safety and health conditions and practices in the workplace. The officer will point out to the employer any unsafe or unhealthful working conditions as they are observed and should propose some possible corrective actions.

After the inspection tour, there is a closing conference between the compliance officer and the employer or employer representative. All unsafe or unhealthful conditions will be discussed, as well as all apparent violations for which a citation may be issued or recommended. The compliance officer does not indicate any proposed penalties at the closing conference. Only the OSHA area director has the authority to issue penalties, and only after having received a full report. If requested, a closing discussion will be held with the employees or their representative to discuss matters of direct interest to them. The employee representative may be present at the closing conference.

CITATIONS, VIOLATIONS, AND PENALTIES

The OSHA area director issues citations and decides what, if any, penalties will be proposed. Citations inform the employer and employees of the regulations and standards alleged to have been violated and of the proposed length of time they have to fix the problems. Citations and notices of proposed penalties are sent by certified mail. The employer must post a copy of each citation at or near the place the violation occurred. The citation must be posted for 3 days or until the violation is fixed, whichever is longer.

The various types of violations include:

Other Than Serious Violations—A violation directly related to job safety and health, but one that would probably not cause death or serious physical harm. A proposed penalty of up to $7,000 may be issued for each violation. The penalty for this type of violation may be adjusted downward by as much as 95%, depending on the employer's demonstrated efforts to comply with the Standard.

Serious Violation—A violation with substantial probability that death or serious physical harm could result and that the employer knew, or should have known, about. A mandatory penalty of $7,000 for each violation is proposed. This penalty may also be adjusted downward, depending on the employer's good faith, history of previous violations, the gravity of the alleged violation, and the size of the business.

Willful Violation—A violation that the employer committed intentionally and knowingly. Penalties of up to $70,000 may be proposed for each willful violation, with a minimum penalty of $5,000 for each violation. This penalty may also be adjusted downward, but rarely for good faith efforts (how often are willful violations committed in good faith?). Employers can also be punished by a court-imposed fine or by imprisonment for up to 6 months, or both, if a willful violation results in the death of an employee.

Repeat Violation—A violation of a standard where, upon reinspection, a similar violation is found. Repeat violations can bring a fine of up to $70,000 for each violation.

Failure to Correct Prior Violation—A civil penalty of up to $7,000 may be imposed for each day the violation continues beyond the prescribed date for its correction.

At $70,000 a pop for willful and repeat violations, it doesn't take long for hospitals, clinics, or offices to reach several hundred thousand dollars worth of fines. What may be even more damaging than fines is the fact that OSHA violations and proposed penalties are not confidential and therefore are often reported in the media. Reporting in the newspaper or on TV that a major hospital had a $250,000 OSHA violation for failing to follow safety regulations is a serious public relations nightmare.

APPEALS

Employees may not contest citations, penalties, or lack of penalties. If an inspection was initiated due to an employee complaint, that employee, or an authorized employee representative, may request an informal review of a decision not to issue a citation.

An employer may request an informal meeting with the OSHA area director to discuss citations. The area director has the authority to settle agreements and revise citations and penalties. If employers have shown good faith efforts to correct the problem, penalties are often reduced.

Once citations are received, the employer has a prescribed date by which time the violation must be corrected. Factors beyond the employer's reasonable control may prevent the completion of corrections by the prescribed date. In this case, employers who have made a good faith effort to comply and correct the violation may file for a petition for modification of abatement (i.e., a request for changing the date prescribed for correction).

If an employer decides to contest a citation, she or he has 15 working days from the time the citation and proposed penalty was received to notify the area director in writing. The written Notice of Contest is forwarded by the area director to the Occupational Safety and Health Review Commission (OSHRC), an independent agency not associated with OSHA or the Department of Labor. The commission assigns the case to an administrative law judge who decides if a hearing is appropriate and then rules on the case. This ruling may be reviewed by OSHRC, whose ruling on the case may be appealed to the appropriate U.S. court of appeals.

ENFORCEMENT DURING THE STANDARD'S FIRST YEAR

The OSHA Office of Health Compliance Assistance reported the results of the first year of bloodborne pathogens enforcement activity in May 1993. The report covered the dates from March 1, 1992 through the end of February 1993; therefore, it does not cover a complete year of full Standard implementation (the Standard was phased in over a 5-month period ending on July 6, 1992.) This report includes the first data to show OSHA's enforcement activity related to the Standard.

During March 1992–February 1993, OSHA performed 984 total inspections relating to the Bloodborne Pathogens Standard (data were collected only from the 27 states that have federal, rather than state, OSHA plans). Of these, 757 (or 77%) were the result of specific employee complaints (unprogrammed inspections), whereas 227 (or 22%) were programmed (planned) inspections. OSHA estimated that over 500,000 separate workplace establishments would be affected by the Standard. Fewer than 1,000 inspections were performed in this first year, so only around one in 500 estimated workplaces affected by the Standard was inspected. During this year, 371 hospitals (of an estimated 6,197, or about one in 17), 23 funeral homes (19,890 estimated, or about one in 850), 103 dentist's offices (100,174 estimated, or about one in 1,000), and 87 doctor's offices (122,104 estimated, or about one in 1400), were inspected. What this means is that, for states with federal OSHA enforcement

- Hospitals had a relatively high chance of having an OSHA inspection
- Funeral homes and dentist's and doctor's offices had a relatively low chance of being inspected

Smaller, nonunionized workplaces have historically had fewer OSHA inspections than larger, unionized workplaces, possibly because union workers may feel more empowered to complain to OSHA. An employee in a small doctor's office with 15 employees would probably be less likely to file a complaint with OSHA than an employee in a union who works at a hospital with 5,000 employees.

During the first year of federal OSHA BBPS enforcement, paragraph (c) (Exposure Control) was cited 728 times for all industries, and 223 of these violations occurred in industries related to health care. The highest number of violations in health care industries was for paragraph (d) (Methods of Compliance) violations (approximately 400 violations). For health care industries, three of the next five most frequently cited standards were for standards other than the BBPS (the Hazard Communication Standard communication program was cited 324 times,[1] failure to maintain an illness and injury log was cited 200 times, and HAZCOM training and information requirements was cited 198 times).

What does all this mean?

For health care industries, only about half of the six most frequently cited

---

1. HAZCOM, the Hazard Communication Standard, must be in place whenever employees work with any hazardous chemical, but this does not include biological hazards.

violations deal with bloodborne pathogens. The other half deal with HAZCOM and illness and injury reporting requirements. For health care industries, citations specifically related to the Bloodborne Pathogens Standard, listed in order of decreasing frequency of citations, were as follows:

Methods of compliance (~400)
Exposure control plan (223)
Information and training (203)
Housekeeping (158)
PPE (140)
HBV vaccination (81)
Engineering and work practices (78)
Eye wash (77)
HBV declination statement (42)

After reviewing these data on the first year of the enforcement of the Blood-borne Pathogen Standard, the OSHA office of Health Compliance Assistance concluded that general industry should focus on exposure control plans and training for designated first-aid providers. They stated that the health care industry should focus on methods of compliance (including needle recapping, sharps containers, regulated waste, and PPE), hepatitis B vaccination, and training.

I would caution the reader against overinterpreting these data. The best approach, quite simply, is to make sure your workplace is in compliance with all aspects of the Standard. And don't forget that the vast majority of OSHA inspections related to bloodborne pathogens result from employee complaints. Probably the best ways to avoid an OSHA inspection are to deal openly with and stay in compliance with this regulation, while also educating employees and letting them know that they can discuss perceived problems with a caring employer.

Chapter 16

Legal Implications

Commonly physicians, like beer, are best when they are old; and lawyers, like bread, when they are young and new.

—Thomas Fuller
The Holy State

There are probably thousands of health care workers infected with HIV. The vast majority of these are nonoccupational infections; probably less than 1% are the result of occupational infection. It would be practically impossible to get adequate data on health care workers' HIV infection rates in this population, mainly because those who know they are HIV-positive, and those at risk, would most likely refuse to participate in a screening program. Thus, the very people whose status is of interest to us would have removed themselves from the study. (This is a good example of what is called "selection bias" in a study—those we are most interested in select themselves out of, or into, a study.)

For reasons of simplification, my discussion of legal implications will deal only with HIV, even though HBV infection causes much more occupational illness and death than HIV. The vast majority of HBV infections do not result in serious illness, whereas most HIV infections do. We might draw an analogy here between this situation and the fear of transportation-related death: People are afraid to fly in airplanes, yet they have no such fears about automobile travel. Though most commercial airplane crashes result in deaths, a far smaller percent of total car crashes are fatal. Nevertheless, the total number of deaths from car crashes is astoundingly high—approximately 50,000 per year—because there are so many more automobile accidents than plane crashes. The fear of flying and the fear of occupationally acquired HIV both produce maximum fear from minimal risk, and it is maximum fear that drives the legal system.

Because OSHA places the responsibility of protecting workers on the employer, it is the employer who has the most to lose in legal terms by not fully implementing the requirements of the Standard. As of July 1992, employers who do not comply with the Standard have everything to lose legally, while employers who comply with the Standard have everything to win medically. On the other hand, employees have everything to win legally when employers do not comply with the Standard and everything to lose medically.

Let's look at some examples of HIV-infected workers:

1. An emergency room physician who knows he is already at risk because he has engaged in risky homosexual activity[1] works at a hospital that did not start annual Bloodborne Pathogens training until 1994. In October 1994, after having received his first BBPS training, he has a needlestick exposure incident and reports it to his employer. On baseline HIV testing, he is found to be HIV-positive. He states, however, that he has had numerous needlesticks over the last 2 years, including one in January 1993 from a suspected AIDS patient. He did not report the incident because he had been stuck quite frequently and did not know he had to report such incidents.

Although this physician knows he is at risk for HIV infection, he has not gotten tested because of ethical concerns about what happens if he knows he's positive. (This is not a far-fetched scenario; I personally know physicians who have not been tested because of their fear of what they'd find out.) He has now had enlarged lymph nodes for about a year and suspects he's HIV-infected, so he finally gets an anonymous test at a local HIV clinic and tests positive for HIV. He knows that the hospital should have started BBPS training a year and a half ago. So he conveniently remembers getting stuck in January 1993, after the Standard came into effect and before the hospital initiated the training.

The legal trial would find that the employer was negligent for not making employees aware of the requirements of the Standard, since all employees should have been trained within the first year. There would be no way to prove or disprove the physician's route of infection, and he could not be blamed for not reporting needlesticks because he had not yet received the training and did not know they had to be reported. The question about route of infection is unanswerable; there is

---

1. He is not at risk because he's gay, he is at risk because he has engaged in risky activities. Many gay men are at less risk of acquiring HIV infection than heterosexual women who engage in unprotected vaginal intercourse with men who may be infected with HIV.

no question, however, that the employer did not follow the requirements of the Standard. Fault would therefore lie with the employer, who would be liable in this case, even though the physician may not have been occupationally infected. This example illustrates the fact that **employers who do not comply with the Standard may be liable for nonoccupationally infected employees.**

The following example shows that employers who do comply with the Standard are protected from liability for nonoccupationally infected employees, even though there are probably 100 times more nonoccupationally infected employees than those occupationally infected:

2. A nurse named Pat (gender unimportant, though Pat has engaged in risky sexual activity) has an exposure incident and reports it. The employer has provided annual BBPS training and fully instituted the requirements of the Standard. The nurse declines postexposure baseline testing. A year later, Pat develops symptoms consistent with HIV infection and is now found to be HIV-positive. Even if Pat decides to sue the hospital, stating that the occupational exposure incident caused the infection, there would be no way to correlate infection with the incident, so Pat would lose. In this case, the employer is protected by following the Standard's requirements. Thus, **employers who comply with the Standard are not liable for nonoccupational infections.**

3. A research lab worker accidentally breaks a vial of blood, and blood spills on her hands, which have a severe dermatitis. There were no biohazard warning signs at the entrance to the work area, and gloves were on back order. Although the lab worker's baseline testing was HIV-negative, follow-up testing 6 months later showed that she had converted to HIV-positive. The employer would be liable for not providing biohazard warning signs and for not providing appropriate PPE. Thus, **employers who do not comply with the Standard are liable for occupationally infected employees.**

4. A trained phlebotomist drawing blood on a seizing patient accidentally gets a needlestick when the patient violently thrashes his arm. The employer had complied with the Standard, so the phlebotomist was wearing gloves and had been fully trained. The employer would be liable for workers' compensation payments to the employee, which have a set limit, but would not be liable for negligence, which may not have set limits. The infection, though occupational, could not be specifically blamed on the employer, because it is assumed that there is some innate risk in performing the duties of a phlebotomist. The employer did what was legally required and would not be responsible for any payments beyond those provided by workers' compensation. Thus, **employers who comply with the Standard are less liable for occupationally infected employees.**

To sum up the preceding scenarios:

Employers who do not comply with the Standard are more liable for both nonoccupational and occupational HIV infection, whereas employers who comply are not liable for nonoccupational infections and are less liable for occupational infections.

Given that many more infections occur in nonoccupational settings, it becomes much clearer that employers are legally better off if they comply with the Standard. If they do not comply, they may incur legal liability for nonoccupational infections in their employees.

Do not underestimate your employees' knowledge of their HIV status, especially if they are health care workers. In my experience in the U.S. Air Force, which performs mandatory HIV screening, about half the members who were informed that they tested HIV-positive had previous knowledge of their HIV status. You can reasonably assume that health care workers at risk for nonoccupational HIV infection are aware of their status. If they don't know their status, they will find out before they consent to postexposure blood testing. Employees who know they are at risk are probably less likely to have postexposure testing performed, because if they were positive, it would most likely affect their job.[2] I even know of a health care worker who was at risk for nonoccupational HIV infection and submitted someone else's blood as his own for HIV testing. To avoid this scenario, hospitals might consider testing postexposure blood for blood type and ensuring that it matches the employee's. They might also consider keeping the blood sample for future testing or comparison with the 6-month follow-up sampling.

It has been estimated that even with full compliance with the Standard, only about half of the occupational HIV infections can be prevented (as compared to well over 95% of the HBV infections, mainly because vaccination is so successful in preventing infection). So unless a really effective needle covering device is developed (which seems unlikely at this time), HIV infections in workers will

2. I am not personally concerned about the infectious nature of health care workers who are HIV-positive. What I am worried about, though, is the performance of HIV-infected health care workers. My concern about being operated on by an HIV-positive surgeon does not center on fears of my being infected. My concern is about the surgeon losing fine motor control or central nervous system functions because of direct effects of HIV.

continue—and may even increase in the future as more patients become infected. In sum:

It is to the advantage of employers and employees, both medically and legally, to comply fully with the requirements of OSHA's Bloodborne Pathogens Standard.

Chapter 17

The Future

Time wounds all heels.

—Jane Ace

If employers and employees complied fully with the requirements of the Standard, over 95% of possible future occupational HBV infections could be prevented. This is due to the greater than 90% effectiveness of HBV vaccination and an estimated 50% decrease in exposure due to engineering, administrative, and work practice controls, as well as PPE use. Vaccinating employees and other high-risk groups will also decrease the total number of infected individuals, resulting in a decreasing risk from each exposure incident because fewer people will actually be infected.

Even with full compliance, only an estimated 50% of possible future HIV infections could probably be prevented. The decrease in HIV infection would be entirely due to control measures, since no HIV vaccine is currently available, and none is likely to be available in the near future. This decrease is based on the assumption that the number of infectious individuals will stay the same. Unfortunately, we can fully expect the number of HIV-infected individuals to continue to increase. Furthermore, with advances in medical care, those who are HIV-infected will live longer, thus increasing occupational risk as they continue to come into contact with workers. Thus, the number of occupational HIV infections can be expected to increase in the future, even with BBPS compliance, since the possible 50% decrease in occupational exposure will be offset by an absolute increase in numbers of infectious individuals and their longer survival time. The increase may be small, but any increase would be significant.

Throughout this book I have emphasized that HBV is a more significant occupational risk than HIV. Nevertheless, specifically because of OSHA's Bloodborne Pathogens Standard, HIV will become more of a concern, relatively, than HBV in the future. People did not worry as much about cancer in the 1930s, since a lot more of them died of infectious diseases; but once antibiotics reduced the infectious disease death rates, cancer death rates increased (you have to die of something.) The relative decrease in HBV infections, versus the increase in HIV infections, will shift the focus to HIV.

As the number of HIV infections has increased, so has the occupational risk to workers from tuberculosis (TB). Since the Standard only deals with bloodborne pathogens, I have postponed any discussion of the TB problem to this final chapter.

Tuberculosis is a significant occupational risk not only to health care workers, but to all workers.

TB is a risk mainly because it can be casually transmitted. A TB exposure incident is as simple as breathing the same air breathed by an infected individual.

After decades of decreasing numbers of TB infections, in 1986 the rate started to increase. The number has grown ever year since, until around 1993, when a small decline was seen. The growing number of TB infections was due mainly to an increase in the number of AIDS patients who were developing full-blown tuberculosis. Those who are HIV-positive and also TB-infected develop active TB at a rate of approximately 10% per year. Immune-competent patients (i.e., people with normal functioning immune systems) who are TB-infected develop active TB at a rate of less than 1% per year. TB infection is analogous to HBV infection in that the vast majority of those infected have no significant symptoms. However, in contrast to HBV, which causes symptoms within 6 months or so of infection, TB may remain latent in the body and not produce symptoms until many years after infection.

Though an increasing number of people with AIDS have active TB, it is often overlooked or not diagnosed because health care professionals are much more concerned about *Pneumocystis pneumonia* infection. Thus, the diagnosis of active TB is often delayed because of concerns about other more life-threatening infections, and also because TB may have an atypical presentation in those who are immunocompromised (they may be more likely to have nonpulmonary infections, or their pulmonary infections might be located somewhere in the lung other than the typical top part).

People with AIDS have also developed atypical strains of TB, strains like *Mycobacterium kansasaii* and *Mycobacterium avium intracellulare,* in addition to

Mycobacterium tuberculosis (the type that causes regular TB). These cases are resistant to many of the drugs normally used. AIDS patients have started dying quite rapidly from multidrug-resistant strains of TB (MDR TB). Some health care workers have become infected and died from MDR TB, which may be more virulent and resistant to treatment.

TB has spread to health care workers from AIDS patients. In some HIV, internal medicine, or pulmonary floors, from 30% to over 50% of the health care workers converted to TB antibody–positive (only a small percentage eventually develop disease, but it is still an occupational infection). TB has also increased among IV drug users, in prisons and inner cities, and in other places where people are in close contact and may be immunocompromised. TB has now spread outside of the HIV-infected realm and is claiming a growing number of victims.

Health care workers, unless they are HIV-infected, do not normally develop active TB within the first year of infection. They may, however, develop active TB years later, which could cause significant morbidity. MDR TB has caused at least six deaths in workers in recent years. All of these workers, however, were immune-compromised (most were HIV-positive, and one, a prison guard, was immune-suppressed because of a transplant). One could argue that significant TB morbidity and mortality occurs only in those who are already somewhat ill. However, TB infection is still a significant concern in healthy workers who may develop active TB years down the road, or infect hundreds of others if they have active, yet asymptomatic, infections.

Occupational TB concerns are so strong at this time that OSHA is currently working on TB guidelines and a possible TB standard. Because it can be casually transmitted to workers and the general population, TB may, in the long term, present a greater threat than HIV. To summarize, in the future, I see occupational HBV infection becoming less important, with occupational HIV infection and occupational TB infection becoming more important.

Whether or not you think that OSHA is a four-letter word, the goals that OSHA has set—to prevent and decrease the risk of occupational illness and injury in workers—are important ones. The Bloodborne Pathogens Standard, though costly to implement in terms of both money and time involved, finally places full emphasis on the prevention of illness and injuries in health care and other workers whose occupations place them at risk of exposure to infectious diseases.

OSHA Bloodborne Pathogens Standard Regulatory Text[1]

(a) SCOPE AND APPLICATION

This section applies to all occupational exposure to blood or other potentially infectious materials as defined by paragraph (b) of this section.

(b) DEFINITIONS

For purposes of this section, the following shall apply:

Assistant Secretary means the Assistant Secretary of Labor for Occupational Safety and Health, or designated representative.

Blood means human blood, human blood components, and products made from human blood.

---

1. As published in the *Federal Register,* Friday, December 6, 1991, which states:

Part 1910 of title 29 of the Code of Federal Regulations is amended as follows:

Part 1910—[Amended]

Subpart Z—[Amended]

1. The general authority citation for subpart Z of 29 CFR part 1910 continues to read as follows and a new citation for 1910.1030 is added:

Authority: Secs. 6 and 8, Occupational Safety and Health Act, 29 U.S.C. 655, 657, Secretary of Labor's Orders Nos. 12-71 (36 CFR 8754), 8-76 (41 CFR 25059), or 9-83 (48 CFR 35736), as applicable; and 29 CFR part 1911.

Section 1910.1030 also issued under 29 U.S.C. 853.

*   *   *

2. Section 1910.1030 is added to read as follows:

1910.1030 Bloodborne Pathogens.

Bloodborne Pathogens means pathogenic microorganisms that are present in human blood and can cause disease in humans. These pathogens include, but are not limited to, Hepatitis B Virus [HBV] and Human Immunodeficiency Virus [HIV].

Clinical Laboratory means a workplace where diagnostic or other screening procedures are performed on blood or other potentially infectious materials.

Contaminated means the presence or the reasonably anticipated presence of blood or other potentially infectious materials on an item or surface.

Contaminated Laundry means laundry which has been soiled with blood or other potentially infectious materials or may contain sharps.

Contaminated Sharps means any contaminated object that can penetrate the skin including, but not limited to, needles, scalpels, broken glass, broken capillary tubes, and exposed ends of dental wires.

Decontamination means the use of physical or chemical means to remove, inactivate, or destroy bloodborne pathogens on a surface or item to the point where they are no longer capable of transmitting infectious particles and the surface or item is rendered safe for handling, use, or disposal.

Director means the Director of the National Institute for Occupational Safety and Health, U.S. Department of Health and Human Services, or designated representative.

Engineering Controls means controls (e.g., sharps disposal containers, self-sheathing needles) that isolate or remove the bloodborne pathogens hazard from the workplace.

Exposure Incident means a specific eye, mouth, other mucous membrane, non-intact skin, or parenteral contact with blood or other potentially infectious materials that results from the performance of an employee's duties.

Handwashing Facilities means a facility providing an adequate supply of running potable water, soap, and single-use towels or hot air drying machines.

Licensed Health Care Professional is a person whose legally permitted scope of practice allows him or her to independently perform the activities required by paragraph (f) Hepatitis B vaccination and Post-Exposure Evaluation and Follow-Up.

HBV means Hepatitis B Virus.

HIV means Human Immunodeficiency Virus.

Occupational Exposure means reasonably anticipated skin, eye, mucous membrane, or parenteral contact with blood or other potentially infectious materials that may result from the performance of an employees duties.

Other Potentially Infectious Materials means

(1) The following human body fluids: semen, vaginal secretions, cerebrospinal fluid, synovial fluid, pleural fluid, pericardial fluid, peritoneal fluid, amniotic fluid, saliva in dental procedures, any body fluid that is visibly contaminated with blood, and all body fluids in situations where it is difficult or impossible to differentiate between body fluids;

(2) Any unfixed tissue or organ (other than intact skin) from a human (living or dead); and

(3) HIV-containing cell or tissue cultures, organ cultures, and HIV- or HBV-containing culture medium or other solutions; and blood, organs, or other tissues from experimental animals infected with HIV or HBV.

Parenteral means piercing mucous membranes or the skin barrier through such events as needlesticks, human bites, cuts, and abrasions.

Personal Protective Equipment is specialized clothing or equipment worn by an employee for protection against a hazard. General work clothes (e.g., uniforms, pants, shirts, or blouses) not intended to function as protection against a hazard are not considered to be personal protective equipment.

Production Facility means a facility engaged in industrial-scale, large-volume, or high-concentration production of HIV or HBV.

Regulated Waste means liquid or semi-liquid blood or other potentially infectious materials; contaminated items that would release blood or other potentially infectious materials in a liquid or semi-liquid state if compressed; items that are caked with dried blood or other potentially infectious materials and are capable of releasing these materials during handling; contaminated sharps; and pathological and microbiological wastes containing blood or other potentially infectious materials.

Research Laboratory means a laboratory producing or using research-laboratory–scale amounts of HIV or HBV. Research laboratories may produce high concentrations of HIV or HBV but not in the volume found in production facilities.

Source Individual means any individual, living or dead, whose blood or other potentially infectious materials may be a source of occupational exposure to the employee. Examples include, but are not limited to, hospital and clinic patients; clients in institutions for the developmentally disabled; trauma victims; clients of drug and alcohol treatment facilities; residents of hospices and nursing homes; human remains; and individuals who donate or sell blood or blood components.

Sterilize means the use of a physical or chemical procedure to destroy all microbial life including highly resistant bacterial endospores.

Universal Precautions is an approach to infection control. According to the concept of Universal Precautions, all human blood and certain human body fluids are treated as if known to be infectious for HIV, HBV, and other bloodborne pathogens.

Work Practice Controls means controls that reduce the likelihood of exposure by altering the manner in which a task is performed (e.g., prohibiting recapping of needles by a two-handed technique).

(c) EXPOSURE CONTROL

(1) *Exposure Control Plan*

(i) Each employer having an employee(s) with occupational exposure as defined by paragraph (b) of this section shall establish a written Exposure Control Plan designed to eliminate or minimize employee exposure.

(ii) The Exposure Control Plan shall contain at least the following elements:

(A) The exposure determination required by paragraph (c)(2);

(B) The schedule and method of implementation for paragraphs (d) Methods of Compliance, (e) HIV and HBV Research Laboratories and Production Facilities, (f) Hepatitis B Vaccination and Post-Exposure Evaluation and Follow-Up, (g) Communication of Hazards to Employees, and (h) Recordkeeping of this standard; and

(C) The procedure for the evaluation of circumstances surrounding exposure incidents as required by paragraph (f)(3)(i) of this standard.

(iii) Each employer shall ensure that a copy of the Exposure Control Plan is accessible to employees in accordance with 29 CFR 1910.20(e).

(iv) The Exposure Control Plan shall be reviewed and updated at least annually and whenever necessary to reflect new or modified tasks and procedures which affect occupational exposure and to reflect new or revised employee positions with occupational exposure.

(v) The Exposure Control Plan shall be made available to the Assistant Secretary and the Director upon request for examination and copying.

(2) *Exposure Determination*

(i) Each employer who has an employee(s) with occupational exposure as defined by paragraph (b) of this section shall prepare an exposure determination. This exposure determination shall contain the following:

(A) A list of all job classifications in which all employees in those job classifications have occupational exposure;

(B) A list of job classifications in which some employees have occupational exposure; and

(C) A list of all tasks and procedures or groups of closely related task and procedures in which occupational exposures occur and that are performed by employees in job classifications listed in accordance with the provisions of paragraph (c)(2)(i)(B) of this standard.

(ii) This exposure determination shall be made without regard to the use of personal protective equipment.

(d) METHODS OF COMPLIANCE

(1) *General*

Universal precautions shall be observed to prevent contact with blood or other potentially infectious materials. Under circumstances in which differentiation between body fluid types is difficult or impossible, all body fluids shall be considered potentially infectious materials.

(2) *Engineering and Work Practice Controls*

(i) Engineering and work practice controls shall be used to eliminate or minimize employee exposure. Where occupational exposure remains after institution of these controls, personal protective equipment shall also be used.

(ii) Engineering controls shall be examined and maintained or replaced on a regular schedule to ensure their effectiveness.

(iii) Employers shall provide handwashing facilities which are readily accessible to employees.

(iv) When provision of handwashing facilities is not feasible, the employer shall provide either an appropriate antiseptic hand cleanser in conjunction with clean cloth/paper towels or antiseptic towelettes. When antiseptic hand cleansers or towelettes are used, hands shall be washed with soap and running water as soon as feasible.

(v) Employers shall ensure that employees wash their hands immediately or as soon as feasible after removal of gloves or other personal protective equipment.

(vi) Employers shall ensure that employees wash hands and any other skin with soap and water, or flush mucous membranes with water immediately or as soon as feasible following contact of such body areas with blood or other potentially infectious materials.

(vii) Contaminated needles and other contaminated sharps shall not be bent, recapped, or removed except as noted in paragraphs (d)(2)(vii)(A) and (d)(2)(vii)(B) below. Shearing or breaking of contaminated needles is prohibited.

    (A) Contaminated needles and other contaminated sharps shall not be recapped or removed unless the employer can demonstrate that no alternative is feasible or that such action is required by a specific medical procedure.

    (B) Such recapping or needle removal must be accomplished through the use of a mechanical device or a one-handed technique.

(viii) Immediately or as soon as possible after use, contaminated reusable sharps shall be placed in appropriate containers until properly reprocessed. These containers shall be:

    (A) Puncture-resistant;

    (B) Labeled or color-coded in accordance with this standard;

    (C) Leakproof on the sides and bottom; and

    (D) In accordance with the requirements set forth in paragraph (d)(4)(ii)(E) for reusable sharps.

(ix) Eating, drinking, smoking, applying cosmetics or lip balm, and handling contact lenses are prohibited in work areas where there is a reasonable likelihood of occupational exposure.

(x) Food and drink shall not be kept in refrigerators, freezers, shelves, cabinets or on countertops or benchtops where blood or other potentially infectious materials are present.

(xi) All procedures involving blood or other potentially infectious materials shall be performed in such a manner as to minimize splashing, spraying, spattering, and generation of droplets of these substances.

(xii) Mouth pipetting/suctioning of blood or other potentially infectious materials is prohibited.

(xiii) Specimens of blood or other potentially infectious materials shall be placed in a container which prevents leakage during collection, handling, processing, storage, transport, or shipping.

    (A) The container for storage, transport, or shipping shall be labeled or color-coded according to paragraph (g)(1)(i) and closed prior to being stored, transported, or shipped. When a facility utilizes Universal Precautions in the handling of all specimens, the labeling/color-coding of specimens is not necessary provided containers are recognizable as containing specimens. This exemption only applies while such specimens/containers remain within the facility. Labeling or color-coding in accordance with paragraph (g)(1)(i) is required when such specimens/containers leave the facility.

(B) If outside contamination of the primary container occurs, the primary container shall be placed within a second container which prevents leakage during handling, processing, storage, transport, or shipping and is labeled or color-coded according to the requirements of this standard.

(C) If the specimen could puncture the primary container, the primary container shall be placed within a secondary container which is puncture-resistant in addition to the above characteristics.

(xiv) Equipment which may become contaminated with blood or other potentially infectious materials shall be examined prior to servicing or shipping and shall be decontaminated as necessary, unless the employer can demonstrate that decontamination of such equipment or portions of such equipment is not feasible.

(A) A readily observable label in accordance with paragraph (g)(1)(i)(H) shall be attached to the equipment stating which portions remain contaminated.

(B) The employer shall ensure that this information is conveyed to all affected employees, the servicing representative, and/or the manufacturer, as appropriate, prior to handling, servicing, or shipping so that appropriate precautions will be taken.

(3) *Personal Protective Equipment*

(i) Provision. When there is occupational exposure, the employer shall provide, at no cost to the employee, appropriate personal protective equipment such as, but not limited to, gloves, gowns, laboratory coats, face shields or masks and eye protection, and mouthpieces, resuscitation bags, pocket masks, or other ventilation devices. Personal protective equipment will be considered "appropriate" only if it does not permit blood or other potentially infectious materials to pass through to or reach the employees work clothes, street clothes, undergarments, skin, eyes, mouth, or other mucous membranes under normal conditions of use and for the duration of time which the protective equipment will be used.

(ii) Use. The employer shall ensure that the employee uses appropriate personal protective equipment unless the employer shows that the employee temporarily and briefly declined to use personal protective equipment when, under rare and extraordinary circumstances, it was the employee's professional judgment that in the specific instance its use would have prevented the delivery of health care or public safety services or would have posed an increased hazard to the safety of the worker or coworker. When the employee makes this judgment, the circumstances shall be investigated and documented in order to determine whether changes can be instituted to prevent such occurrences in the future.

(iii) Accessibility. The employer shall ensure that appropriate personal protective equipment in the appropriate sizes is readily accessible at the worksite or is issued to employees. Hypoallergenic gloves, glove liners, powderless gloves, or other similar alternatives shall be readily accessible to those employees who are allergic to the gloves normally provided.

(iv) Cleaning, Laundering, and Disposal. The employer shall clean, launder, and dispose of personal protective equipment required by paragraphs (d) and (e) of this standard, at no cost to the employee.

(v) Repair and Replacement. The employer shall repair or replace personal protective equipment as needed to maintain its effectiveness, at no cost to the employee.

(vi) If a garment(s) is penetrated by blood or other potentially infectious materials, the garment(s) shall be removed immediately or as soon as feasible.

(vii) All personal protective equipment shall be removed prior to leaving the work area.

(viii) When personal protective equipment is removed it shall be placed in an appropriately designated area or container for storage, washing, decontamination, or disposal.

(ix) Gloves. Gloves shall be worn when it can be reasonably anticipated that the employee may have hand contact with blood, other potentially infectious materials, mucous membranes, and non-intact skin; when performing vascular access procedures except as specified in paragraph (d)(3)(ix)(D); and when handling or touching contaminated items or surfaces.

(A) Disposable (single-use) gloves such as surgical or examination gloves, shall be replaced as soon as practical when contaminated or as soon as feasible if they are torn, punctured, or when their ability to function as a barrier is compromised.

(B) Disposable (single-use) gloves shall not be washed or decontaminated for re-use.

(C) Utility gloves may be decontaminated for reuse if the integrity of the glove is not compromised. However, they must be discarded if they are cracked, peeling, torn, punctured, or exhibit other signs of deterioration or when their ability to function as a barrier is compromised.

(D) If an employer in a volunteer blood donation center judges that routine gloving for all phlebotomies is not necessary then the employer shall:

(1) Periodically reevaluate this policy;

      (2) Make gloves available to all employees who wish to use them for phlebotomy;

      (3) Not discourage the use of gloves for phlebotomy; and

      (4) Require that gloves be used for phlebotomy in the following circumstances:

         (i) When the employee has cuts, scratches, or other breaks in his or her skin;

         (ii) When the employee judges that hand contamination with blood may occur, for example, when performing phlebotomy on an uncooperative source individual; and

         (iii) When the employee is receiving training in phlebotomy.

(x) Masks, Eye Protection, and Face Shields. Masks in combination with eye protection devices, such as goggles or glasses with solid side shields, or chin-length face shields, shall be worn whenever splashes, spray, spatter, or droplets of blood or other potentially infectious materials may be generated and eye, nose, or mouth contamination can be reasonably anticipated.

(xi) Gowns, Aprons, and Other Protective Body Clothing. Appropriate protective clothing such as, but not limited to, gowns, aprons, lab coats, clinic jackets, or similar outer garments shall be worn in occupational exposure situations. The type and characteristics will depend upon the task and degree of exposure anticipated.

(xii) Surgical caps or hoods and/or shoe covers or boots shall be worn in instances when gross contamination can reasonably be anticipated (e.g., autopsies, orthopedic surgery).

(4) *Housekeeping*

    (i) General. Employers shall ensure that the worksite is maintained in a clean and sanitary condition. The employer shall determine and implement an appropriate written schedule for cleaning and method of decontamination based upon the location within the facility, type of surface to be cleaned, type of soil present, and tasks or procedures being performed in the area.

    (ii) All equipment and environmental and working surfaces shall be cleaned and decontaminated after contact with blood or other potentially infectious materials.

      (A) Contaminated work surfaces shall be decontaminated with an appropriate disinfectant after completion of procedures; immediately or as soon as feasible when surfaces are overtly contaminated or after any spill of blood or other potentially infectious materials; and at the end of the work shift if the surface may have become contaminated since the last cleaning.

      (B) Protective coverings, such as plastic wrap, aluminum foil, or imperviously backed absorbent paper used to cover equipment and environmental surfaces, shall be removed and replaced as soon as feasible when they become overtly contaminated or at the end of the work shift if they may have become contaminated during the shift.

(C) All bins, pails, cans, and similar receptacles intended for reuse which have a reasonable likelihood for becoming contaminated with blood or other potentially infectious materials shall be inspected and decontaminated on a regularly scheduled basis and cleaned and decontaminated immediately or as soon as feasible upon visible contamination.

(D) Broken glassware which may be contaminated shall not be picked up directly with the hands. It shall be cleaned up using mechanical means, such as a brush and dustpan, tongs, or forceps.

(E) Reusable sharps that are contaminated with blood or other potentially infectious materials shall not be stored or processed in a manner that requires employees to reach by hand into the containers where these sharps have been placed.

(iii) Regulated Waste.

  (A) Contaminated Sharps Discarding and Containment.

  (1) Contaminated sharps shall be discarded immediately or as soon as feasible in containers that are:

   (i) Closable;

   (ii) Puncture-resistant;

   (iii) Leakproof on sides and bottom; and

   (iv) Labeled or color-coded in accordance with paragraph (g)(1)(i) of this standard.

  (2) During use, containers for contaminated sharps shall be:

   (i) Easily accessible to personnel and located as close as is feasible to the immediate area where sharps are used or can be reasonably anticipated to be found (e.g., laundries);

   (ii) Maintained upright throughout use; and

   (iii) Replaced routinely and not be allowed to overfill.

  (3) When moving containers of contaminated sharps from the area of use, the containers shall be:

   (i) Closed immediately prior to removal or replacement to prevent spillage or protrusion of contents during handling, storage, transport, or shipping;

   (ii) Placed in a secondary container if leakage is possible. The second container shall be:

    (A) Closable;

    (B) Constructed to contain all contents and prevent leakage during handling, storage, transport, or shipping; and

(**C**) Labeled or color-coded according to paragraph (g)(1)(i) of this standard.

(**4**) Reusable containers shall not be opened, emptied, or cleaned manually or in any other manner which would expose employees to the risk of percutaneous injury.

(**B**) Regulated Waste Containment.

(**1**) Regulated waste shall be placed in containers that are:

(**i**) Closable;

(**ii**) Constructed to contain all contents and prevent leakage of fluids during handling, storage, transport, or shipping;

(**iii**) Labeled or color-coded in accordance with paragraph (g)(1)(i) of this standard; and

(**iv**) Closed prior to removal to prevent spillage or protrusion of contents during handling, storage, transport, or shipping.

(**2**) If outside contamination of the regulated waste container occurs, it shall be placed in a second container. The second container shall be:

(**i**) Closable;

(**ii**) Constructed to contain all contents and prevent leakage of fluids during handling, storage, transport, or shipping;

(**iii**) Labeled or color-coded in accordance with paragraph (g)(1)(i) of this standard; and

(**iv**) Closed prior to removal to prevent spillage or protrusion of contents during handling, storage, transport, or shipping.

(**C**) Disposal of all regulated waste shall be in accordance with applicable regulations of the United States, States and Territories, and political subdivisions of States and Territories.

(**iv**) Laundry.

(**A**) Contaminated laundry shall be handled as little as possible with a minimum of agitation.

(**1**) Contaminated laundry shall be bagged or containerized at the location where it was used and shall not be sorted or rinsed in the location of use.

(**2**) Contaminated laundry shall be placed and transported in bags or containers labeled or color-coded in accordance with paragraph (g)(1)(i) of this standard. When a facility utilizes Universal Precautions in the handling of all soiled laundry, alternative labeling or color-coding is sufficient if it permits all employees to recognize the containers as requiring compliance with Universal Precautions.

(**3**) Whenever contaminated laundry is wet and presents a reasonable likelihood of soak-through of or leakage from the bag or container, the laundry shall be placed and transported in bags or containers which prevent soak-through and/or leakage of fluids to the exterior.

(B) The employer shall ensure that employees who have contact with contaminated laundry wear protective gloves and other appropriate personal protective equipment.

(C) When a facility ships contaminated laundry off-site to a second facility which does not utilize Universal Precautions in the handling of all laundry, the facility generating the contaminated laundry must place such laundry in bags or containers which are labeled or color-coded in accordance with paragraph (g)(1)(i).

(e) HIV AND HBV RESEARCH LABORATORIES AND PRODUCTION FACILITIES

(1) *This paragraph applies to research laboratories and production facilities* engaged in the culture, production, concentration, experimentation, and manipulation of HIV and HBV. It does not apply to clinical or diagnostic laboratories engaged solely in the analysis of blood, tissues, or organs. These requirements apply in addition to the other requirements of the standard.

(2) *Research laboratories and production facilities shall meet the following criteria:*

(i) Standard microbiological practices. All regulated waste shall either be incinerated or decontaminated by a method such as autoclaving known to effectively destroy bloodborne pathogens.

(ii) Special practices:

(A) Laboratory doors shall be kept closed when work involving HIV or HBV is in progress.

(B) Contaminated materials that are to be decontaminated at a site away from the work area shall be placed in a durable, leakproof, labeled or color-coded container that is closed before being removed from the work area.

(C) Access to the work area shall be limited to authorized persons. Written policies and procedures shall be established whereby only persons who have been advised of the potential biohazard, who meet any specific entry requirements, and who comply with all entry and exit procedures shall be allowed to enter the work areas and animal rooms.

(D) When other potentially infectious materials or infected animals are present in the work area or containment module, a hazard warning sign incorporating the universal biohazard symbol shall be posted on all access doors. The hazard warning sign shall comply with paragraph (g)(1)(ii) of this standard.

(E) All activities involving other potentially infectious materials shall be conducted in biological safety cabinets or other physical-containment devices within the containment module. No work with these other potentially infectious materials shall be conducted on the open bench.

(F) Laboratory coats, gowns, smocks, uniforms, or other appropriate protective clothing shall be used in the work area and animal rooms. Protective clothing shall not be worn outside of the work area and shall be decontaminated before being laundered.

(G) Special care shall be taken to avoid skin contact with other potentially infectious materials. Gloves shall be worn when handling infected animals and when making hand contact with other potentially infectious materials is unavoidable.

(H) Before disposal all waste from work areas and from animal rooms shall either be incinerated or decontaminated by a method such as autoclaving known to effectively destroy bloodborne pathogens.

(I) Vacuum lines shall be protected with liquid disinfectant traps and high efficiency particulate air (HEPA) filters or filters of equivalent or superior efficiency and which are checked routinely and maintained or replaced as necessary.

(J) Hypodermic needles and syringes shall be used only for parenteral injection and aspiration of fluids from laboratory animals and diaphragm bottles. Only needle-locking syringes or disposable syringe-needle units (i.e., the needle is integral to the syringe) shall be used for the injection or aspiration of other potentially infectious materials. Extreme caution shall be used when handling needles and syringes. A needle shall not be bent, sheared, replaced in the sheath or guard, or removed from the syringe following use. The needle and syringe shall be promptly placed in a puncture-resistant container and autoclaved or decontaminated before reuse or disposal.

(K) All spills shall be immediately contained and cleaned up by appropriate professional staff or others properly trained and equipped to work with potentially concentrated infectious materials.

(L) A spill or accident that results in an exposure incident shall be immediately reported to the laboratory director or other responsible person.

(M) A biosafety manual shall be prepared or adopted and periodically reviewed and updated at least annually or more often if necessary. Personnel shall be advised of potential hazards, shall be required to read instructions on practices and procedures, and shall be required to follow them.

(iii) Containment Equipment

    (A) Certified biological safety cabinets (Class II, III, or IV) or other appropriate combinations of personal protection or physical containment devices, such as special protective clothing, respirators, centrifuge safety cups, sealed centrifuge rotors, and containment caging for animals, shall be used for all activities with other potentially infectious materials that pose a threat of exposure to droplets, splashes, spills, or aerosols.

    (B) Biological safety cabinets shall be certified when installed, whenever they are moved, and at least annually.

(3) *HIV and HBV research laboratories shall meet the following criteria:*

    (i) Each laboratory shall contain a facility for handwashing and an eye wash facility which is readily available within the work area.

    (ii) An autoclave for decontamination of regulated waste shall be available.

(4) *HIV and HBV production facilities shall meet the following criteria:*

    (i) The work areas shall be separated from areas that are open to unrestricted traffic flow within the building. Passage through two sets of doors shall be the basic requirement for entry into the work area from access corridors or other contiguous areas. Physical separation of the high-containment work area from access corridors or other areas or activities may also be provided by a double-doored clothes-change room (showers may be included), airlock, or other access facility that requires passing through two sets of doors before entering the work area.

    (ii) The surfaces of doors, walls, floors, and ceilings in the work area shall be water-resistant so that they can be easily cleaned. Penetrations in these surfaces shall be sealed or capable of being sealed to facilitate decontamination.

    (iii) Each work area shall contain a sink for washing hands and readily available eye wash facility. The sink shall be foot, elbow, or automatically operated and shall be located near the exit door of the work area.

    (iv) Access doors to the work area or containment module shall be self-closing.

    (v) An autoclave for decontamination of regulated waste shall be available within or as near as possible to the work area.

    (vi) A ducted exhaust-air ventilation system shall be provided. This system shall create directional airflow that draws air into the work area through the entry area. The exhaust air shall not be recirculated to any other area of the building, shall be discharged to the outside, and shall be dispersed away from occupied areas and air intakes. The proper direction of the airflow shall be verified (i.e., into the work area).

(5) Training Requirements.

Additional training requirements for employees in HIV and HBV research laboratories and HIV and HBV production facilities are specified in paragraph (g)(2)(ix).

(f) HEPATITIS B VACCINATION AND POST-EXPOSURE EVALUATION AND FOLLOW-UP

(1) General

   (i) The employer shall make available the Hepatitis B vaccine and vaccination series to all employees who have occupational exposure, and post-exposure evaluation and follow-up to all employees who have had an exposure incident.

   (ii) The employer shall ensure that all medical evaluations and procedures including the Hepatitis B vaccine and vaccination series and post-exposure evaluation and follow-up, including prophylaxis, are:

      (A) Made available at no cost to the employee;

      (B) Made available to the employee at a reasonable time and place;

      (C) Performed by or under the supervision of a licensed physician or by or under the supervision of another licensed health care professional; and

      (D) Provided according to recommendations of the U.S. Public Health Service current at the time these evaluations and procedures take place, except as specified by this paragraph (f).

   (iii) The employer shall ensure that all laboratory tests are conducted by an accredited laboratory at no cost to the employee.

(2) Hepatitis B Vaccination

   (i) Hepatitis B vaccination shall be made available after the employee has received the training required in paragraph (g)(2)(vii)(1) and within 10 working days of initial assignment to all employees who have occupational exposure unless the employee has previously received the complete Hepatitis B vaccination series, antibody testing has revealed that the employee is immune, or the vaccine is contraindicated for medical reasons.

   (ii) The employer shall not make participation in a prescreening program a prerequisite for receiving Hepatitis B vaccination.

   (iii) If the employee initially declines Hepatitis B vaccination but at a later date while still covered under the standard decides to accept the vaccination, the employer shall make available Hepatitis B vaccination at that time.

(iv) The employer shall assure that employees who decline to accept Hepatitis B vaccination offered by the employer sign the statement in Appendix A1.

(v) If a routine booster dose(s) of Hepatitis B vaccine is recommended by the U.S. Public Health Service at a future date, such booster dose(s) shall be made available in accordance with section (f)(1)(ii).

(3) *Post-Exposure Evaluation and Follow-Up*

Following a report of an exposure incident, the employer shall make immediately available to the exposed employee a confidential medical evaluation and follow-up, including at least the following elements:

(i) Documentation of the route(s) of exposure, and the circumstances under which the exposure incident occurred;

(ii) Identification and documentation of the source individual, unless the employer can establish that identification is infeasible or prohibited by state or local law:

  (A) The source individual's blood shall be tested as soon as feasible and after consent is obtained in order to determine HBV and HIV infectivity. If consent is not obtained, the employer shall establish that legally required consent cannot be obtained. When the source individual's consent is not required by law the source individual's blood, if available, shall be tested and the results documented.

  (B) When the source individual is already known to be infected with HBV or HIV, testing for the source individual's known HBV or HIV status need not be repeated.

  (C) Results of the source individual's testing shall be made available to the exposed employee, and the employee shall be informed of applicable laws and regulations concerning disclosure of the identity and infectious status of the source individual.

(iii) Collection and testing of blood for HBV and HIV serological status:

  (A) The exposed employee's blood shall be collected as soon as feasible and tested after consent is obtained.

  (B) If the employee consents to baseline blood collection, but does not give consent at that time for HIV serologic testing, the sample shall be preserved for at least 90 days. If, within 90 days of the exposure incident, the employee elects to have the baseline sample tested, such testing shall be done as soon as feasible.

(iv) Post-exposure prophylaxis, when medically indicated, as recommended by the U.S. Public Health Service;

(v) Counseling; and

(vi) Evaluation of reported illnesses.

(4) *Information Provided to the Health Care Professional*
- **(i)** The employer shall ensure that the health care professional responsible for the employees Hepatitis B vaccination is provided a copy of this regulation.
- **(ii)** The employer shall ensure that the health care professional evaluating an employee after an exposure incident is provided the following information:
  - **(A)** A copy of this regulation;
  - **(B)** A description of the exposed employees duties as they relate to the exposure incident;
  - **(C)** Documentation of the route(s) of exposure and circumstances under which the exposure occurred;
  - **(D)** Results of the source individual's blood testing, if available; and
  - **(E)** All medical records relevant to the appropriate treatment of the employee including vaccination status which are the employer's responsibility to maintain.

(5) *Health Care Professional's Written Opinion*

The employer shall obtain and provide the employee with a copy of the evaluating health care professional's written opinion within 15 days of the completion of the evaluation.
- **(i)** The health care professional's written opinion for Hepatitis B vaccination shall be limited to whether Hepatitis B vaccination is indicated for an employee, and if the employee has received such vaccination.
- **(ii)** The health care professional's written opinion for post-exposure evaluation and follow-up shall be limited to the following information:
  - **(A)** That the employee has been informed of the results of the evaluation; and
  - **(B)** That the employee has been told about any medical conditions resulting from exposure to blood or other potentially infectious materials which require further evaluation or treatment.
- **(iii)** All other findings or diagnoses shall remain confidential and shall not be included in the written report.

(6) *Medical Recordkeeping*

Medical records required by this standard shall be maintained in accordance with paragraph (h)(1) of this section.

(g) COMMUNICATION OF HAZARDS TO EMPLOYEES

(1) *Labels and Signs*
- **(i)** Labels

(A) Warning labels shall be affixed to containers of regulated waste; refrigerators and freezers containing blood or other potentially infectious material; and other containers used to store, transport, or ship blood or other potentially infectious materials, except as provided in paragraph (g)(1)(i)(E), (F), and (G).

(B) Labels required by this section shall include the BIOHAZARD legend:

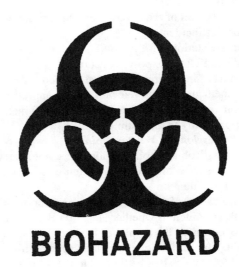

BIOHAZARD

(C) These labels shall be fluorescent orange or orange-red or predominantly so, with lettering or symbols in contrasting color.

(D) Labels required be affixed as close as feasible to the container by string, wire, adhesive, or other method that prevents their loss or unintentional removal.

(E) Red bags or red containers may be substituted for labels.

(F) Containers of blood, blood components, or blood products that are labeled as to their contents and have been released for transfusion or other clinical use are exempted from labeling requirements of paragraph (g).

(G) Individual containers of blood or other potentially infectious materials that are placed in a labeled container during storage, transport, shipment, or disposal are exempted from the labeling requirement.

(H) Labels required for contaminated equipment shall be in accordance with this paragraph and shall also state which portions of the equipment remain contaminated.

(I) Regulated waste that has been decontaminated need not be labeled or color-coded.

(ii) Signs.

(A) The employer shall post signs at the entrance to work areas specified in paragraph (e), HIV and HBV Research Laboratory and Production Facilities, which shall bear the [BIOHAZARD] legend:

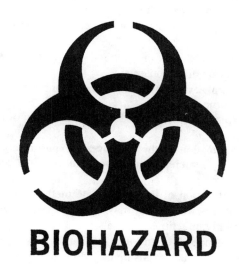

BIOHAZARD

(Name of the Infectious Agent)

(Special requirements for entering the area) (Name, telephone number of the laboratory director or other responsible person)

(B) These signs shall be fluorescent orange-red or predominantly so, with lettering or symbols in a contrasting color.

(2) Information and Training

(i) Employers shall ensure that all employees with occupational exposure participate in a training program which must be provided at no cost to the employee and during working hours.

(ii) Training shall be provided as follows:

(A) At the time of initial assignment to tasks where occupational exposure may take place;

(B) Within 90 days after the effective date of the standard; and

(C) At least annually thereafter.

(iii) For employees who have received training on bloodborne pathogens in the year preceding the effective date of the standard, only training with respect to the provisions of the standard which were not included need be provided.

(iv) Annual training for all employees shall be provided within one year of their previous training.

(v) Employers shall provide additional training when changes such as modification of tasks or procedures or institution of new tasks or procedures affect the employees occupational exposure. The additional training may be limited to addressing the new exposures created.

(vi) Material appropriate in content and vocabulary to educational level, literacy, and language of employees shall be used.

(vii) The training program shall contain at a minimum the following elements:

(A) An accessible copy of the regulatory text of this standard and an explanation of its contents;

(B) A general explanation of the epidemiology and symptoms of bloodborne diseases;

(C) An explanation of the modes of transmission of bloodborne pathogens;

(D) An explanation of the employer's exposure control plan and the means by which the employee can obtain a copy of the written plan;

(E) An explanation of the appropriate methods for recognizing tasks and other activities that may involve exposure to blood and other potentially infectious materials;

(F) An explanation of the use and limitations of methods that will prevent or reduce exposure including appropriate engineering controls, work practices, and personal protective equipment;

(G) Information on the types, proper use, location, removal, handling, decontamination, and disposal of personal protective equipment;

(H) An explanation of the basis for selection of personal protective equipment;

(I) Information on the Hepatitis B vaccine, including information on its efficacy, safety, method of administration, the benefits of being vaccinated, and that the vaccine and vaccination will be offered free of charge;

(J) Information on the appropriate actions to take and persons to contact in an emergency involving blood or other potentially infectious materials;

(K) An explanation of the procedure to follow if an exposure incident occurs, including the method of reporting the incident and the medical follow-up that will be made available;

(L) Information on the post-exposure evaluation and follow-up that the employer is required to provide for the employee following an exposure incident;

(M) An explanation of the signs and labels and/or color-coding required by paragraph (g)(1); and

(N) An opportunity for interactive questions and answers with the person conducting the training session.

(viii) The person conducting the training shall be knowledgeable in the subject matter covered by the elements contained in the training program as it relates to the workplace that the training will address.

(ix) Additional Initial Training for Employees in HIV and HBV Laboratories and Production Facilities. Employees in HIV or HBV research laboratories and HIV or HBV production facilities shall receive the following initial training in addition to the above training requirements:

(A) The employer shall assure that employees demonstrate proficiency in standard microbiological practices and techniques and in the practices and operations specific to the facility before being allowed to work with HIV or HBV.

(B) The employer shall assure that employees have prior experience in the handling of human pathogens or tissue cultures before working with HIV or HBV.

(C) The employer shall provide a training program to employees who have no prior experience in handling human pathogens. Initial work activities shall not include the handling of infectious agents. A progression of work activities shall be assigned as techniques are learned and proficiency is developed. The employer shall assure that employees participate in work activities involving infectious agents only after proficiency has been demonstrated.

(h) RECORDKEEPING

(1) *Medical Records*

(i) The employer shall establish and maintain an accurate record for each employee with occupational exposure, in accordance with 29 CFR 1910.20.

(ii) This record shall include:

(A) The name and social security number of the employee;

(B) A copy of the employee's Hepatitis B vaccination status including the dates of all the Hepatitis B vaccinations and any medical records relative to the employee's ability to receive vaccination as required by paragraph (f)(2);

        (C) A copy of all results of examinations, medical testing, and follow-up procedures as required by paragraph (f)(3);

        (D) The employer's copy of the health care professional's written opinion as required by paragraph (f)(5); and

        (E) A copy of the information provided to the health care professional as required by paragraphs (f)(4)(ii)(B), (C), and (D).

    (iii) Confidentiality. The employer shall ensure that employee medical records required by paragraph (h)(1) are:

        (A) Kept confidential; and

        (B) Not disclosed or reported without the employee's express written consent to any person within or outside the workplace except as required by this section or as may be required by law.

    (iv) The employer shall maintain the records required by paragraph (h) for at least the duration of employment plus 30 years in accordance with 29 CFR 1910.20.

(2) *Training Records*

    (i) Training records shall include the following information:

        (A) The dates of the training sessions;

        (B) The contents or a summary of the training sessions;

        (C) The names and qualifications for the persons conducting the training; and

        (D) The names and job titles of all persons attending the training sessions.

    (ii) Training records shall be maintained for 3 years from the date on which the training occurred.

(3) *Availability*

    (i) The employer shall ensure that all records required to be maintained by this section shall be made available upon request to the Assistant Secretary and Director for examination and copying.

    (ii) Employee training records required by this paragraph shall be provided upon request for examination and copying to employees, to employee representatives, to the Director, and to the Assistant Secretary in accordance with 29 CFR 1910.20.

    (iii) Employee medical records required by this paragraph shall be provided upon request for examination and copying to the subject employee, to anyone having written consent of the subject employee, to the Director, and to the Assistant Secretary in accordance with 29 CFR 1910.20.

(4) *Transfer of Records*

    (i) The employer shall comply with the requirements involving transfer of records set forth in 29 CFR 1910.20(h).

    (ii) If the employer ceases to do business and there is no successor employer to receive and retain the records for the prescribed period, the employer shall notify the Director, at least 3 months prior to their disposal and transmit them to the Director, if required by the Director to do so, within that 3-month period.

(i) DATES

(1) Effective Date. The standard shall become effective on March 6, 1992.
(2) The Exposure Control Plan required by paragraph (c)(1) of this section shall be completed on or before May 5, 1992.
(3) Paragraph (g)(2) Information and Training and (h) Recordkeeping shall take effect on or before June 4, 1992.
(4) Paragraphs (d)(2) Engineering and Work Practice Controls, (d)(3) Personal Protective Equipment, (d)(4), Housekeeping, (e) HIV and HBV Research Laboratories and Production Facilities, (f) Hepatitis B Vaccination and Post-Exposure Evaluation and Follow-Up, and (g)(1) Labels and Signs shall take effect July 6, 1992.

APPENDIX A1 TO SECTION 1910.1030—
HEPATITIS B VACCINE DECLINATION (MANDATORY)

I understand that due to my occupational exposure to blood or other potentially infectious materials I may be at risk of acquiring Hepatitis B Virus (HBV) infection. I have been given the opportunity to be vaccinated with Hepatitis B vaccine, at no charge to myself. However, I decline Hepatitis B vaccination at this time. I understand that by declining this vaccine, I continue to be at risk of acquiring Hepatitis B, a serious disease. If in the future I continue to have occupational exposure to blood or other potentially infectious materials and I want to be vaccinated with Hepatitis B vaccine, I can receive the vaccination series at no charge to me.

Universal Precautions for Prevention of Transmission of Human Immunodeficiency Virus, Hepatitis B Virus, and Other Bloodborne Pathogens in Health Care Settings[1]

INTRODUCTION

The purpose of this report is to clarify and supplement the CDC publication entitled "Recommendations for Prevention of HIV Transmission in Health-Care Settings" (1).[2]

In 1983, CDC published a document entitled "Guideline for Isolation Precautions in Hospitals" (2) that contained a section entitled "Blood and Body Fluid Precautions." The recommendations in this section called for blood and body fluid precautions when a patient was known or suspected to be infected with bloodborne pathogens. In August 1987, CDC published a document entitled "Recommendations for Prevention of HIV Transmission in Health-Care Settings" (1). In contrast to the 1983 document, the 1987 document recommended that blood and body fluid precautions be consistently used for all patients regardless of their bloodborne infection status. This extension of blood and body fluid precautions to *all* patients is referred to as "Universal Blood and Body Fluid Precautions" or "Universal Precautions." Under universal precautions, blood and certain body fluids of all patients are considered potentially infectious for human

---

1. Centers for Disease Control, *MMWR* 1988;37 (no. 24):377–382; 387–388.

2. See Appendix I for general information and specific recommendations not addressed in this update.

immunodeficiency virus (HIV), hepatitis B virus (HBV), and other bloodborne pathogens.

Universal precautions are intended to prevent parenteral, mucous membrane, and nonintact skin exposures of health-care workers to bloodborne pathogens. In addition, immunization with HBV vaccine is recommended as an important adjunct to universal precautions for health-care workers who have exposures to blood (3,4).

Since the recommendations for universal precautions were published in August 1987, CDC and the Food and Drug Administration (FDA) have received requests for clarification of the following issues: 1) body fluids to which universal precautions apply, 2) use of protective barriers, 3) use of gloves for phlebotomy, 4) selection of gloves for use while observing universal precautions, and 5) need for making changes in waste management programs as a result of adopting universal precautions.

BODY FLUIDS TO WHICH UNIVERSAL PRECAUTIONS APPLY

Universal precautions apply to blood and to other body fluids containing visible blood. Occupational transmission of HIV and HBV to healthcare workers by blood is documented (4,5). **Blood is the single most important source of HIV, HBV, and other bloodborne pathogens in the occupational setting. Infection control efforts for HIV, HBV, and other bloodborne pathogens must focus on preventing exposures to blood as well as on delivery of HBV immunization.**

Universal precautions also apply to semen and vaginal secretions. Although both of these fluids have been implicated in the sexual transmission of HIV and HBV, they have not been implicated in occupational transmission from patient to health-care worker. This observation is not unexpected, since exposure to semen in the usual health-care setting is limited, and the routine practice of wearing gloves for performing vaginal examinations protects health-care workers from exposure to potentially infectious vaginal secretions.

Universal precautions also apply to tissues and to the following fluids: cerebrospinal fluid (CSF), synovial fluid, pleural fluid, peritoneal fluid, pericardial fluid, and amniotic fluid. The risk of transmission of HIV and HBV from these fluids is unknown; epidemiologic studies in the health-care and community setting are currently inadequate to assess the potential risk to health-care workers from occupational exposures to them. However, HIV has been isolated from CSF, synovial, and amniotic fluid (6,8), and HBsAg has been detected in synovial fluid, amniotic fluid, and peritoneal fluid (9–11). One case of HIV transmission was reported after a percutaneous exposure to bloody pleural fluid obtained by needle aspiration (12). Whereas aseptic procedures used to obtain these fluids for diagnostic or therapeutic purposes protect health-care workers from skin exposures, they cannot prevent penetrating injuries due to contaminated needles or other sharp instruments.

BODY FLUIDS TO WHICH UNIVERSAL PRECAUTIONS DO NOT APPLY

Universal precautions do not apply to feces, nasal secretions, sputum, sweat, tears, urine, and vomitus unless they contain visible blood. The risk of transmission of HIV and HBV from these fluids and materials is extremely low or nonexistent. HIV has been isolated and HBsAg has been demonstrated in some of these fluids; however, epidemiologic studies in the health-care and community setting have not implicated these fluids or materials in the transmission of HIV and HBV infections (13,14). Some of the above fluids and excretions represent a potential source for nosocomial and community-acquired infections with other pathogens, and recommendations for preventing the transmission of non-bloodborne pathogens have been published (2).

PRECAUTIONS FOR OTHER BODY FLUIDS IN SPECIAL SETTINGS

Human breast milk has been implicated in perinatal transmission of HIV, and HBsAg has been found in the milk of mothers infected with HBV (10,13). However, occupational exposure to human breast milk has not been implicated in the transmission of HIV nor HBV infection to health-care workers. Moreover, the health-care worker will not have the same type of intensive exposure to breast milk as the nursing neonate. Whereas universal precautions do not apply to human breast milk, gloves may be worn by health-care workers in situations where exposures to breast milk might be frequent, for example, in breast milk banking.

Saliva of some persons infected with HBV has been shown to contain HBV-DNA at concentrations 1/1,000 to 1/10,000 of that found in the infected person's serum (15). HBsAg-positive saliva has been shown to be infectious when injected into experimental animals and in human bite exposures (16–18). However, HBsAg-positive saliva has not been shown to be infectious when applied to oral mucous membranes in experimental primate studies (18) or through contamination of musical instruments or cardiopulmonary resuscitation dummies used by HBV carriers (19,20). Epidemiologic studies of nonsexual household contacts of HIV-infected patients, including several small series in which HIV transmission failed to occur after bites or after percutaneous inoculation or contamination of cuts and open wounds with saliva from HIV-infected patients, suggest that the potential for salivary transmission of HIV is remote (5,13,14,21,22). One case report from Germany has suggested the possibility of transmission of HIV in a household setting from an infected child to a sibling through a human bite (23). The bite did not break the skin or result in bleeding. Since the date of seroconversion to HIV was not known for either child in this case, evidence of the role of saliva in the transmission of virus is unclear (23). Another case report suggested the possibility of transmission of HIV from husband to wife by contact with saliva during kissing (24). However, followup studies did not confirm HIV infection in the wife (21).

Universal precautions do not apply to saliva. General infection control practices already in existence—including the use of gloves for digital examination of mucous membranes and endotracheal suctioning, and handwashing after exposure to saliva should further minimize the minute risk, if any, for salivary transmission of HIV and HBV (1,25). Gloves need not be worn when feeding patients and when wiping saliva from skin.

Special precautions, however, are recommended for dentistry (1). Occupationally acquired infection with HBV in dental workers has been documented (4), and two possible cases of occupationally acquired HIV infection involving dentists have been reported (5,26). During dental procedures, contamination of saliva with blood is predictable, trauma to health-care workers' hands is common, and blood spattering may occur. Infection control precautions for dentistry minimize the potential for nonintact skin and mucous membrane contact of dental health-care workers to blood-contaminated saliva of patients. In addition, the use of gloves for oral examinations and treatment in the dental setting may also protect the patient's oral mucous membranes from exposures to blood, which may occur from breaks in the skin of dental workers' hands.

USE OF PROTECTIVE BARRIERS

Protective barriers reduce the risk of exposure of the health-care worker's skin or mucous membranes to potentially infective materials. For universal precautions, protective barriers reduce the risk of exposure to blood, body fluids containing visible blood, and other fluids to which universal precautions apply. Examples of protective barriers include gloves, gowns, masks, and protective eyewear. Gloves should reduce the incidence of contamination of hands, but they cannot prevent penetrating injuries due to needles or other sharp instruments. Masks and protective eyewear or face shields should reduce the incidence of contamination of mucous membranes of the mouth, nose, and eyes.

Universal precautions are intended to supplement rather than replace recommendations for routine infection control, such as handwashing and using gloves to prevent gross microbial contamination of hands (27). Because specifying the types of barriers needed for every possible clinical situation is impractical, some judgment must be exercised.

The risk of nosocomial transmission of HIV, HBV, and other bloodborne pathogens can be minimized if healthcare workers use the following general guidelines:[3]

1. Take care to prevent injuries when using needles, scalpels, and other sharp instruments or devices; when handling sharp instruments after procedures; when cleaning used instruments; and when disposing of used needles. Do not recap used needles by hand; do not remove used needles from disposable syringes by hand; and do not bend, break, or otherwise manipulate used needles by hand. Place used disposable syringes and needles, scalpel blades, and other sharp items in puncture-resistant containers for disposal. Locate the puncture-resistant containers as close to the use area as is practical.

2. Use protective barriers to prevent exposure to blood, body fluids containing visible blood, and other fluids to which universal precautions apply. The type of protective barrier(s) should be appropriate for the procedure being performed and the type exposure anticipated.

3. Immediately and thoroughly wash hands and other skin surfaces that are contaminated with blood, body fluids containing visible blood, or other body fluids to which universal precautions apply.

GLOVE USE FOR PHLEBOTOMY

Gloves should reduce the incidence of blood contamination of hands during phlebotomy (drawing blood samples), but they cannot prevent penetrating injuries caused by needles or other sharp instruments. The likelihood of hand contamination with blood containing HIV, HBV, or other bloodborne pathogens

---

3. See Appendix I for general information and specific recommendations not addressed in this update.

during phlebotomy depends on several factors: 1) the skill and technique of the health-care worker, 2) the frequency with which the health-care worker performs the procedure (other factors being equal, the cumulative risk of blood exposure is higher for a health-care worker who performs more procedures), 3) whether the procedure occurs in a routine or emergency situation (where blood contact may be more likely), and 4) the prevalence of infection with bloodborne pathogens in the patient population. The likelihood of infection after skin exposure to blood containing HIV or HBV will depend on the concentration of virus (viral concentration is much higher for hepatitis B than for HIV), the duration of contact, the presence of skin lesions on the hands of the health-care worker, and for HBV the immune status of the health-care worker. Although not accurately quantified, the risk of HIV infection following intact skin contact with infective blood is certainly much less than the 0.5% risk following percutaneous needlestick exposures (5). In universal precautions, *all* blood is assumed to be potentially infective for bloodborne pathogens, but in certain settings (e.g., volunteer blood donation centers) the prevalence of infection with some bloodborne pathogens (e.g., HIV, HBV) is known to be very low. Some institutions have relaxed recommendations for using gloves for phlebotomy procedures by skilled phlebotomists in settings where the prevalence of bloodborne pathogens is known to be very low.

Institutions that judge that routine gloving for *all* phlebotomies is not necessary should periodically reevaluate their policy. Gloves should always be available to health-care workers who wish to use them for phlebotomy. In addition, the following general guidelines apply:

1. Use gloves for performing phlebotomy when the health-care worker has cuts, scratches, or other breaks in his/her skin.
2. Use gloves in situations where the health-care worker judges that hand contamination with blood may occur, for example, when performing phlebotomy on an uncooperative patient.
3. Use gloves for performing finger and/or heel sticks on infants and children.
4. Use gloves when persons are receiving training in phlebotomy.

SELECTION OF GLOVES

The Center for Devices and Radiological Health, FDA, has responsibility for regulating the medical glove industry. Medical gloves include those marketed as sterile surgical or nonsterile examination gloves made of vinyl or latex. General purpose utility ("rubber") gloves are also used in the healthcare setting, but they are not regulated by FDA since they are not promoted for medical use. There are no reported differences in barrier effectiveness between intact latex and intact vinyl used to manufacture gloves. Thus, the type of gloves selected should be appropriate for the task being performed.

The following general guidelines are recommended:

1. Use sterile gloves for procedures involving contact with normally sterile areas of the body.
2. Use examination gloves for procedures involving contact with mucous membranes, unless otherwise indicated, and for other patient care or diagnostic procedures that do not require the use of sterile gloves.
3. Change gloves between patient contacts.
4. Do not wash or disinfect surgical or examination gloves for reuse. Washing with surfactants may cause "wicking," i.e., the enhanced penetration of liquids through undetected holes in the glove. Disinfecting agents may cause deterioration.
5. Use general-purpose utility gloves (e.g., rubber household gloves) for housekeeping chores involving potential blood contact and for instrument cleaning and decontamination procedures. Utility gloves may be decontaminated and reused but should be discarded if they are peeling, cracked, or discolored, or if they have punctures, tears, or other evidence of deterioration.

WASTE MANAGEMENT

Universal precautions are not intended to change waste management programs previously recommended by CDC for health-care settings (1). Policies for defining, collecting, storing, decontaminating, and disposing of infective waste are generally determined by institutions in accordance with state and local regulations. Information regarding waste management regulations in healthcare settings may be obtained from state or local health departments or agencies responsible for waste management.

Reported by: Center for Devices and Radiological Health, Food and Drug Administration. Hospital Infections Program, AIDS Program, and Hepatitis Branch, Division of Viral Diseases, Center for Infectious Diseases, National Institute for Occupational Safety and Health, CDC.

Editorial Note: Implementation of universal precautions does not eliminate the need for other category- or disease-specific isolation precautions, such as enteric precautions for infectious diarrhea or isolation for pulmonary tuberculosis (1,2). In addition to universal precautions, detailed precautions have been developed for the following procedures and/or settings in which prolonged or intensive exposures to blood occur: invasive procedures, dentistry, autopsies or morticians' services, dialysis, and the clinical laboratory. These detailed precautions are found in the August 21, 1987, "Recommendations for Prevention of HIV Transmission in Health-Care Settings", (1). In addition, specific precautions have been developed for research laboratories (28).

REFERENCES

1. Centers for Disease Control. Recommendations for prevention of HIV transmission in healthcare settings. *MMWR* 1987;36(suppl 2S).
2. Garner JS, Simmons BP. Guideline for isolation precautions in hospitals. *Infect Control* 1983;4:245–325.
3. Immunization Practices Advisory Committee. Recommendations for protection against viral hepatitis. *MMWR* 1985;34:313–24, 329–35.
4. Department of Labor, Department of Health and Human Services. *Joint advisory notice: protection against occupational exposure to hepatitis B virus (HBV) and human immunodeficiency virus (HIV).* Washington, DC: U.S. Department of Labor, U.S. Department of Health and Human Services, 1987.
5. Centers for Disease Control. Update: acquired immunodeficiency syndrome and human immunodeficiency virus infection among health-care workers. *MMWR* 1988;37:229–34, 239.
6. Hollander H, Levy JA. Neurologic abnormalities and recovery of human immunodeficiency virus from cerebrospinal fluid. *Ann Intern Med* 1987;106:692–5.
7. Wirthrington RH, Cornes P, Harris JRW, et al. Isolation of human immunodeficiency virus from synovial fluid of a patient with reactive arthritis. *Br Med J* 1987;294:484.
8. Mundy DC, Schinazi RF, Gerber AR, Nahmias AJ, Randall HW. Human immunodeficiency virus isolated from amniotic fluid. *Lancet* 1987;2:459–60.
9. Onion DK, Crumpacker CS, Gilliland BC. Arthritis of hepatitis associated with Australia antigen. *Ann Intern Med* 1971;75:29–33.
10. Lee AKY, Ip HMH, Wong VCW. Mechanisms of maternal–fetal transmission of hepatitis B virus. *J Infect Dis* 1978 138:668–71.
11. Bond WW, Petersen NJ, Gravelle CR, Favero MS. Hepatitis B virus in peritoneal dialysis fluid: A potential hazard. *Dialysis and Transplantation* 1982;11:592–600.
12. Oskenhendler E, Harzic M, Le Roux J-M, Rabian C, Clauvel JP. HIV infec-

tion with seroconversion after a superficial needlestick injury to the finger [Letter]. *N Engl J Med* 1986;315:582.

13. Lifson AR. Do alternate modes for transmission of human immunodeficiency virus exist? A review. *JAMA* 1988;259:1353–6.
14. Friedland GH, Saltzman BR, Rogers MF, et al. Lack of transmission of HTLV-III/LAV infection to household contacts of patients with AIDS or AIDS-related complex with oral candidiasis. *N Engl J Med* 1986;314:344–9.
15. Jenison SA, Lemon SM, Baker LN, Newbold JE. Quantitative analysis of hepatitis B virus DNA in saliva and semen of chronically infected homosexual men. *J Infect Dis* 1987;156: 299–306.
16. Cancio-Bello TP, de Medina M, Shorey J, Valledor MD, Schiff ER. An institutional outbreak of hepatitis B related to a human biting carrier. *J Infect Dis* 1982;146:652–6.
17. MacQuarrie MB, Forghani B, Wolochow DA. Hepatitis B transmitted by a human bite. *JAMA* 1974;230 :723–4.
18. Scott RM, Snitbhan R, Bancroft WH, Alter HJ, Tingpalapong M. Experimental transmission of hepatitis B virus by semen and saliva. *J Infect Dis* 1980;142:67–71.
19. Glaser JB, Nadler JP. Hepatitis B virus in a cardiopulmonary resuscitation training course: Risk of transmission from a surface antigen-positive participant. *Arch Intern Med* 1985;145:1653–5.
20. Osterholm MT, Bravo ER, Crosson JT, et al. Lack of transmission of viral hepatitis type B after oral exposure to HBsAg-positive saliva. *Br Med J* 1979;2:1263-4.
21. Curran JW, Jaffe HW, Hardy AM, et al. Epidemiology of HIV infection and AIDS in the United States. *Science* 1988;239:610–6.
22. Jason JM, McDougal JS, Dixon G, et al. HTLV-III/LAV antibody and immune status of household contacts and sexual partners of persons with hemophilia. *JAMA* 1986;255:212–5.
23. Wahn V, Kramer HH, Voit T, Bruster HT, Scrampical B, Scheid A. Horizontal transmission of HIV infection between two siblings [Letter]. *Lancet* 1986;2:694.
24. Salahuddin SZ, Groopman JE, Markham PD, et al. HTLV-III in symptom-free seronegative persons. *Lancet* 1984;2:1418–20.
25. Simmons BP, Wong ES. *Guideline for prevention of nosocomial pneumonia.* Atlanta: U.S. Department of Health and Human Services, Public Health Service, Centers for Disease Control, 1982.
26. Klein RS, Phelan JA, Freeman K., et al. Low occupational risk of human immunodeficiency virus infection among dental professionals. *N Engl J Med* 1988;318:86–90.
27. Garner JS, Favero MS. *Guideline for handwashing and hospital environmental control. 1985.* Atlanta: U.S. Department of Health and Human Ser-

vices, Public Health Service, Centers for Disease Control, 1985: HHS publication no. 99–1117.

28. Centers for Disease Control. 1988 Agent summary statement for human immunodeficiency virus and report on laboratory-acquired infection with human immunodeficiency virus. *MMWR* 7988;37(suppl S4):1S–22S.

Enforcement Procedures for the Occupational Exposure to Bloodborne Pathogens Standard 29 CFR 1910.1030[1]

A. PURPOSE

This instruction establishes policies and provides clarifications to ensure uniform inspection procedures are followed when conducting inspections to enforce the Occupational Exposure to Bloodborne Pathogens Standard.

B. SCOPE

This instruction applies OSHA-wide.

C. CANCELLATION

This instruction cancels OSHA Instruction CPL 2–2.44B, February 27, 1990, (except as noted at M.9. of this instruction).

---

1. OSHA Office of Health Compliance Assistance, March 6, 1992.

D. REFERENCES

1. OSHA Instruction CPL 2.45B, June 15, 1989, The Revised Field Operations Manual (FOM).
2. OSHA Instruction ADM 1–1.12B, December 29, 1989, The Integrated Management Information System (IMIS) Forms Manual.
3. Centers for Disease Control. *Morbidity and Mortality Weekly Report:* "Recommendations for Prevention of HIV Transmission in Health Care Settings." August 1987; Vol. 36, No. S-2. (See Appendix I.)
4. Centers for Disease Control. *Morbidity and Mortality Weekly Report:* 1988 Agent Summary Statement for Human Immunodeficiency Virus and Report on Laboratory-Acquired Infection with Human Immunodeficiency Virus. April 1, 1988; Vol. 37, No. S-4.
5. Centers for Disease Control. *Morbidity and Mortality Weekly Report:* "Guidelines for Prevention of Transmission of HIV and HBV to Health Care and Public Safety Workers." June 23, 1989; Vol. 38, No. S-6. (See Appendix H.)
6. Centers for Disease Control. *Morbidity and Mortality Weekly Report:* "Update: Universal Precautions for the Prevention of Transmission of HIV, HBV and Other Bloodborne Pathogens in Health Care Settings." June 24, 1988; Vol. 37, No. 24. (See Appendix B.)
7. Centers for Disease Control. *Morbidity and Mortality Weekly Report:* "Public Health Service Statement on Management of Occupational Exposure to Human Immunodeficiency Virus, Including Consideration Regarding Zidovudine Postexposure Use." January 1990; Vol. 139, No. RR2. (See Appendix G.)
8. Centers for Disease Control. *Morbidity and Mortality Weekly Report:* "Protection Against Viral Hepatitis, Recommendations of the Immunization Practices Advisory Committee." February 1990; Vol. 39, No. S-2. (See Appendix F.)
9. U.S. Department of Health and Human Services: *Biosafety in Microbiological and Biomedical Laboratories,* publication no. (NIH) 88-8395, May 1988.

E. ACTION

OSHA Regional Administrators and Area Directors shall use the guidelines in this instruction to ensure uniform enforcement of the Bloodborne Pathogens Standard. The Directorate of Compliance Programs will provide support as necessary to assist the Regional Administrators and Area Directors in enforcing the Bloodborne Pathogens Standard.

F. FEDERAL PROGRAM CHANGE

This instruction describes a Federal program change which affects State programs. Each Regional Administrator shall:

1. Ensure that this change is promptly forwarded to each State designee, using a format consistent with the Plan Change Two-Way Memorandum in Appendix P of OSHA Instruction STP 2.22A CH-3.
2. Explain the technical content of this change to the State designee as requested.
3. Ensure that State designees are asked to acknowledge receipt of this Federal program change in writing to the Regional Administrator as soon as the State's intention is known, but not later than 70 calendar days after the date of issuance (10 days for mailing and 60 days for response). This acknowledgment must include the State's intention to follow OSHA's policies and procedures described in this instruction, or a description of the State's alternative policy and/or procedure which is "at least as effective" as the Federal policy.
4. Ensure that the State designees submit a plan supplement, in accordance with OSHA Instruction STP 2.22A, Ch-3, as appropriate, following the established schedule that is agreed upon by the State and Regional Administrator to submit non-Field Operations Manual/Technical Manual Federal Program Changes.
    a. If a State intends to follow the revised inspection procedures described in this instruction, the State must submit either a revised version of this instruction, adapted as appropriate to reference State law, regulations and administrative structure, or a cover sheet describing how references in this instruction correspond to the State's structure. The State's acknowledgment letter may fulfill the plan supplement requirement if the appropriate documentation is provided.
    b. If the State adopts an alternative to Federal enforcement inspection procedures, the State's plan supplement must identify and provide a rationale for all substantial differences from Federal procedures in order for OSHA to judge whether a different State procedure is as effective as the comparable procedure.
5. After Regional review of the State plan supplement and resolution of any comments thereon, forward the State submission to the National Office in accordance with established procedures. The Regional Administrator shall provide a judgment on the relative effectiveness of each substantial difference in the State plan change and an overall assessment thereon with a recommendation for approval or disapproval by the Assistant Secretary.
6. Advise State designees that the State is also responsible for extending coverage under its procedures for addressing occupational exposure to bloodborne pathogens to the public sector, such as police, firefighters, ambulance and other emergency response employees.

7. Review policies, instructions and guidelines issued by the State to determine that this change has been communicated to State program personnel.

G. BACKGROUND

In September 1986, OSHA was petitioned by various unions representing health care employees to develop an emergency temporary standard to protect employees from occupational exposure to bloodborne diseases. The agency decided to pursue the development of a Section 6(b) of the Act standard and published a proposed rule on May 30, 1989.

1. The agency also concluded that the risk of contracting the hepatitis B virus (HBV) and human immunodeficiency virus (HIV) among members of various occupations within the health care sector required an immediate response and therefore issued OSHA Instruction CPL 2–2.44, January 19, 1988. That instruction was canceled by CPL 2–2.44A, August 15, 1988, and subsequently, CPL 2–2.44B was issued February 27, 1990.
2. On December 6, 1991, the agency issued its final regulation on occupational exposure to bloodborne pathogens (29 CFR 1910.1030). Based on a review of the information in the rulemaking record, OSHA has determined that employees face a significant health risk as the result of occupational exposure to blood and other potentially infectious materials (OPIM) because they may contain bloodborne pathogens. These pathogens include HBV which causes hepatitis B, a serious liver disease, and HIV, which causes acquired immunodeficiency syndrome (AIDS). The agency further concludes that this hazard can be minimized or eliminated using a combination of engineering and work practice controls, personal protective clothing and equipment, training, medical surveillance, hepatitis B vaccination, signs and labels, and other provisions.

H. INSPECTION SCHEDULING AND SCOPE

1. Inspection scheduling shall be conducted in accordance with the procedures outlined in the FOM, Chapter II, and for Federal agencies, Chapter XIII, except as modified in paragraphs 2, 3, and 4 below.
2. All inspections, programmed or unprogrammed, shall include, if appropriate, a review of the employer's exposure control plan and employee interviews to assess compliance with the standard.
3. Expansion of an inspection to areas involving the hazard of occupational

exposure to body fluids (including on-site health care units and emergency response or first aid personnel) shall be performed when:

  a. The exposure control plan or employee interviews indicate deficiencies in complying with OSHA requirements, as set forth in 29 CFR 1910.1030 or this instruction.
  b. Relevant formal employee complaints are received which are specifically related to occupational exposure to blood or OPIM.
  c. A fatality/catastrophe inspection is conducted as the result of occupational exposure to blood or OPIM.
4. Regional Offices may develop and implement local emphasis programs as a supplement to complaint-generated inspection activities.

I. GENERAL INSPECTION PROCEDURES

The procedures given in the FOM, Chapter III, shall be followed except as modified in the following sections:

1. Where appropriate, the facility administrator, infection control director or occupational health nurse, "in service" education (i.e., training) director, and head of central services and/or housekeeping shall be included in the opening conference or interviewed early in the inspection.
2. If the facility maintains a file of "incident reports" or a first aid log on injuries (e.g., needlesticks), this shall be reviewed as it may contain injuries not included on the OSHA 200 log.
3. Compliance officers shall take necessary precautions to avoid direct contact with body fluids and shall not participate in activities that will require them to come into contact with body fluids, needles or other sharp instruments contaminated with blood. To evaluate such activities, compliance officers normally shall establish the existence of hazards and adequacy of work practices through employee interviews and shall observe them at a safe distance.
4. On occasions when entry into potentially hazardous areas are judged necessary, the compliance officer shall be properly equipped as required by the facility as well as by his/her own professional judgment, after consultation with the supervisor.
5. Compliance officers shall use appropriate caution when entering patient care areas of the facility. When such visits are judged necessary for determining actual conditions in the facility, the privacy of patients shall be respected. Photographs of patients normally will not be necessary and in no event shall identifiable photographs be taken without their consent.

J. Recording of Exposure Incidents

For OSHA 200 recordkeeping purposes, an occupational bloodborne pathogens exposure incident (e.g., needlestick, laceration, or splash) shall be classified as an injury since it is usually the result of an instantaneous event or exposure. It shall be recorded if it meets one of the following recordability requirements:

1. The incident is a work-related injury that involves loss of consciousness, transfer to another job, or restriction of work or motion.
2. The incident results in the recommendation of medical treatment beyond first aid (e.g., gamma globulin, hepatitis B immune globulin, hepatitis B vaccine, or zidovudine) regardless of dosage.
3. The incident results in a diagnosis of seroconversion. The serological status of the employee shall not be recorded on the OSHA 200. If a case of seroconversion is known, it shall be recorded on the OSHA 200 as an injury (e.g., "needlestick" rather than "seroconversion") in the following manner:
    a. If the date of the event or exposure is known, the original injury shall be recorded with the date of the event or exposure in column B.
    b. If there are multiple events or exposures, the most recent injury shall be recorded with the date that seroconversion is determined in column B.

K. MULTI-EMPLOYER WORKSITE

The following citation guidelines apply in multi-employer worksites (See FOM, Chapter V, F.):

1. Employers shall be cited for violations of the standard to which their own employees are exposed.
2. They shall also be cited for violations to which employees of other employers on their premises are exposed to the extent that they control the hazard. For example, they shall be cited for not providing personal protective equipment to unprotected employees of other employers on their premises.
3. Physicians who are members of professional corporations are generally considered to be employees of that corporation. Therefore, the corporation may be cited for violations affecting those physicians, such as failure to provide the hepatitis B vaccine. Also, the hospitals where they work may be cited for violations to which they are exposed.
4. No citation shall be issued where the only persons exposed are physicians who

are sole practitioners or partners, and thus not employees under the Occupational Safety and Health Act.

L. FEDERAL AGENCY FACILITIES

Agencies of the Federal Government are covered by this instruction.

M. CLARIFICATION OF THE STANDARD ON OCCUPATIONAL EXPOSURE TO BLOODBORNE PATHOGENS 29 CFR 1910.1030

The guidance that follows relates to specific provisions of 29 CFR 1910.1030 and is provided to assist compliance officers in conducting inspections where the standard may be applicable:

> NOTE: Compliance officers shall refer to 29 CFR 1910.1030 regulatory text and preamble for further information.

M.1.
1. **Scope and Application—29 CFR 1910.1030(a).** This section defines the range of employees covered by the standard.

M.1.a.
a. Since there is no population that is risk-free for HIV or HBV infectivity, any employee who has occupational exposure to blood or other potentially infectious material will be included within the scope of this standard.

M.1.b.
b. Although a list is included below of a number of job classifications that may be associated with tasks that have occupational exposure to blood and other potentially infectious materials, the scope of this standard is in no way limited to employees in these jobs. The hazard of exposure to infectious materials affects employees in many types of employment and is not restricted to the health care industry. At the same time, employees in the following jobs are not automatically covered unless they have occupational exposure:

Physicians, physician's assistants, nurses, nurse practitioners, and other health care employees in clinics and physicians' offices;

Employees of clinical and diagnostic laboratories;

Housekeepers in health care facilities;

Personnel in hospital laundries or commercial laundries that service health care or public safety institutions;

Tissue bank personnel;

Employees in blood banks and plasma centers who collect, transport, and test blood;

Freestanding clinic employees (e.g., hemodialysis clinics, urgent care clinics, health maintenance organization [HMO] clinics, and family planning clinics);

Employees in clinics in industrial, educational, and correctional facilities (e.g., those who collect blood, and clean and dress wounds);

Employees assigned to provide emergency first aid;

Dentists, dental hygienists, dental assistants and dental laboratory technicians;

Staff of institutions for the developmentally disabled;

Hospice employees;

Home health care workers;

Staff of nursing homes and long-term care facilities;

Employees of funeral homes and mortuaries;

HIV and HBV research laboratory and production facility workers;

Employees handling regulated waste;

Medical equipment service and repair personnel;

Emergency medical technicians, paramedics, and other emergency medical service providers; and

Firefighters, law enforcement personnel, and correctional officers (employees in the private sector, the Federal Government, or a State or local government in a State that has an OSHA-approved State plan).

INSPECTION GUIDELINES. The scope section of this standard states that it "applies to all occupational exposure to blood or other potentially infectious materials as defined by paragraph (b)." The compliance officer must take careful note of the phrase "as defined by paragraph (b)" when determining coverage. Definitions of particular importance that the compliance officer must clearly understand before beginning an inspection are: Blood, Bloodborne Pathogens, Contaminated, Exposure Incident, Occupational Exposure, Other Potentially Infectious Materials, and Regulated Waste. These will be of use in determining if an employee in either a health care or a non-health care setting is covered by this standard.

NOTES: 1. Part-time, temporary, and health care workers known as "per diem" employees are covered by this standard.

2. If an employee is trained in first aid and designated by the employer as responsible for rendering medical assistance as part of his/her job duties, that employee is covered by the standard.

3. Employees in the construction and maritime industries who have occupational exposure to blood or OPIM are covered by the standard.

M.2.

2. Definitions—29 CFR 1910.1030(b). The following provides further clarifications of some definitions found in this section:

M.2.a.

a. **"Blood":** The term **"human blood components"** includes plasma, platelets, and serosanguineous fluids (e.g., exudates from wounds).

M.2.b.

b. **"Bloodborne Pathogens":** While HBV and HIV are specifically identified in the standard, the term includes any pathogenic microorganism that is present in human blood and can infect and cause disease in persons who are exposed to blood containing the pathogen. Other examples include hepatitis C, malaria, syphilis, babesiosis, brucellosis, leptospirosis, arboviral infections, relapsing fever, Creutzfeld-Jakob disease, Human T-lymphotrophic Virus Type 1, and viral hemorrhagic fever.

M.2.c.

c. **"Exposure Incident":** **"Non-intact skin"** includes skin with dermatitis, hangnails, cuts, abrasion, chafing, etc.

M.2.d.

d. **"Occupational Exposure":** The term **"reasonably anticipated"** includes the potential for exposure as well as actual exposure. Lack of history of blood exposures among first aid personnel of a particular manufacturing site, for instance, does not preclude coverage.

NOTE: This definition does not cover "Good Samaritan" acts which result in exposure to blood or other potentially infectious materials from assisting a fellow employee, although OSHA encourages employers to offer follow-up procedures in such cases.

M.2.e.

e. **"Other Potentially Infectious Materials"** (OPIM): Coverage under this definition also extends to blood and tissues of animals who are deliberately infected with HIV or HBV.

M.2.f.

f. **"Parenteral":** This definition includes human bites that break the skin, which are most likely to occur in violent situations such as may be encountered by prison personnel and police and in emergency rooms or psychiatric wards.

M.2.g.

g. **"Regulated Waste":** This definition is covered in detail at M.4.d.(3) of this instruction.

M.3.

3. **Exposure Control Plan—29 CFR 1910.1030(c).** This section requires the employer to identify those tasks and procedures in which occupational exposure may occur and to identify the positions whose duties include those tasks and procedures identified with occupational exposure. The exposure control plan required by section (c)(1) is a key provision of the standard because it requires the employer to identify the individuals who will receive the training, protective equipment, vaccination, and other benefits of the standard.

INSPECTION AND CITATION GUIDELINES. The compliance officer shall review the facility's written exposure control plan. While the plan may be part of a larger document, such as one addressing all health and safety hazards in the workplace, in order for the plan to be accessible to employees, it must be a cohesive entity by itself or there must be a guiding document which states the overall policy goals and references the elements of existing separate policies that comprise the plan.

The compliance officer shall determine whether the plan is reviewed annually and updated to reflect significant modifications in tasks or procedures which may result in occupational exposure as required in section (c)(1)(iv).

The content of the exposure control plan shall be reviewed for at least the following elements:

M.3.a.

a. **Sections (c)(1)(ii)(A) and (c)(2)(i).** The exposure determination requires employers to identify and document:

M.3.a.(1)

(1) Those job classifications in which all employees have occupational exposure, and

M.3.a.(2)

(2) Those job classifications in which some employees have occupational exposure.

M.3.a.(2)(a)

    (a) In the latter case, the specific tasks and procedures, or groups of closely related tasks and procedures, which are associated with occupational exposure must be delineated. For example, only some of the employees in a hospital laundry room might be assigned the task of handling contaminated laundry.

M.3.a.(2)(b)

    (b) The tasks and procedures that are grouped must be related; i.e., they must share a common activity such as "vascular access procedures," handling of contaminated sharps," or "handling of deceased persons," etc.

M.3.a.(3)

    (3) The exposure determination shall have been made without taking into consideration the use of personal protective clothing or equipment.

M.3.b.

    b. Section (c)(1)(ii)(B). The schedule and method of implementation for sections (d)–(h) in a manner appropriate to the circumstances of the particular workplace must be addressed in the exposure control plan. An annotated copy of the final standard may be adequate for small facilities. An employer may state on a copy of the final standard when and how he/she will implement the provisions of the standard. Larger facilities could develop a broad facility-wide program incorporating provisions from the standard that apply to their establishments.

M.3.c.

    c. Section (c)(1)(ii)(C). The exposure control plan shall include the procedure for evaluating the circumstances surrounding exposure incidents, including an evaluation of the policies and "failures of control" at the time of the exposure incident. Also to be considered are the engineering controls and work practices in place, as well as protective equipment or clothing used, at the time of the exposure incident.

M.3.d.

    d. Sections (c)(1)(iii). The location of the plan may be adapted to the circumstances of a particular workplace provided that the employee can access a copy at the workplace, during the work shift (e.g., if the plan is maintained solely on computer, employees must be trained to operate the computer). In accordance with 29 CFR 1910.20, a hard copy of the exposure control plan shall be made available to the employee within 15 working days of the employee's request.

M.3.e.

 e. **Sections (c)(2)(i)(A) and (B).** As previously discussed in the exposure control plan, the employer is required to list the job classifications covered by the plan. The list is part of the exposure determination. If a job classification, task, or procedure with occupational exposure is omitted from the list, but all employees in the job or performing the task or procedure have been included in all other aspects of the plan (i.e., vaccinations, training, etc.), it is to be considered an other-than-serious violation.

M.4.

 4. **Methods of Compliance—29 CFR 1910.1030(d).** Section (d) sets forth the methods by which employers shall protect their employees from the hazards of bloodborne pathogens and comply with this standard through the use of universal precautions, engineering controls, work practice controls, personal protective equipment, proper housekeeping and handling of regulated waste.

M.4.a.

 a. **Universal Precautions—(d)(1).** Universal precautions is OSHA's accepted method of control to protect employees from exposure to all human blood and OPIM. The term "universal precautions" refers to a concept of bloodborne disease control which requires that all human blood and OPIM be treated as if known to be infectious for HIV, HBV, or other bloodborne pathogens regardless of the perceived "low risk" of a patient or patient population.

M.4.a.(1)

 (1) Another method of infection control is called Body Substance Isolation (BSI). This method defines all body fluids and substances as infectious. BSI incorporates not only the fluids and materials covered by this standard but expands coverage to include all body fluids and substances.

M.4.a.(2)

 (2) BSI is an acceptable alternative to universal precautions provided facilities utilizing BSI adhere to all other provisions of this standard.

 CITATION GUIDELINES. If the employer has a policy of treating the blood or OPIM of some patients as potentially infectious and the blood or OPIM of others (e.g., the elderly or children) as not infectious, a violation of this provision exists.

M.4.b.

 b. **Engineering Controls and Work Practices—(d)(2).**
 This section requires the employer to institute engineering and work

practice controls as the primary means of eliminating or minimizing employee exposure. In those circumstances in which occupational exposure remains after institution of engineering and work practice controls, employers must provide, and ensure that employees use, personal protective equipment as additional protection.

INSPECTION GUIDELINES. The compliance officer shall determine through interviews or observation of work involving the use of needles whether proper engineering controls and work practices, such as immediate disposal of used needles into a sharps container, are used.

Most preferable is the use of devices which offer an alternative to needles being used to perform the procedure. Examples of such devices include stopcocks (on-off switch), needle-protected systems or needleless systems which can be used in place of open needles to connect intravenous lines. Other devices which are integral to the syringe, such as self-sheathing needles, allow both hands to remain behind the needle and require very little manipulation to isolate the needle safely.

When a health care worker must recap, such as during intermittent administration of various drugs during certain procedures, and when it is not feasible to use self-sheathing needle syringes, the employee must use some type of device that protects the hand or allows a safe one-handed recapping method. A proper one-handed scoop method is a work practice which may also be used in these circumstances. (See M.4.b.(3)(b) of this instruction on section (d)(2)(vii) for details.) The compliance officer shall evaluate the work practices used by health care providers to determine that they ensure the effectiveness of engineering controls. For example, some devices provide a fixed barrier between the hands and the needle after use. While some finger/hand shields available on the market offer full protection of the hand holding the needle sheath from accidental puncture, some do not. They may leave much of the hand area uncovered and are not considered acceptable protection for use in a two-handed recapping procedure. Both the shield and the cap must be constructed so that an employee is not exposed to puncture from a needle protruding from the side or end of the cap.

The compliance officer should note that sharps may include more than the traditional needles or scalpels. They also include anything that might produce a puncture wound which would expose employees to blood or OPIM (e.g., the ends of contaminated orthodontia wires or broken glass).

CITATION GUIDELINES. Section (d)(2) shall be cited for failure to use engineering/work practice controls. A citation for the appropriate section of (g)(2)(vii) shall be grouped with it, if the compliance officer determines that inadequate training caused the failure to use such controls.

Citations shall be issued if engineering or work practice controls are not used to eliminate or minimize employee exposure.

While employers do not automatically have to institute the most sophisticated engineering controls (e.g., needleless IV connectors, self-sheathing needles), it is the employer's responsibility to evaluate the effectiveness of existing controls and to review the feasibility of instituting more advanced engineering controls.

M.4.b.(1)

(1) **Section (d)(2)(ii).** This section requires that engineering controls be examined and maintained or replaced on a regular schedule to ensure their effectiveness. Regularly scheduled inspections are required to confirm, for instance, that engineering controls such as protective shields have not been removed or broken, that sharps disposal containers are being replaced in sufficiently frequent intervals and that other physical, mechanical or replacement-dependent controls are functioning as intended.

CITATION GUIDELINES. It is the employer's responsibility to regularly examine and repair and/or replace engineering controls as often as necessary to ensure that each control is maintained and that it provides the protection intended. If the compliance officer finds that there is no system for regular checking of the engineering controls, section (d)(2)(ii) shall be cited.

If there is a check system, but the compliance officer finds, for example, that the biosafety cabinet is not functional, filters are overloaded (in research laboratories or production facilities), disposal containers are overfilled, or a hematron splash shield is broken or missing, section (d)(2)(ii) shall be cited if an effective monitoring system would have uncovered the deficiency.

Additionally, if there is unprotected employee exposure, section (d)(2)(i) shall be cited for failure to use personal protective equipment after institution of engineering controls.

M.4.b.(2)

(2) **Sections (d)(2)(iii) through (d)(2)(vi).** These sections require employers to provide handwashing facilities which are readily

accessible to employees. Handwashing with soap and at least tepid running water must be performed as soon as feasible, particularly in cases of gross contamination, to adequately flush contaminated material from the skin.

M.4.b.(2)(a)

(a) **Section (d)(2)(iv).** This section allows the use of alternative handwashing methods as an interim measure when soap and water are not a feasible means of washing the hands or other parts of the body. Antiseptic hand cleaner, in conjunction with clean cloth or paper towels, or antiseptic towelettes are examples of alternative methods.

M.4.b.(2)(a)1

1 When these types of alternatives are used, employees shall wash their hands (or other affected area) with soap and running water as soon as feasible thereafter.

M.4.b.(2)(a)2

2 The compliance officer may see these types of alternative washing methods used by ambulance-based paramedics and emergency medical technicians (EMTs), firefighters, police, and mobile blood collection personnel who are exposed to blood or OPIM with no means of washing up with running water.

M.4.b.(2)(b)

(b) **Section (d)(2)(v).** This section requires employers to ensure that employees wash their hands immediately or as soon as feasible after removal of gloves or other PPE. There is no requirement for handwashing upon leaving the work area unless contact with blood or OPIM has occurred or gloves/PPE have been removed.

CITATION GUIDELINES. If the compliance officer finds that required handwashing facilities are not being provided, section (d)(2)(iii) shall be cited unless the employer demonstrates that handwashing facilities are not feasible. If unfeasibility is demonstrated, section (d)(2)(iv) shall be cited when the required alternatives are not used. If handwashing is not performed by the employees after exposures or removal of gloves, sections (d)(2)(iv), (v), or (vi) shall be cited. This may be grouped with the pertinent training sections of (g)(2) if employees have not been adequately trained in handwashing procedures.

At a fixed establishment, if employees need to perform handwashing, they must have a location for washing available at a reasonable distance from their normal work area; i.e., no further than what would be considered reasonable for location of restrooms.

If an employee must thread his/her way through doorways and/or stairs to wash with appropriate frequency so that there is a reasonable chance of resultant environmental surface contamination, a violation of section (d)(2)(iii) exists.

M.4.b.(3)

(3) **Section (d)(2)(vii).** Shearing or breaking of contaminated needles is completely prohibited by this section. Bending, recapping, or removing contaminated needles by hand is prohibited as a general practice. However, certain circumstances may exist in which these actions are necessary; e.g., when performing blood gas analyses, inoculating a blood culture bottle, administering incremental doses of a medication such as an anesthetic to the same patient, or removing the needle from a phlebotomy collection apparatus (e.g., vacutainer).

M.4.b.(3)(a)

(a) In these procedures, if the employer can demonstrate that no alternative is feasible or that such action is required by a specific medical procedure, recapping is allowed by some method other than the traditional two-handed procedure; e.g., by means of resheathing instruments or forceps.

M.4.b.(3)(b)

(b) The use of the properly performed one-handed scoop method (in which the hand holding the sharp is used to scoop up the cap from a flat surface) for recapping is a recognized and acceptable method; however, the scoop method must be performed in a safe manner and must be limited to situations in which recapping is necessary.

M.4.b.(3)(c)

(c) An acceptable means of demonstrating that no alternative is feasible would be a written justification included as part of the exposure control plan and stating that the particular medical procedure requires, for example, the bending of the needle and the use of forceps to accomplish this.

M.4.b.(4)

(4) **Section (d)(2)(viii).** Since reusable sharps, such as large-bore needles, scalpels, and saws, pose the same percutaneous exposure hazard as disposable sharps, they must be contained in a manner that eliminates or minimizes the hazard until they are reprocessed. Therefore, the containers for reusable sharps must meet the same requirements as containers for disposable sharps

(See M.4.d.(3)(b) of this instruction on section (d)(4)(iii)(A)(1), with the exception that they are not required to be closeable since it is anticipated that containers used for collecting and holding reusable sharps will, themselves, be reused. (See M.4.d.(2)(e) of this instruction on section (d)(4)(ii)(E) for the manner in which these reusable sharps are to be stored and processed, and M.4.d.(3)(g) on section (d)(4)(iii)(A)(4) on the requirements for cleaning and processing of these reusable containers.)

M.4.b.(5)

(5) **Sections (d)(2)(ix) and (x).** These sections are intended primarily to eliminate or minimize indirect transmission of HBV from contaminated environmental surfaces.

M.4.b.(5)(a)

(a) Hand cream is not considered a "cosmetic" and is permitted. It should be noted that:

M.4.b.(5)(a)1

1 Some petroleum-based hand creams can adversely affect glove integrity, and

M.4.b.(5)(a)2

2 The handwashing requirements of section (d)(2)(v) and (d)(2)(vi) shall be followed.

M.4.b.(5)(b)

(b) The term "work area" means the area where work involving exposure or potential exposure to blood or OPIM exists, along with the potential contamination of surfaces. Employees are permitted to eat and drink in an ambulance cab, for example, as long as the employer has implemented procedures to permit employees to wash up and change contaminated clothing prior to entering the ambulance cab, and to ensure that patients and contaminated material remain behind the separating partition.

INSPECTION GUIDELINES. In addition to direct contamination of food or drink by blood or OPIM, the compliance officer must keep in mind that containers of food and beverage may also become contaminated, resulting in unsuspected contamination of the hands. The key to this section is whether food and drink may be contaminated by such processes as leakage/spilling of specimen containers, contact with contaminated items, or the performance of activities (e.g., laboratory analysis) that could generate splashes, sprays, or droplets of blood.

CITATION GUIDELINES. Deficiencies of sections (d)(2)(iv) through (x) shall be cited in conjunction with the appropriate section of (g)(2) if inadequate training exists.

M.4.b.(6)

(6) **Section (d)(2)(xi).** The intent of this section is not only to decrease the chances of direct employee exposure through spraying or splashing of infectious materials onto employees, but also to reduce contamination of surfaces in the general work area.

M.4.b.(6)(a)

(a) Surgical power tools, lasers, and electrocautery devices may generate aerosols. However, OSHA does not believe that the data currently support the mandatory use of respiratory protection for exposure to aerosols, nor is there an effective engineering control to address aerosol exposure or approved respirator and filter cartridges.

M.4.b.(6)(b)

(b) Particularly hazardous is the use of sprays, brushes, and high pressure in equipment lines.

M.4.b.(6)(c)

(c) Typically, spattering or generation of droplets would necessitate use of eye protection and mask or a face shield. (See M.4.c.(8) of this instruction on section (d)(3)(x).)

CITATION GUIDELINES. A citation shall normally be issued for section (d)(2)(xi) if cleaning procedures unnecessarily cause splashing, spraying, spattering, and generation of droplets of blood or OPIM.

M.4.b.(7)

(7) **Section (d)(2)(xii).** While this section prohibits mouth pipetting/suctioning, the agency allows a recognized emergency care method of clearing an infant's airways called "DeLee suctioning" in the following situation:

M.4.b.(7)(a)

(a) In an emergency,

M.4.b.(7)(b)

(b) When no other method is available; and

M.4.b.(7)(c)

(c) Provided that a trap which prevents suctioned fluid from reaching the employee's mouth is inserted in-line between the infant and the employee.

M.4.b.(8)

(8) **Sections (d)(2)(xiii)—(d)(2)(xiii)(C).** These sections deal with the containerization and labeling of specimens with the intent to eliminate or minimize the possibility of inadvertent employee

contact with blood or OPIM which have leaked out of the container, contaminated exterior surfaces of the container, and/or surrounding surfaces. The labeling requirement warns employees that these substances are present so that proper handling precautions can be taken.

M.4.b.(8)(a)

(a) The labeling exemption listed in section (d)(2)(xiii)(A) applies to facilities which handle all specimens (not just those specimens which contain blood or OPIM) with universal precautions.

M.4.b.(8)(a)1

1 This exemption applies only while these specimens remain within the facility.

M.4.b.(8)(a)2

2 All employees who will have contact with the specimens must be trained to handle all specimens with universal precautions.

M.4.b.(8)(a)3

3 If the specimens leave the facility (e.g., during transport, shipment, or disposal) a label or red color coding would be required.

M.4.b.(8)(b)

(b) Extracted teeth are subject to the containerization and labeling provisions of the standard.

M.4.b.(8)(c)

(c) The use of pneumatic tube systems for transport of small materials in hospitals now includes transmittal of laboratory specimens and other more fragile items. The primary concern in the transportation of clinical specimens in a pneumatic tube system is leakage of the specimen into the carrier and potentially into the system tubing. Some systems have virtually eliminated breakage as a cause of leakage by means of padded inserts for carriers and soft delivery of the carrier. Leakage generally results from improper packaging and/or the use of primary containers that do not prevent leakage during transport.

M.4.b.(8)(c)1

1 All workers who might potentially open a carrier shall be trained to regard the contents as biohazardous in nature. Employees who open biohazard carriers shall wear gloves in accordance with section (d)(3) when removing specimens from the tube system carrier, as it may be contaminated with leakage. They shall be

M.4.b.(8)(c)2

trained in decontamination of the carrier and, if need be, the tube system in accordance with section (g)(2).

2 All precautions and standards for manual transport of specimens also apply to the automated transport of specimens (e.g., containerization and tagging/labeling).

INSPECTION GUIDELINES. The compliance officer must observe or document work practices to determine whether a secondary container is being used when necessary. If a bloody glove contaminates the outside of a primary container while the employee is placing a specimen, the employee would need to use a secondary container. Also, primary containers which may be punctured by their contents, including such items as pointed bone slivers, must be placed in a puncture-resistant secondary contain.

M.4.b.(9)

(9) Section (d)(2)(xiv). When it is not possible to decontaminate equipment prior to servicing or shipping (e.g., highly technical or sensitive equipment and/or limited access to contaminated parts), at least partial decontamination, such as flushing lines and wiping the exterior, shall be accomplished.

INSPECTION AND CITATION GUIDELINES. The compliance officer shall ensure that the employer's program makes provision for the required equipment labels. A label shall be attached to equipment stating which portions of the equipment remain contaminated in order to inform downstream servicing/repair employees of the hazard and precautions they need to take.

M.4.b.(9)(a)

(a) Before citing (d)(2)(xiv), the compliance officer shall document that equipment is being shipped and/or serviced.

M.4.b.(9)(b)

(b) Compliance officers shall observe or document work practices used when employees are decontaminating equipment. (See M.4.b.(6) of this instruction on section (d)(2)(xi) for use of high-pressure equipment.)

M.4.b.(9)(c)

(c) When decontaminating reusable equipment that is heavily soiled, the employee will have to perform some prewashing before proceeding with decontamination because most disinfectants/sterilants cannot sufficiently penetrate the organic material that may remain on such heavily soiled equipment. (See M.4.d.(2)(e) of this instruction for details.)

M.4.c.

c. Personal Protective Equipment—(d)(3). PPE must be used to prevent blood or OPIM from passing through to, or contacting the employees' work or street clothes, undergarments, skin, eyes, mouth, or other mucous membranes, unless engineering controls and work practices have eliminated occupational exposure.

M.4.c.(1)

(1) Section (d)(3)(i). The type and amount of PPE shall be chosen to protect against contact with blood or OPIM based upon the type of exposure and quantity of these substances which can be reasonably anticipated to be encountered during the performance of a task or procedure.

INSPECTION AND CITATION GUIDELINES. The financial responsibility for purchasing and providing PPE rests with the employer. The employer is not obligated under this standard to provide general work clothes to employees, but is responsible for providing PPE. If laboratory coats or uniforms are intended to protect the employee's body from contamination, they are to be provided by the employer.

M.4.c.(1)(a)

(a) Laboratory coats, uniforms, and the like that are used as PPE shall be laundered by the employer and not sent home with the employee for cleaning. (See M.4.c.(4) of this instruction on section (d)(3)(iv).)

M.4.c.(1)(b)

(b) Scrubs are usually worn in a manner similar to street clothing, and normally should be covered by appropriate gowns, aprons, or laboratory coats when splashes to skin or clothing are anticipated.

M.4.c.(1)(b)1

1 If a pullover scrub (as opposed to scrubs with snap closures) becomes minimally contaminated, employees should be trained in accordance with section (g)(2)(vii)(G) to remove the pullover scrub in such a way as to avoid contact with the outer surface; e.g., rolling up the garment as it is pulled toward the head for removal.

M.4.c.(1)(b)2

2 However, if the amount of blood exposure is such that the blood penetrates the scrub and contaminates the inner surface, not only is it impossible to remove the scrub without exposure to blood, but the penetration itself would constitute exposure. It may be prudent to train employees to cut such a contaminated scrub to aid removal and prevent exposure to the face.

M.4.c.(1)(c)

(c) A gown which is frequently ripped or falls apart under normal use would not be considered "appropriate PPE."

M.4.c.(1)(d)

(d) Resuscitator devices are to be readily available and accessible to employees who can reasonably be expected to resuscitate a patient.

M.4.c.(1)(d)1

1 Emergency ventilation devices also fall under the scope of PPE and hence must be provided by the employer for use in resuscitation (e.g., masks, mouthpieces, resuscitation bags, shields/overlay barriers).

M.4.c.(1)(d)2

2 Improper use of these devices shall be cited as a violation of section (d)(3)(ii). In addition, section (g)(2)(vii)(G) which requires employees to be trained in the types, proper use, location, etc., of the PPE shall be cited if inadequate training exists. Improper use includes failure to follow the manufacturer's instructions and/or accepted medical practice.

NOTE: The American Society for Testing Materials is currently (at the publication date of this document) testing and evaluating methods to be used for assessing the quality of PPE that is available for medical use.

M.4.c.(2)

(2) Section (d)(3)(ii). This section requires the use of PPE. It also provides for a limited exemption from the use of PPE, based on situations in which use of PPE would prevent the proper delivery of health care or public safety services, or would pose an increased hazard to the personal safety of the worker. The following represents examples of when such a situation could occur:

M.4.c.(2)(a)

(a) A sudden change in patient status occurs such as when an apparently stable patient unexpectedly begins to hemorrhage profusely, putting the patient's life in immediate jeopardy;

M.4.c.(2)(b)

(b) A firefighter rescues an individual who is not breathing from a burning building and discovers that his/her resuscitation equipment is lost/damaged and he/she must administer CPR;

M.4.c.(2)(c)

    (c) A bleeding suspect unexpectedly attacks a police officer with a knife, threatening the safety of the officer and/or coworkers.

NOTE: An employee's decision not to use PPE is to be made on a case-by-case basis and must have been prompted by legitimate and truly extenuating circumstances. In such cases, no citation shall be issued when the employee temporarily and briefly abandons use of PPE. This does not relieve the employer of the responsibility to ensure that PPE is readily accessible at all times. The employer shall document why PPE was not used in each case and evaluate the circumstances surrounding the incident to reduce the likelihood of a future (unprotected) incident.

CITATION GUIDELINES. Section (d)(3)(ii) shall be cited if PPE is not being used properly. Improper use would include wearing the wrong PPE (e.g., wearing a laboratory coat when a rubber apron is needed) or wearing the wrong size PPE.

In addition, section (g)(2)(vii)(G) shall also be cited if the employees have not been adequately trained.

Unless all elements of the exemption, including the documentation requirements are met, the employer shall not receive the benefit of this exemption and section (d)(3)(ii) shall be cited.

M.4.c.(3)

    (3) Section (d)(3)(iii). This section requires that the employer provide PPE in appropriate sizes and accessible locations. In addition, hypoallergenic gloves, glove liners, powderless gloves, or other similar alternatives shall be readily accessible to those employees who are allergic to the gloves normally provided. The compliance officer shall review the employer's program and, through employee interviews, ensure that these provisions have been met.

CITATION GUIDELINES. If PPE is not provided, the compliance officer shall cite section (d)(3)(i). If PPE is not readily available, the compliance officer shall cite section (d)(3)(iii). For example, the clothing of paramedics out on an emergency call may become blood-soaked. If they are unable to change before the next emergency call because a second set of clothing is located at the ambulance's home base, and the ambulance does not return to base for prolonged periods, a violation of section (d)(3)(iii) would exist.

If it is common practice that PPE is not utilized during certain situations or procedures where exposure to blood or OPIM is anticipated, then a violation of section (d)(3)(ii) would exist. If inaccessibility of PPE exists, section (d)(3)(iii) shall also be cited.

M.4.c.(4)

(4) Section (d)(3)(iv). It is the employer's responsibility not only to provide PPE, but to clean, maintain, and/or dispose of it.

M.4.c.(4)(a)

(a) While many employees have traditionally provided and laundered their own uniforms or laboratory coats or the like, if the item's intended function is to act as PPE, then it is the employer's responsibility to provide, clean, repair, replace, and/or dispose of it.

M.4.c.(4)(b)

(b) Home laundering is not permitted since the employer cannot guarantee that proper handling or laundering procedures are being followed; it could also lead to the migration of contaminants to the home.

M.4.c.(4)(c)

(c) If the employee wishes to choose, wear, and maintain his/her own uniform or laboratory coat, then he/she would need to don additional employer-handled and employer-controlled PPE when performing tasks where it is reasonable to anticipate exposure to blood or OPIM.

CITATION GUIDELINES. If PPE is not cleaned/ laundered/disposed of by the employer, or if the employer cleans the PPE but there is a charge to the employee, then section (d)(3)(iv) shall be cited. If PPE is not repaired and/or replaced by the employer at no cost to the employee then section (d)(3)(v) shall be cited.

If PPE is not removed when penetrated by blood or OPIM, the compliance officer shall cite section (d)(3)(vi).

If the PPE is not changed, and additional PPE was available, section (g)(2)(vii)(G) may also be cited if employees have not been adequately trained.

M.4.c.(5)

(5) Section (d)(3)(vii). To minimize migration of contamination beyond the work area, employees who are provided designated lunchrooms or break rooms are permitted to eat/ drink/smoke in these areas as long as the employees wash up and change any contaminated clothing prior to entry.

INSPECTION AND CITATION GUIDELINES. The "work area" shall be evaluated on a case-by-case basis. While it is not the intent of the standard to require employees to change PPE when traveling, for example, from one hospital laboratory area to another, the compliance officer shall evaluate on a case-by-case basis whether the employee received adequate training in accordance with section (g)(2)(vii)(F) to ensure that no surface contamination occurs during the employee's movement. A violation would exist for the following:

> An employee wearing contaminated gloves exits from a pathology laboratory to use a public telephone located in a public hallway of the hospital. Under such circumstances, it can be reasonably anticipated that another employee, without benefit of gloves or knowledge of the potential surface contamination, could use the phone and unwittingly become contaminated.

M.4.c.(6)

(6) **Section (d)(3)(ix)(A)–(C).** These sections discuss the use of gloves. Gloves of appropriate sizes must be made available in accordance with section (d)(3)(iii). Studies have shown that gloves provide a barrier, but that neither vinyl nor latex procedure gloves are completely impermeable. Thus, hand washing after glove removal is required.

M.4.c.(6)(a)

(a) While disposable gloves shall be replaced as soon as practical when contaminated, obviously some critical procedures (i.e., surgery, delivery) cannot be interrupted to change gloves. The key words to evaluate are "practical" and "feasible."

M.4.c.(6)(b)

(b) Disinfecting agents may cause deterioration of the glove material; washing with surfactants could result in "wicking," or enhanced penetration of liquids into the glove via undetected pores thereby transporting potentially infectious materials into contact with the hand. For this reason, disposable (single-use) gloves may not be washed and reused.

M.4.c.(6)(c)

(c) The compliance officer should note that certain solutions, such as iodine, may cause discoloration of gloves without affecting their integrity and function.

M.4.c.(6)(d)

(d) At a minimum, gloves shall be used where there is reasonable anticipation of employee hand contact with blood, OPIM, mucous membranes, or nonintact skin; when performing vascular access procedures; or when handling or touching contaminated surfaces or items.

M.4.c.(7)

(7) Section (d)(3)(ix)(D). The exemption regarding the use of gloves during phlebotomy procedures applies only to employees of volunteer donor blood collection centers, and does not apply to phlebotomy conducted in other settings such as plasmapheresis centers or hospitals.

INSPECTION GUIDELINES. Where an employer in a volunteer donor blood collection center does not require routine gloving for all phlebotomies, the compliance officer shall document that the employer has fulfilled the requirements of sections (d)(3)(ix)(D)(1) through (d)(3)(ix)(D)(4)(iii), and that employees have received the training necessary to make an informed decision on the wearing of gloves.

CITATION GUIDELINES. Section (d)(3)(ix)(D) shall not be cited. Rather, the other sections of (d)(3) shall be cited if such an employer violates them and if the employer has not demonstrated fulfillment of all the requirements of the exemptions.

M.4.c.(8)

(8) Section (d)(3)(x). This section requires protection for the mucous membranes of the face and upper respiratory tract from droplet spattering. Minimum protection would consist of a mask in conjunction with eyeglasses with solid side shields or a chin-length face shield.

M.4.c.(8)(a)

(a) The employer would not necessarily have to provide prescription eyewear for employees. They could provide and mandate the use of side shields, goggles, and/or protective face shields, and provide proper training in decontamination procedures.

M.4.c.(8)(b)

(b) During microsurgery, when it is not reasonably anticipated that there would be any spattering, it would not constitute a violation for the surgeon, while observing surgery through a microscope, not to wear other eye protection.

M.4.c.(9)

(9) **Section (d)(3)(xi)-(xii).** Use of protective body clothing, such as gowns, aprons, laboratory coats, clinic jackets, surgical caps, or shoe covers, and the degree to which such PPE must resist penetration, are performance-based. The employer must evaluate the task and the type of exposure expected and, based on the determination, select the "appropriate" personal protective clothing in accordance with section (d)(3)(i). For example, laboratory coats or gowns with long sleeves shall be used for procedures in which exposure of the forearm to blood or OPIM is reasonably anticipated to occur.

INSPECTION GUIDELINES. The compliance officer will need to evaluate the task being performed and the degree of anticipated exposure by direct observation, employee interview, or review of written standard operating procedures.

NOTE: There are no currently available standardized methods of testing and classification of performance specifications for resistance of clothing to biological hazards.

M.4.d.

d. **Housekeeping—(d)(4).** The term "worksite" in this section refers not only to permanent fixed facilities such as hospitals, dental/medical offices, clinics, etc., but also covers temporary non-fixed workplaces. Examples of such facilities include but are not limited to ambulances, bloodmobiles, temporary blood collection centers, and any other non-fixed worksites which have a reasonable possibility of becoming contaminated with blood or OPIM.

M.4.d.(1)

(1) **Section (d)(4)(i).** Cleaning schedules and methods will vary according to the factors outlined in this section. While extraordinary attempts to disinfect or sterilize environmental surfaces such as walls or floors are rarely indicated, routine cleaning and removal of soil are required.

M.4.d.(1)(a)

(a) The employer must determine and implement an appropriate written schedule of cleaning and decontamination based upon the location within the facility (e.g., surgical operatory versus patient room), type of surface to be cleaned (e.g., hard-surfaced flooring versus carpeting), type of soil present (e.g., gross contamination versus minor splattering), and tasks and procedures being performed (e.g., laboratory analyses versus normal patient care).

M.4.d.(1)(b)

(b) The particular disinfectant used, as well as the frequency with which it is used, will depend upon the circumstances in which the housekeeping task occurs.

INSPECTION AND CITATION GUIDELINES. Compliance officers should consult the Environmental Protection Agency (EPA) lists of registered sterilants (representing the highest level of antimicrobial activity which destroys all viruses), tuberculocidal disinfectants (effective against tuberculosis bacteria and the specific viruses named on the product label as well as the hepatitis B virus), and antimicrobial with HIV-efficacy claims for verification that the disinfectant used is appropriate. These lists are available from the Regional bloodborne pathogens coordinators.

NOTE: Products registered by the EPA as HIV-effective are not necessarily tuberculocidal and are therefore not necessarily effective against HBV which is more resistant to inactivation than is HIV. To determine the overall effectiveness of a particular product with an HIV-efficacy claim for use in a cleanup where HBV or other bloodborne pathogens are also of concern, the compliance officer must compare the listing of HIV-effective products with the other two listings to check if they overlap for the product of interest.

M.4.d.(2)

(2) Section (d)(4)(ii). Since environmental contamination is an effective method of disease transmission for HBV (the CDC states that HBV can survive for at least one week in dried blood on environmental surfaces or contaminated needles and instruments), section (d)(4)(ii) provides the minimum requirements for the cleaning and decontamination of equipment and environmental and working surfaces that come into contact with blood or OPIM.

M.4.d.(2)(a)

(a) In section (d)(4)(ii)(A), cleaning of contaminated work surfaces after completion of procedures is required to ensure that employees are not unwittingly exposed to blood or OPIM remaining on a surface from previous procedures.

M.4.d.(2)(a)1

1 Where procedures are performed on a continual basis throughout a shift or a day, as may be the case with a clinical laboratory technician performing blood analyses, it is not the agency's intent for the work surface to be decontaminated before the technician can proceed to the next analysis; rather for contaminated work surfaces to be decontaminated after the procedures are completed which in the above example, would include a set of analyses. The completion of procedures might also occur when the employee is going to leave the work area for a period of time.

M.4.d.(2)(a)2

2   Decontamination is not automatically required after each patient care procedure, rather only after procedures resulting in surface contamination.

M.4.d.(2)(a)3

3   There may be some instances in which "immediate" decontamination of overt contamination and spills may not be practical as with, for example, an operating table during surgery.

M.4.d.(2)(a)4

4   The third instance of mandated work surface decontamination is to be performed at the end of the work shift if the work surface may have become contaminated since the last cleaning by, for example, setting down contaminated instruments or specimens. This requirement is based upon the existence of a contaminated work surface rather than a particular worksite location. It does not, for example, encompass desks, countertops, and so forth that remain uncontaminated.

M.4.d.(2)(b)

(b) The use of protective coverings described in section (d)(4)(ii)(B) is an acceptable alternative for protecting items and surfaces against contamination and is particularly useful in situations in which a piece of equipment would be difficult to decontaminate but could be protected by a cover.

M.4.d.(2)(b)1

1   If this option is chosen, the covering must be removed and replaced at the stated minimum intervals; e.g., as soon as feasible following overt contamination or at the end of a work shift if they may have become contaminated during the shift.

M.4.d.(2)(b)2

2   More stringent decontamination rules, such as cleaning equipment or changing coverings between patients, may

be prudent infection control policy but do not fall under OSHA's jurisdictional mandate to safeguard employee (not patient) health.

M.4.d.(2)(c)

(c) Section d(4)(ii)(C) requires both the inspection and decontamination on a regularly scheduled basis of cans, bins, pails, and so forth which are intended for reuse.

M.4.d.(2)(c)1

1 Since these containers may be used in a manner which presents the potential for their becoming contaminated with blood or OPIM, they must be cleaned immediately or as soon as feasible upon visible contamination. For example, a reusable metal trashcan may be lined with a disposable plastic regulated waste bag which leaks and contaminates the can. In addition, regular decontamination will prevent the can from leaking, spilling, or contaminating the outside of successive bags.

M.4.d.(2)(c)2

2 Disinfection of these containers is not necessary to ensure their safety for their intended use; it may be possible to achieve their proper decontamination by means of a soap and water wash.

M.4.d.(2)(d)

(d) Since contaminated broken glass is capable of inflicting percutaneous injury and direct inoculation of bloodborne pathogens into the bloodstream, section (d)(4)(ii)(D) stipulates that broken glassware which may be contaminated shall not be picked up directly with the hands. The tools which are used in cleanup must be properly decontaminated or discarded after use and the broken glass placed in a sharps container and employees must be given specific information and training with respect to this task in accordance with the requirements of section (g)(2). Vacuum cleaners are not appropriate for cleanup of contaminated broken glass.

M.4.d.(2)(e)

(e) Section (d)(4)(ii)(E) prohibits employers from allowing employees to place their hands into containers whose contents include reusable sharps contaminated with blood or OPIM. (See M.4.d.(3)(g) of this instruction on section (d)(4)(iii)(A)(4).

NOTE: The final standard recognizes that proper decontamination of reusable equipment, such as glassware or hand instruments, cannot be achieved in the presence of organic debris (e.g., blood) as it interferes with the efficacy of the disinfecting/sterilizing process and the number of products which can successfully penetrate a heavy bioburden is limited.

M.4.d.(2)(f)

    (f) Violations of sections (d)(4)(ii) and (d)(4)(ii)(A)–(E) may result from a failure to adequately train employees in proper housekeeping procedures. If the compliance officer determines this is the case, violations should be grouped with the appropriate section(s) of (g)(2).

M.4.d.(3)

    (3) Regulated Waste—(d)(4)(iii). This section requires regulated waste to be properly contained and disposed of, so as not to become a means of transmission of disease to workers.

M.4.d.(3)(a)

    (a) To eliminate the implication that OSHA has determined the "infectivity" of certain medical wastes, the bloodborne pathogens standard uses the term "regulated waste" to refer to the following categories of waste which require special handling, at a minimum:

M.4.d.(3)(a)1

    1 Liquid or semi-liquid blood or OPIM.

M.4.d.(3)(a)2

    2 Items contaminated with blood or OPIM and which would release these substances in a liquid or semiliquid state if compressed.

M.4.d.(3)(a)3

    3 Items that are caked with dried blood or OPIM and are capable of releasing these materials during handling.

M.4.d.(3)(a)4

    4 Contaminated sharps.

M.4.d.(3)(a)5

    5 Pathological and microbiological wastes containing blood or OPIM.

INSPECTION AND CITATION GUIDELINES. The compliance officer shall not use the actual volume of blood as the determining factor as to whether or not a particular material is to be considered regulated waste since 10 ml of blood on a disposable bed sheet would appear as a spot (not regulated waste), while the same amount of blood on a cotton ball would likely cause saturation and dripping (regulated waste). Similarly, an item may adequately contain these materials when in a static state yet liberate them when compacted in the waste container.

Rather, the potential for dripping of liquid blood or OPIM, or flaking off of dried blood or OPIM should be considered.

Under no circumstances should a bag of waste be squeezed or shaken to determine this. The compliance officer shall exercise professional judgment to make a determination based on visual factors such as a pool of liquid in the bottom of the container or dried blood flaking or falling off during handling, or based on employee interviews.

NOTES: 1. The compliance officer should keep in mind that while OSHA specifies certain features of the regulated waste containers, including appropriate tagging, the ultimate disposal method (landfilling, incinerating, and so forth) for medical waste falls under the purview of the EPA and possibly State and local regulations.

2. The EPA's Standard for the Tracking and Management of Medical Waste and a number of State regulations consider used needles to be regulated medical waste regardless of the presence of infectious agents. Failing information to the contrary, the compliance officer should consider a used needle to be contaminated.

M.4.d.(3)(b)

(b) Section (d)(4)(iii)(A)(1). The construction of the sharps containers must meet at least four criteria, two of which will be easily discernible. The compliance officer shall examine a container, preferably empty, to check that it is closable and color-coded or labeled.

M.4.d.(3)(b)1

1 Sharps containers are made from a variety of products, from cardboard to plastic. As long as they meet the definition of a sharps container, the compliance officer should consider them to be acceptable no matter what the composition.

M.4.d.(3)(b)2

2 At the time of publication of this instruction, the American Biological Safety Association was in the process of developing a standard for puncture-resistance of sharps disposal containers.

M.4.d.(3)(b)2 a

a If questions arise, the compliance officer shall consult the manufacturer's literature or contact the manufacturer directly to determine if the container is leakproof on the sides and bottom, as well as puncture-resistant.

M.4.d.(3)(b)2 b

b If the container is considered puncture-resistant by the manufacturer, but there is evidence, through observation or employee statements, that sharps have been protruding through a container, section (d)(4)(iii)(A)(1)(ii) shall be cited.

M.4.d.(3)(b)3

3 The sharps container should not create additional hazards. Some sharps containers have unwinders that are used to separate needles from syringes.

M.4.d.(3)(b)3 a

a If this situation is encountered, the compliance officer shall determine if the circumstances warrant needle removal. If they do not, section (d)(2)(vii)(A) which prohibits needle removal unless no alternative is feasible or it is required by a specific medical procedure, shall be cited.

M.4.d.(3)(b)3 b

b If needle removal must be accomplished, the employee shall be trained in the correct procedure as required by (g)(2)(vii)(F).

M.4.d.(3)(b)4

4 The needle sheath is not to be considered a "waste container" because it is viewed as a temporary measure. Self-sheathing needle products must be disposed of in a sharps container.

M.4.d.(3)(b)4 a

a Some self-sheathing devices contain a fast-curing colored liquid adhesive which is released inside the sheath after completion of administration of a substance through the needle. This product is intended to permanently adhere all components of the syringe needle and needle sheath, rendering the syringe and needle assembly inoperable and incapable of causing injury.

M.4.d.(3)(b)4 b

b These devices shall still be disposed of in sharps containers since there is no guarantee of correct usage or proper functioning of the device.

M.4.d.(3)(b)5

5 Duct tape may be used to secure a sharps container lid but is not acceptable if it serves as the lid itself.

M.4.d.(3)(c)

(c) **Section (d)(4)(iii)(A)(2)(1).** The compliance officer shall ensure that the sharps container is as close as feasible to where sharps are used or can be reasonably anticipated to be found.

M.4.d.(3)(c)1

1 If an employee must travel to a remote location to discard a sharp, it will increase the possibility of an accidental needlestick and increase the chances that needles and sharps will be improperly discarded and create potential hazards for other staff members.

M.4.d.(3)(c)1 a

a Areas such as correctional facilities, psychiatric units, or pediatric units may have difficulty placing containers in the immediate use area. If a mobile cart is used by health care workers in these units, an alternative would be to lock a sharps container in the cart.

M.4.d.(3)(c)1 b

b The determination of whether or not the container is as close as feasible shall be made on a case-by-case basis. After interviewing employees, if the compliance officer believes there is a better location for the container, management shall be given the opportunity to explain the present location of the container. The acceptability of the new site shall also be discussed. The compliance officer shall then decide if a violation of this section exists.

M.4.d.(3)(c)2

2 Laundries shall also have sharps containers easily accessible due to the incidence of needles being mixed with laundry. Facilities that handle shipments of waste which may contain contaminated sharps, shall also have sharps containers available in the event a package accidentally opens and releases sharps.

M.4.d.(3)(d)

(d) **Section (d)(4)(iii)(A)(2)(iii).** The compliance officer shall ensure the employer's exposure control plan specifies how and when the sharps containers will be replaced and that the program is followed.

M.4.d.(3)(d)1

1 The employer's plan must include the method by which sharps containers will be determined to need to be

replaced, such as sharps containers which have a transparent window or are at a height which allows employees to see if the container needs to be replaced.

M.4.d.(3)(d)2

2 If the employer has a plan but it is not followed, a citation for inadequate training on work practices, (g)(2)(vii)(F), shall be grouped with this section if a training violation exists.

M.4.d.(3)(e)

(e) Section (d)(4)(iii)(A)(3)(i) and (ii). If work practice violations of these sections exist (e.g., not closing the container prior to movement or not placing the container in a secondary container if leakage is possible), they shall be grouped with (g)(2)(vii)(F) if employees have not received adequate training.

M.4.d.(3)(f)

(f) Section (d)(4)(iii)(A)(3)(ii)(B). It is reasonable to presume that some sharps containers will contain residual liquids. If the container cannot be sealed to prevent leakage, it must be placed in a secondary container.

M.4.d.(3)(g)

(g) Section (d)(4)(iii)(A)(4). A sharps container system will be acceptable if it does not expose employees to the risk of percutaneous injury. No system involving the manual opening, emptying, or cleaning of the containers will be allowed. The only acceptable system is a fully automated container cleaning system that eliminates employee exposure to sharps.

M.4.d.(3)(h)

(h) Section (d)(4)(iii)(B). While this section requires that regulated waste containers be closable, simply being closed does not ensure that wastes will be contained. Waste-containing bags may break and spill their contents, including liquid blood, while, for example, being loaded onto incinerator hoppers, thus contaminating both the employees and the work area.

M.4.d.(3)(h)1

1 Also, small medical offices which generate only a small volume of regulated waste may place that waste in a large holding container until the container is filled. In such a case, the design of the container must be such that it is able to retain the waste over an extended period of time between pickups by a specialized waste service.

M.4.d.(3)(h)2

    2 The compliance officer should, therefore, check for visual signs of leakage of fluids during handling, storage, transport, or shipping.

M.4.d.(3)(h)3

    3 Any failures to comply with the container construction requirements would be cited under this section. If the compliance officer determines that the employee was not properly trained to recognize the problem or use the containers correctly, a citation for the appropriate section of (g)(2) should be grouped with violations of paragraph (d).

M.4.d.(3)(i)

  (i) **Sections (d)(4)(iii)(B)(1)(iii) and (2)(iii).** Regulated waste containers are required to be labeled with the biohazard symbol or color-coded to warn employees who may have contact with the containers of the potential hazard posed by their contents.

M.4.d.(3)(i)1

    1 Even if a facility considers all of its waste to be regulated waste, the waste containers must still bear the required label or color-coding in order to protect new employees, who would not normally come into contact with wastes, and employees from outside the facility. This requirement is in contrast to the labeling alternative allowed when laundries use universal precautions for the handling of all soiled laundry. (See M.4.d.(4)(a) of this instruction on section (d)(4)(iv)(A)(2).)

M.4.d.(3)(i)2

    2 Regulated waste that has been decontaminated need not be labeled or color-coded. The compliance officer in such a case shall verify that the employer's exposure control plan states the decontamination procedures to be followed.

M.4.d.(3)(i)2 a

    a In order to ensure that the decontamination process is successful, the employer must monitor factors such as the content, volume, density, configuration, and organic content of the load of waste. (See M.7.a.(2) of this instruction on section (g)(1)(i)(I).)

M.4.d.(3)(i)2 b

    b The temperature needed for the complete breakdown of plastics, as required by EPA, is sufficient to decontaminate regulated waste.

M.4.d.(3)(i)2 c

    <u>c</u> Autoclave efficiency can be verified by means of biological or chemical indicators. While most disposal bags used will contain an indicative color strip, if this is not the case a review may be made of the documentation kept for the sterilizer. Such documentation should include (1) date, time, and operator of each run, (2) type and approximate amount of waste tracked, (3) post-treatment reading of temperature-sensitive tape, (4) dates and results of calibration of the sterilizer, and (5) results of routine spore testing.

M.4.d.(3)(i)2 d

    <u>d</u> For a more detailed discussion of chemical decontamination, see guidelines at M.4.d.(1) of this instruction.

M.4.d.(3)(i)3

    <u>3</u> Although these sections contain label requirements, failure to label can also be cited under section (g)(1)(i).

M.4.d.(3)(j)

  (j) **Section (d)(4)(iii)(B)(2).** A second container is required to be used when outside contamination of the first waste container occurs. This provision does not require routine double-bagging but rather requires double-bagging in such circumstances as a waste container being splashed with blood during surgery or autopsy, when a container has been handled by an employee with bloody gloves, or when a waste bag leaks blood or OPIM onto an adjacent bag.

M.4.d.(4)

  (4) **Laundry—(d)(4)(iv).** This section reduces employee exposure to bloodborne pathogens by reducing the amount of manual handling of contaminated laundry. Restricting the sorting to the laundry area will also reduce contamination of additional surfaces.

INSPECTION AND CITATION GUIDELINES. Sections (d)(4)(iv)(A) and (A)(1) limit the handling of laundry to removal and bagging or containerization. The compliance officer shall check the laundry collection program as well as the training of the employees assigned to these tasks.

M.4.d.(4)(a)

(a) **Section (d)(4)(iv)(A)(2̲).** The employer has been given the choice, by this section, to either:

M.4.d.(4)(a)1̲

1̲ Label or color-code according to section (g)(1)(i), or

M.4.d.(4)(a)2̲

2̲ Utilize universal precautions in the handling of all soiled (i.e., used) laundry.

M.4.d.(4)(a)2̲ a

a̲ If universal precautions are used for handling all soiled laundry, the employer may use an alternative color or label for the bags/containers, as long as all employees are trained to recognize them as containing soiled laundry which requires the use of universal precautions.

M.4.d.(4)(a)2̲ b

b̲ Training violations would be cited under the appropriate section of (g)(2)(vii).

M.4.d.(4)(a)3̲

3̲ Refer to M.4.d.(4)(d) on section (d)(4)(iv)(C) for labeling when laundry is shipped off-site.

M.4.d.(4)(b)

(b) **Section (d)(4)(iv)(A)(3̲).** The material for the bags or containers used in laundry collection must prevent soak-through or leakage of fluids to the exterior, if the contaminated laundry is wet and presents a reasonable likelihood of soak-through or leakage. Not all contaminated laundry must be placed in such bags or containers, only laundry wet enough to leak or soak through and expose workers handling the bags/containers to blood or OPIM.

M.4.d.(4)(c)

(c) **Section (d)(4)(iv)(B).** Employees having direct contact with contaminated laundry must wear protective gloves and any other appropriate personal protective equipment, in order to prevent or reduce contact exposure to blood or OPIM. Any other personal protective equipment required must be determined on a case-by-case basis. Gowns, aprons, eyewear, and masks may be necessary to prevent employee exposure.

M.4.d.(4)(d)

(d) **Section (d)(4)(iv)(C).** The generator of the laundry must have determined if the facility to which it is shipped utilizes universal precautions. If not, all bags or containers of contaminated laundry must be labeled or color-coded in accordance with section (g)(1)(i). In this instance, if the generator of the laundry chooses to color-code rather than label, the color of the bag must be red.

INSPECTION AND CITATION GUIDELINES. The compliance officer shall check the employer's program to determine if laundry is shipped to another facility for cleaning and shall evaluate the methods used to ship contaminated laundry (CL) to a facility that does not utilize universal precautions in the handling of all soiled laundry. The following are unacceptable shipment methods and constitute violations of this section:

M.4.d.(4)(d)1

1 The CL is not shipped labeled or in a red bag. Section (d)(4)(iv)(C) would be cited and grouped with the applicable subsection of (g)(l)(i).

M.4.d.(4)(d)2

2 The CL is shipped with an improper label. Section (d)(4)(iv)(C) would be cited and grouped with the applicable subsections of (g)(1)(i)(B),(C), and/or (D).

M.4.d.(4)(d)3

3 The CL is shipped in a bag color-coded for in-house use (in a color other than red). Section (d)(4)(iv)(C) would be cited and grouped with section (g)(1)(i)(E).

M.5.

5. HIV and HBV Research Laboratories and Production Facilities—29 CFR 1910.1030(e). This section includes additional requirements that must be met by research laboratories and production facilities engaged in the culture, production, concentration, and manipulation of HIV and HBV.

"Research laboratory" means a laboratory which produces or uses research laboratory scale amounts of HIV or HBV. Although research laboratories may not have the volume found in production facilities, they deal with solutions containing higher viral titers than those normally found in patients' blood. Academic research laboratories are included in this definition. Laboratories that conduct research unrelated to HIV or HBV on blood and other body fluids, or who use unconcentrated blood or blood components as the source of HIV or HBV, are not considered research laboratories for the purpose of this section.

"Production facilities" are those engaged in industrial-scale, large-volume, or high-concentration production of HIV or HBV.

NOTES: 1. Employers in such a facilities remain responsible for complying with the entire standard. Requirements stated elsewhere in the standard are not repeated.

2. These requirements are based largely on information from published guidelines of the Centers for Disease Control (CDC) and the National Institutes of Health (NIH) (See D.9. of this instruction, "Biosafety in Microbiological and Biomedical Laboratories.")

INSPECTION AND CITATION GUIDELINES. The compliance officer shall review the covered facility's plan, interview a sufficient number of employees, and observe work practices as necessary to determine if the requirements of this section are met. Care shall be taken to ensure the compliance officer understands the special practices and precautions in place at the facility, so that the compliance officer is not placed at risk. Specific requirements include:

M.5.a.

    a. **Section (e)(2)(i).** The term "regulated waste" refers to the OSHA definition as found in section (b) of this standard. The purpose of decontaminating regulated waste is to prevent the accidental exposure of other employees to the concentrated virus.

M.5.b.

    b. **Sections (e)(2)(ii) (A) through (M).** Sections (A), (C), and (D) limit access to the laboratory and warn of the hazards associated with bloodborne pathogens. The compliance officer must review the written policies and procedures to determine if they are adequate to ensure that unauthorized individuals are not placed at risk nor that they can distract or otherwise interfere with the work of the authorized employees. Interviews with employees should be used to determine if the policies are followed.

M.5.b.(1)

    (1) **Section (e)(2)(ii)(E).** The "other physical containment device" must be sufficient to ensure that virus-containing material will be kept away from the worker's mucous membranes, unprotected skin, and breathing zone.

M.5.b.(2)

    (2) **Sections (e)(2)(ii)(H) and (I).** These sections prevent the spread of contamination to other work areas. Section (I) allows for an alternative to a HEPA filter as long as it is of equivalent or superior efficiency. HEPA filters may be ineffective in humid atmospheres.

M.5.b.(2)(a)

    (a) The employer must also have made provisions for routine maintenance and/or replacement of all filters and traps.

M.5.b.(2)(b)

    (b) If the compliance officer suspects that the engineering controls are failing to prevent the spread of the virus, the manufacturer should be contacted to establish the limits and required maintenance of the filters and traps.

M.5.b.(3)

    (3) Section (e)(2)(ii)(J). The compliance officer shall determine if the use of needles and syringes is kept to a minimum and that they are properly handled as required, paying particular attention to establishing if the puncture-resistant containers are properly autoclaved or decontaminated before being discarded, reused, or incinerated.

M.5.b.(4)

    (4) Section (e)(2)(ii)(M). This section ensures that any necessary additional procedures are developed to protect employees in situations unique to a research/production facility. The biosafety manual required by this section shall be reviewed and updated annually or more often if necessary. The facility will thus be required to review its procedures and determine if they are adequate to protect workers.

M.5.c.

    c. Section (e)(2)(iii). Specific containment equipment is required by this section to minimize or eliminate exposure to the viruses.

M.5.c.(1)

    (1) If the compliance officer determines that biological safety cabinets (BSC) have been chosen as the means of containment, they must be certified (Class I, Class II, or Class III) when installed or moved, and at least annually.

M.5.c.(1)(a)

    (a) The compliance officer shall check that a dated tag is affixed to the BSC indicating who performed the certification. Alternatively, a certification report attesting to a minimum inward face velocity of at least 75 linear feet per minute and the integrity of the HEPA filters shall be reviewed by the compliance officer. The report must be dated and signed by the trained technician performing the measurements and integrity tests.

M.5.c.(1)(b)

    (b) See Appendix C1 for details on biological safety cabinets.

M.5.c.(2)

     (2) In the alternative, appropriate combinations of PPE or physical containment devices (examples listed in the standard) will be accepted.

M.5.d.

    d. Sections (e)(3)(i) and (e)(4)(iii). The handwashing facility must be supplied with at least tepid water, soap, and hand towels. The eyewash must supply a sufficient quantity of water to completely flush the eyes. A 15-minute supply of continuous free-flowing water is acceptable. The hands must be free to hold the eyelids open to aid in the complete flushing of the eyes. Portable facilities are acceptable only if they meet these requirements.

M.5.e.

    e. Section (e)(4) covers additional requirements for production facilities only. The requirement in section (e)(4)(v) minimizes the potential for accidental exposure to other employees from the transport of culture fluids, plasticware, and other contaminated equipment.

M.5.f.

    f. Training Requirements—(e)(5). The additional training requirements are specified in section (g)(2)(ix). Any violations found would be cited under that section of the standard. (See M.7.b.(5) of this instruction for details.)

M.6.

    6. Hepatitis B Vaccination and Post-Exposure Evaluation and Follow-up—29 CFR 1910.1030 (f). This section provides a means to protect employees from infection caused by the hepatitis B virus by requiring employers to make the hepatitis B vaccination available to employees with occupational exposure to blood or OPIM. It also ensures that employees receive appropriate medical follow-up after each specific exposure incident. Appendix D provides general algorithms for these requirements.

M.6.a

    a. General—(f)(1). This section refers to the hepatitis B vaccination as both the hepatitis B vaccine and vaccination series. These are to be made available to all occupationally exposed employees. In addition, a post-exposure evaluation and follow-up procedures are to be made available to all employees who experience an exposure incident. While it is OSHA's intent to have the employer remove, as much as possible, obstacles to the employee's acceptance of the vaccine, the term "made available" emphasizes that it is the employee's option to participate in the vaccination and follow-up programs.

INSPECTION GUIDELINES. The compliance officer shall examine the employer's program to determine if the vaccination series and post-exposure follow-up procedures meet the requirements of section (f)(1)(ii).

M.6.a.(1)

(1) Section (f)(1)(ii)(A). The term "no cost to the employee" means no "out of pocket" expense to the employee.

M.6.a.(1)(a)

(a) The employer may not require the employee to use his/her health care insurance to pay for the series unless the employer pays all of the cost of the health insurance and unless there is no cost to the employee in the form of deductibles, copayments, or other expenses. Even partial employee contribution to the insurance premium means the employee could be affected by a rise in the total premium caused by insurance company reaction to widespread hepatitis B vaccinations and is therefore unacceptable.

M.6.a.(1)(b)

(b) The employer may not institute a program in which the employee pays the original cost of the vaccine and is reimbursed by the employer if she/he remains employed for a specified period of time.

M.6.a.(1)(c)

(c) An "amortization contract" which requires employees to reimburse the employer for the cost of the vaccination should they leave his/her employ prior to a specified period of time is similarly prohibited.

M.6.a.(2)

(2) Section (f)(1)(ii)(B). The term "reasonable time and place" requires the medical procedures and evaluations to be convenient to the employee. They shall be offered during normally scheduled work hours. If participation requires travel away from the worksite, the employer must bear the cost.

M.6.a.(3)

(3) Section (f)(1)(ii)(C). The compliance officer may have to contact the Regional bloodborne pathogens coordinator to determine if the State board of nursing licensing allows licensed health care professionals other than physicians to carry out the procedures and evaluations required by section (f).

M.6.a.(4)

(4) Section (f)(1)(ii)(D). This section takes into consideration the changing nature of medical treatment relating to bloodborne pathogens. The CDC is the U.S. Public Health Service (USPHS) agency responsible for issuing guidelines and making recommendations regarding infectious agents. OSHA will accept the CDC guidelines current at the time of the evaluation or procedure. Copies of the current guidelines can be obtained by contacting the Regional bloodborne pathogens coordinator or CDC.

NOTE: This section requires that the current USPHS/CDC guidelines be followed for all vaccinations, evaluations, and follow-up procedures. Any additional requirements (such as obtaining a written health care professional's opinion) specified in section (f) must also be met.

M.6.a.(5)

(5) **Section (f)(1)(iii)** requires that all laboratory tests be conducted by an accredited laboratory. The compliance officer must determine by means of employer documentation (e.g., certificate) that the laboratory is accredited by a national accrediting body (such as CDC or College of American Pathologists) or equivalent State agency which participates in a recognized quality assurance program.

M.6.b.

b. **Hepatitis B Vaccination—(f)(2).** The compliance officer shall determine whether or not all occupationally exposed employees have the hepatitis B vaccination series made available to them after training required by section (g)(2)(vii)(I) and within 10 working days of their initial assignment. The term "made available" includes the health care professional's evaluation and arranging for the administration of the first dose of the hepatitis B vaccination series to begin within the 10 days. This includes all employees with reasonably anticipated occupational exposure, regardless of how often the exposure may occur. Part-time and temporary employees are included in this coverage. The vaccine does not have to be made available if the employer documents (1) the exemption(s) set forth in section (f)(2), or (2) the signature of the employee on the mandatory declination form.

M.6.b.(1)

(1) **Section (f)(2)(i)** states the circumstances under which an employer is exempted from making the vaccination available. If, (a) the complete hepatitis B vaccination series was previously received, or (b) antibody testing shows the employee to be immune, or (c) the vaccine cannot be given for medical reasons, the series does not have to be made available. If the employer claims one of these exemptions, it must be documented in the employee's medical record.

M.6.b.(1)(a)

    (a) The hepatitis B vaccination must be given in the standard dose and through the standard route of administration as recommended in the USPHS/CDC guidelines. At the time of publication of this standard, intradermal inoculation of 0.1 of the normal dose of the hepatitis B vaccine is not recommended by the USPHS and therefore is not an acceptable administration method.

M.6.b.(1)(b)

    (b) Current USPHS guidelines do not recommend routine post-vaccination testing. Therefore, employers are not currently required to routinely test immune status after vaccination has been completed.

M.6.b.(2)

    (2) **Section (f)(2)(ii).** Prevaccination screening for antibody status cannot be required of an employee, although if an employer wishes, he/she can make it available at no cost to employees. An employee may decline the prescreening, and the employer must still make the vaccination series available to the employee.

M.6.b.(3)

    (3) **Section (f)(2)(iii).** The signing of the hepatitis B vaccine declination form by the employee, at the time the vaccination is made available, does not relieve the employer from the requirement to provide the vaccine at a later date if the employee so chooses.

M.6.b.(4)

    (4) **Section (f)(2)(iv).** Although the declination form set forth in 29 CFR 1910.1030, Appendix A, does not have to be reproduced, the declination statement used by the employer must contain the same language as that found in Appendix A—no words may be added or subtracted.

M.6.b.(5)

    (5) **Section (f)(2)(v).** At the time of this publication, the possible need for booster doses of the hepatitis B vaccine is still being assessed. There is no current requirement to provide boosters unless the USPHS recommends it at a later date.

M.6.c.

    c. **Post-Exposure Evaluation and Follow-up—(f)(3).** This section requires the employer to make immediately available a confidential medical evaluation and follow-up to an employee reporting an exposure incident.

NOTE: Employees who do not fall within the scope of this standard may still experience a specific exposure incident at work that is unrelated to the performance of their job duties. In such a case, OSHA strongly encourages their employer to offer them the follow-up procedures set forth in this section.

INSPECTION GUIDELINES. The compliance officer must determine if the employer's plan provides for immediate and confidential procedures. At sites where an exposure incident has occurred, it should be determined if the procedures were properly followed through interviews, incident report reviews, and, if necessary, medical records reviews.

> The word "immediately" is used in the standard to emphasize the importance of prompt medical evaluation and prophylaxis. An exact time was not given in the standard since medical knowledge concerning the effectiveness of post-exposure prophylactic measures is constantly changing. OSHA requires the evaluation and follow-up procedures to be given as soon as possible after exposure.

> If the compliance officer believes that an employer is not properly following accepted post-exposure procedures, or needs specific information about current accepted procedures, the Regional bloodborne pathogens coordinator should be contacted. A health care professional in the National Office will then be consulted.

> The employer must also have established a system that maintains the required medical records in a way that protects the confidentiality of the employee's identity and test results. If the employer has contracted with a clinic or other health care facility to provide the follow-up programs, the confidentiality requirements must be part of the contract.

M.6.c.(1)

    (1) Section (f)(3)(i). Documentation of the circumstances surrounding an exposure incident will help the employer and the compliance officer determine, for example, if PPE is being used or if training is lacking.

M.6.c.(2)

    (2) Section (f)(3)(ii). This section requires the employer to identify the source individual in an exposure incident, unless this is infeasible. The employer must document in writing the identity of, or unfeasibility of identifying, the source individual. Examples of when it may not be feasible to identify the source individual include incidents of needlesticks by unmarked syringes left in laundry or those involving blood samples which are not properly labeled, as well as prohibition by State or local law.

M.6.c.(2)(a)

(a) **Section (f)(3)(ii)(A).** This section requires testing of the source individual's blood after consent is obtained. The employer must ask for consent from the source individual or anyone legally authorized to give consent on his/her behalf. If consent is not obtained, the employer must document this in writing. The compliance officer shall ensure that the employer's plan includes this provision.

M.6.c.(2)(a)1

1 For those jurisdictions that do not require consent of the individual, available blood must be tested. The term "if available" applies to blood samples that have already been drawn from the source individual.

M.6.c.(2)(a)2

2 OSHA does not require redrawing of blood specifically for HBV and HIV testing without consent of the source individual.

M.6.c.(2)(b)

(b) **Section (f)(3)(ii)(C).** This section does not authorize the employer to be informed of the results of source individual or exposed employee testing. However, the results of the source individual's testing must be made available to the exposed employee.

M.6.c.(2)(b)1

1 The boundary between employer and health care professional may be blurred in a medical setting in which, for example, the physician is both the employer and the evaluating health care professional. In such cases, the compliance officer shall ensure that requirements for consent and confidentiality have been followed.

M.6.c.(2)(b)2

2 "Applicable laws and regulations concerning disclosure" refers to State and Federal laws that specifically cover medical privacy and confidentiality.

M.6.c.(2)(c)

(c) **Section (f)(3)(iii).** The compliance officer must determine if the employer's program offers covered employees all of the listed requirements, in the event of an exposure incident. Counseling and evaluation of reported illnesses is not dependent on the employee's electing to have baseline HBV and HIV serological testing.

M.6.c.(2)(c)1

1 **Section (f)(3)(iii)(A).** Although the consent of the em-

ployee must also be obtained before collection of blood and before hepatitis B serological testing, the 90-day holding requirement in section (f)(3)(iii)(B) does not apply.

M.6.c.(2)(c)2

2 **Section (f)(3)(iii)(B).** This section allows employees the opportunity for future testing without the need for an immediate decision.

M.6.c.(2)(c)2 a

a Employees involved in an exposure incident have at least 90 days following baseline blood collection to decide if they wish to have their blood tested for HIV.

M.6.c.(2)(c)2 b

b Employers are required to preserve the blood the employee consented to have drawn, if it was not tested for HIV initially, for at least the 90-day period. Compliance officers shall check that if the employer contracts for post-exposure follow-up, the contractor has been informed of the 90-day requirement.

M.6.c.(2)(d)

(d) **Section (f)(3)(iv).** *(See Appendices G and F for CDC's current guidelines on management of occupational exposure to HIV and HBV.)*

M.6.d.

d. **Information Provided to the Health Care Professional—(f)(4).** This section requires the employer to provide information to the health care professional responsible for the employee's hepatitis B vaccination and post-exposure incident follow-up.

INSPECTION GUIDELINES. The compliance officer must determine if the employer's plan includes providing a copy of this standard to the health care professional responsible for the employee's hepatitis B vaccination.

M.6.d.(1)

(1) In the case of an exposure incident, the plan must provide for the transmission of the information required by (f)(4)(ii)(A–C) and (E) to the health care professional. The information required by (f)(4)(ii)(D) must be provided only if available.

M.6.d.(2)

(2) The employer does not have a specific right to know the actual results of the source individual's blood testing, but must ensure that the information is provided to the evaluating health care professional.

M.6.d.(3)

(3) If the evaluating health care professional is also the employer, the information must still be in the employee's record and made available at the time of a post-exposure incident. All applicable laws and standards of confidentiality apply in this situation.

M.6.e.

e. **Health Care Professional's Written Opinion (f)(5).** The employer is required to obtain and provide a written opinion to the employee within 15 working days of completion of the original evaluation. Employer access is allowed to the health care professional's written opinion.

M.6.e.(1)

(1) **Section (f)(5)(i)** limits the health care professional's written opinion to very specific information regarding the employee's hepatitis B vaccine status, including indication for vaccine and whether such vaccination was completed.

M.6.e.(2)

(2) **Section (f)(5)(ii)** requires documentation that a post-exposure evaluation was performed and that the exposed employee was informed of the results as well as any medical conditions resulting from exposure which require further evaluation and treatment.

M.7.

7. **Employee Information and Training—1910.1030(g).** Section (g) ensures that employees receive sufficient warning through labels, signs, and training to eliminate or minimize their exposure to bloodborne pathogens.

M.7.a.

a. **Labels—(g)(1).** Labels must be provided on containers of regulated waste, on refrigerators and freezers that are used to store blood or OPIM, and on containers used to store, dispose of, transport, or ship blood or OPIM. This requirement alerts employees to possible exposure since the nature of the material or contents will not always be readily identifiable as blood or OPIM. *(See Table C1.)*

NOTE: This does not preempt either the U.S. Postal Service labeling requirements (39 CFR Part III) or the Department of Transportation's Hazardous Materials Regulations (49 CFR Parts 171–180).

INSPECTION AND CITATION GUIDELINES. The compliance officer shall determine that the warning labels in the facility are used as required by sections (g)(1)(i)(A) through ID) and include the term "BIOHAZARD."

Table C1. Labeling requirements

Item	No label required		Biohazard label		Red coler-coded container
Regulated waste container			X	or	X
Reusable contaminated sharps			X	or	X
Refrigerator/freezer holding blood or other potentially infectious materials (OPIM)			X		
Containers used for storage, transport, or shipping of blood or OPIM			X	or	X
Blood/blood products released for clinical use	X[a]	or	X	or	X
Specimens shipped from the primary facility to another facility			X	or	X
Individual containers of blood or OPIM placed in labeled container during storage, transport, shipment, or disposal	X				
Contaminated equipment needing servicing or shipping			X[b]		
Contaminated laundry	X[c]	or	X	or	X
Laundry sent to another facility that does not use Universal Precautions			X	or	X

[a]Labels are not required if Universal Precautions are used in handling all specimens and containers are recognizable as containing specimens.

[b]Specifying, in addition, the location of the contamination.

[c]Alternative label or color code must be used when facility uses Universal Precautions in handling all soiled laundry and employees can recognize containers as required compliance with Universal Precautions.

OSHA does not require nor prohibit the use of warning signs or labels indicating source individuals' or specimens' known infectivity status although, in accordance with universal precautions, the agency strongly recommends against such warning signs.

M.7.a.(1)

(1) **Sections (g)(1)(i)(E) through (G).** These sections list exemp-

tions from the labeling requirements which are additional to those exemptions listed for specimens in section (d)(2)(xiii)(A) and for laundry in section (d)(4)(iv)(A)(2). (See M.4.b.(8)(a) and M.4.d.(4)(a) of this instruction.)

M.7.a.(1)(a)

   (a) Blood and blood products bearing an identifying label as specified by the Food and Drug Administration, which have been screened for HBV and HIV antibodies and released for transfusion or other clinical uses, are exempted from the labeling requirements.

M.7.a.(1)(b)

   (b) When blood is being drawn or laboratory procedures are being performed on blood samples, then the individual containers housing the blood or OPIM do not have to be labeled provided the larger container into which they are placed for storage, transport, shipment, or disposal (e.g., test tube rack) is labeled.

M.7.a.(2)

  (2) **Section (g)(1)(i)(I).** Regulated waste that has been decontaminated by incineration, autoclaving, or chemical means, prior to disposal is not required to bear the BIOHAZARD warning label.

M.7.a.(2)(a)

   (a) Decontamination is discussed at M.4.d.(3)(i)(2) of this instruction.

M.7.a.(2)(b)

   (b) Failure to ensure adequate decontamination procedures prior to removal of the hazard label shall be cited under (g)(1)(i)(A), since the material would still be regulated waste.

M.7.b.

  b. **Information and Training—(g)(2).** All employees with occupational exposure must receive initial and annual training on the hazards associated with blood and OPIM, and the protective measures to be taken to minimize the risk of occupational exposure. Retraining shall take place when changes in procedures or tasks occur which affect occupational exposure. While the provisions for employee training are performance oriented, with flexibility allowed to tailor the program to, for example, the employee's background and responsibilities, the categories of information listed in section (g)(2)(vii) must be covered at a minimum. These requirements include some site-specific information.

INSPECTION GUIDELINES. The compliance officer shall verify that the training is provided at the time of initial employment or on or before June 4, 1992, and at least annually thereafter as well as whenever a change in an employee's responsibilities, procedures, or work situation is such that an employee's occupational exposure is affected. "At the time of initial assignment to tasks where occupational exposure may take place" means that employees shall be trained prior to being placed in positions where occupational exposure may occur.

Employees who received training on bloodborne pathogens within the year preceding March 6, 1992, shall receive information on the sections of the standard which were not included in their training. The annual retraining for these employees shall be provided within one year of their original training.

Part-time and temporary employees, and health care employees known as "per diem" employees are covered and are also to be trained on company time.

The compliance officer shall interview a representative number of employees from different work areas to determine that the training (including written material, oral presentations, films, videos, computer programs, or audiotapes) was presented in a manner that was appropriate to the employee's education, literacy level, and language, and also that the trainer was able to answer questions as needed. If an employee is only proficient in a foreign language, the trainer or an interpreter must convey the information in that foreign language.

M.7.b.(1)

    (1) Sections (g)(2)(vii)(B) and (C). These sections require that HIV and HBV and other bloodborne diseases be described. The employer must convey the idea that a number of bloodborne diseases other than HIV and HBV exist, such as hepatitis C or syphilis. At the same time, the employer need not cover such uncommon diseases as Cruetzfeld-Jacob disease unless, for example, it is appropriate for employees working in a research facility with that particular virus.

M.7.b.(2)

    (2) Section (g)(2)(vii)(J). The word "emergency" in this section refers to blood exposure outside the normal scope of work. This does not refer to hospital emergency rooms or emergency medical technicians' work.

M.7.b.(3)

    (3) Section (g)(2)(vii)(N). This section requires that there be an opportunity for interactive questions and answers with the person conducting the training session.

M.7.b.(3)(a)

    (a) Training the employees solely by means of a film or video without the opportunity for a discussion period would constitute a violation of this section.

M.7.b.(3)(b)

    (b) Similarly, a generic computer program, even an interactive one, is not considered appropriate unless the employer supplements such training with the site-specific information required (e.g., the location of the exposure control plan and the procedures to be followed if an exposure incident occurs) and a person is accessible for interaction.

M.7.b.(4)

    (4) Section (g)(2)(viii). The person conducting the training is required to be knowledgeable in the subject matter covered by the elements contained in the training program as it relates to the workplace that the training will address. In addition to demonstrating expertise in the area of the occupational hazard of bloodborne pathogens, the trainer must be familiar with the manner in which the elements in the training program relate to the particular workplace.

M.7.b.(4)(a)

    (a) The compliance officer shall verify the competency of the trainer based on the completion of specialized courses, degree programs, or work experience, if he/she determines that deficiencies in training exist.

M.7.b.(4)(b)

    (b) Possible trainers include a variety of health care professionals such as infection control practitioners, nurse practitioners, registered nurses, physician's assistants, or emergency medical technicians.

M.7.b.(4)(c)

    (c) Non–health care professionals, such as industrial hygienists, epidemiologists, or professional trainers, may conduct the training provided they can demonstrate evidence of specialized training in the area of bloodborne pathogens.

M.7.b.(4)(d)

    (d) In some workplaces, such as dental or physicians' offices, the individual employer may conduct the training provided he or she is familiar with bloodborne pathogen exposure control and the subject matter required by sections (g)(2)(viii)(A) through (N).

M.7.b.(5)

(5) **Section (g)(2)(ix)(A)–(C).** "Standard microbiological practices" in these sections refer to procedures outlined in "Biosafety in Microbiological and Biomedical Laboratories." (See D.9. of this instruction.)

M.7.b.(5)(a)

(a) The requirement that "proficiency" be demonstrated means that employees who are experienced laboratorians may not need to be retrained in accordance with these sections.

M.7.b.(5)(b)

(b) Education such as a graduate degree in the study of HIV or HBV, or another closely related subject area with a period of related laboratory research experience, would also constitute "proficiency."

M.7.b.(5)(c)

(c) The employer is responsible for evaluating the employee's proficiency and for documenting the mechanism used to determine proficiency.

M.8.

8. **Recordkeeping—1910.1030(h).** Records are required to be kept for each employee covered by this standard for training, as well as for medical evaluations, treatment, and surveillance.

M.8.a.

a. Medical records required by section (h)(1) will be of particular importance to the health care professional in determining vaccination status and courses of treatment to follow in the event of an exposure incident. Although the employer is required to establish and maintain medical records, he/she may contract for the services of a health care professional located off-site and that person or company may retain the records.

NOTE: While section (h)(1)(iii) requires that medical records are to be kept confidential, section (h)(1)(iii)(B) stipulates that disclosure is permitted when required by this standard or other Federal, State, or local regulations.

INSPECTION GUIDELINES. All medical records required to be kept by this standard are also required to be made available to OSHA. The compliance officer must protect the confidentiality of these records. If they are copied for the case file, the provisions of 29 CFR 1913.10 must be followed.

The compliance officer shall review the employer's recordkeeping program to ensure that the required information is collected, and provision has been made to ensure the confidentiality of the medical records in accordance with 29 CFR 1910.20.

M.8.b.

b. Section (h)(2) requires accurate recordkeeping of training sessions, including titles of the employees who attend. The records are necessary to assist the employer and OSHA in determining whether the training program adequately addresses the risks involved in each job. Additionally, this information is helpful in tracking the relationship between exposure incidents (e.g., needlesticks) and various jobs and the corresponding level of training.

M.8.b.(1)

(1) Training records may be stored on-site and therefore the actual documents will be easily accessible for review. In order to ensure that the employee training is complete, all the components of the program required by section (g)(2)(vii) must be covered.

M.8.b.(2)

(2) Training records are not considered to be confidential and may be maintained in any file. They must be retained for 3 years from the training date.

M.9.

9. Dates—1910.1030(I). The effective dates of the requirements of the standard appear in Appendix F[2] of this instruction.

NOTE: OSHA Instruction CPL 2-2.44B shall remain in effect until the effective dates of the requirements of 29 CFR 1910.1030.

N. Interface with Other Standards

1. The hazard communication standard, 29 CFR 1910.1200, applies only to the hazards of chemicals in the workplace and does not apply to biological hazards such as bloodborne diseases.

2. Records concerning employee exposure to bloodborne pathogens and records about HIV and/or HBV status are considered employee medical

---

2. Appendix F of the original compliance guide is not included here, because it merely gives the 6-month phase-in schedule for all the requirements. All paragraphs are in effect as of July 6, 1992, so inclusion of this appendix would be superfluous. Reference paragraph (i) of the regulatory text for the historical phase-in schedule.

records within the meaning of 29 CFR 1910.20. Under 29 CFR 1913.10, the compliance officer may review these records for purposes of determining compliance with 29 CFR 1910.20.

3. Generally, the respiratory protection standard, 29 CFR 1910.134 does not apply since there are no respirators approved for biohazards. However, placing respirators in areas where they could be contaminated by body fluids constitutes a violation of 29 CFR 1910.134(b)(6).

4. The Hazardous Waste Operations and Emergency Response (HAZWOPER) standard, 29 CFR 1910.120, covers three groups of employees—workers at uncontrolled hazardous waste remediation sites; workers at Resource Conservation and Recovery Act (RCRA) permitted hazardous waste treatment, storage and disposal facilities; and those workers expected to respond to emergencies caused by the uncontrolled release of a hazardous substance.

    a. The definition of hazardous substance includes any biological agent or infectious material which may cause disease or death. There are potential scenarios where the bloodborne and HAZWOPER standards may interface such as:

        (1) Workers involved in cleanup operations at hazardous waste sites involving infectious waste;

        (2) Workers responding to an emergency caused by the uncontrolled release of infectious material; e.g., a transportation accident; and

        (3) Workers at RCRA-permitted incinerators that burn infectious waste.

    b. Employers of employees engaged in these types of activities must comply with the requirements in 29 CFR 1910.120 as well as the bloodborne pathogens standard. If there is a conflict or overlap, the provision that is more protective of employee safety and health applies.

O. RECORDING IN THE IMIS

Current instructions for completing the appropriate inspection classification boxes on the OSHA-1, Inspection Report, as found in the IMIS manual, shall be applied when recording bloodborne pathogens inspections:

1. For any inspection which includes an evaluation of the hazards of bloodborne pathogens, Item 42 of the OSHA-1 shall be recorded as follows:

N   02   Blood

2. If local emphasis programs are approved at a later date, Item 25C of the OSHA-1 shall be completed with the appropriate value.

P. REFERRALS

When a complaint or inquiry regarding occupational exposure to bloodborne disease in a State or local government facility is received in a State without an OSHA-approved State plan, the Regional Administrator should refer it to the appropriate State public health agency or local health agency with jurisdiction over the facility.

APPENDIX C1
BIOLOGICAL SAFETY CABINETS[1]

Biological safety cabinets (BSC) are among the most effective, as well as the most commonly used, primary containment devices in laboratories working with infectious agents. Each of the three types—Class I, II, III—has performance characteristics that are described in this appendix. In addition to the design, construction, and performance standards for vertical laminar flow biological safety cabinets (Class II), the National Sanitation Foundation has also developed a list of such products which meet the reference standard. Utilization of this standard and list should be the first step in selection and procurement of a biological safety cabinet.

Class I and II biological safety cabinets, when used in conjunction with good microbiological techniques, provide an effective partial containment system for safe manipulation of moderate- and high-risk microorganisms (i.e., biosafety Level 2 and 3 agents). Both Class I and II biological safety cabinets have comparable inward face velocities (75 linear feet per minute) and provide comparable levels of containment in protecting the laboratory worker and the immediate laboratory environment from infectious aerosols generated within the cabinet.

It is imperative that Class I and II biological safety cabinets are tested and certified in situ at the time of installation within the laboratory, at any time the

1. *Biosafety in Microbiological and Biomedical Laboratories, Washington,* DC: U.S. Department of Health and Human Services, publication no. (NIH) 88-8395, May 1988.

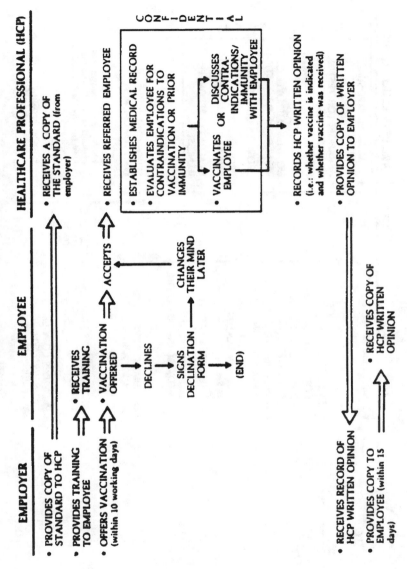

Figure C-1 Hepatitis B Vaccination

POST-EXPOSURE EVALUATION AND FOLLOW-UP

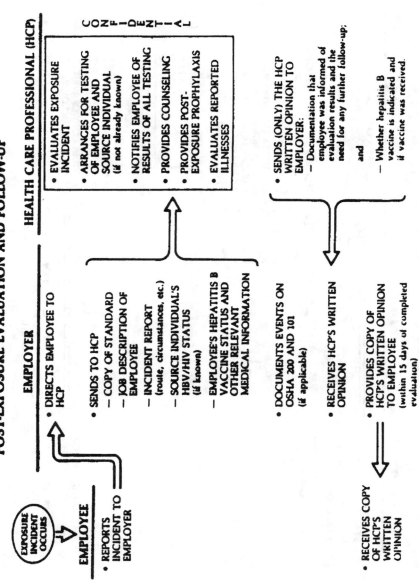

Figure C-2 Post-Exposure Evaluation and Follow-Up

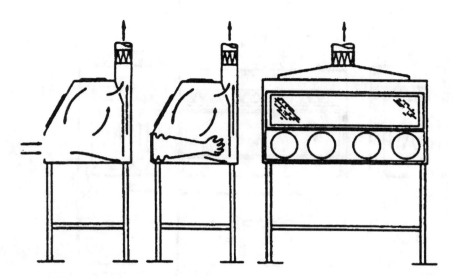

Figure C1-1 Class I Cabinet

BSC is moved, and at least annually thereafter. Certification at locations other than the final site may attest to the performance capability of the individual cabinet or model, but does not supersede the critical certification prior to use in the laboratory.

As with any other piece of laboratory equipment, personnel must be trained in the proper use of the biological safety cabinets. Of particular note are those activities which may disrupt the inward directional airflow through the work opening of Class I and II cabinets. Repeated insertion and withdrawal of the workers' arms in and from the work chamber, opening and closing doors to the laboratory or isolation cubicle, improper placement or operation of materials or equipment within the work chamber, or brisk walking past the BSC while it is in use are demonstrated causes of the escape of aerosolized particles from within the cabinet. Strict adherence to recommended practices for the use of biological safety cabinets is as important in attaining the maximum containment capability of the equipment as is the mechanical performance of the equipment itself.

Horizontal laminar flow "clean benches" are present in a number of clinical, pharmacy, and laboratory facilities. These "clean benches" provide a high-quality environment within the work chamber for manipulation of nonhazardous materials. *Caution:* Since the operator sits in the immediate downstream exhaust from the "clean bench," this equipment must never be used for the handling of toxic, infectious, or sensitizing materials.

The Class I biological safety cabinet (Figure C1-1) is an open-fronted, negative-pressure, ventilated cabinet with a minimum inward face velocity at the

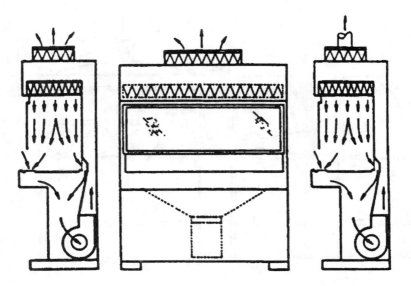

Figure C1-2A Class II Cabinets-Type A

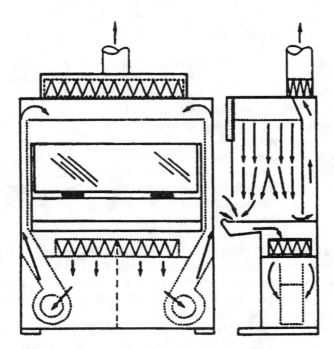

Figure C1-2B Class II Cabinets- Type B

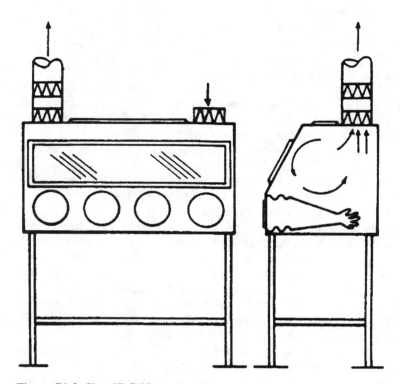

Figure C1-3 Class III Cabinet

work opening of at least 75 feet per minute. The exhaust air from the cabinet is filtered by a high-efficiency particulate air (HEPA) filter. This cabinet may be used in three operational modes: with a full-width open front, with an installed front closure panel not equipped with gloves, and with an installed front closure panel equipped with arm-length rubber gloves.

The Class II vertical laminar-flow biological cabinet (Figure C1-2) is an open-fronted, ventilated cabinet with an average inward face velocity at the work opening of at least 75 feet per minute. This cabinet provides a HEPA-filtered, recirculated mass airflow within the work space. The exhaust air from the cabinet is also filtered by HEPA filters. Design, construction, and performance standards for Class II cabinets have been developed by and are available from the National Sanitation Foundation, Ann Arbor, MI.

The Class III cabinet (Figure C1-3) is a totally enclosed ventilated cabinet of gaslight construction. Operations within the Class III cabinet are conducted through attached rubber gloves. When in use, the Class III cabinet is maintained under negative air pressure of at least 0.5 inches water gauge. Supply air is drawn into the cabinet through HEPA filters. The cabinet exhaust air is filtered by two HEPA filters, installed in series, before discharge outside of the facility. The exhaust fan for the Class III cabinet is generally separate from the exhaust fans of the facility's ventilation system.

Personnel protection provided by Class I and Class II cabinets is dependent on the inward airflow. Since the face velocities are similar, they generally provide an equivalent level of personnel protection. The use of these cabinets alone, however, is not appropriate for containment of highest-risk infectious agents because aerosols may accidentally escape through the open front.

The use of a Class II cabinet in the microbiological laboratory offers the additional capability and advantage of protecting materials contained within it from extraneous airborne contaminants. This capability is provided by the HEPA-filtered, recirculated mass airflow within the work space.

The Class III cabinet provides the highest level of personnel and product protection. This protection is provided by the physical isolation of the space in which the infectious agent is maintained. When these cabinets are required, all procedures involving infectious agents are contained within them. Several Class III cabinets are therefore typically set up as an interconnected system. All equipment required by the laboratory activity, such as incubators, refrigerators, and centrifuges, must be an integral part of the cabinet system. Double-doored autoclaves and chemical dunk tanks are also attached to the cabinet system to allow supplies and equipment to be safely introduced and removed.

Personnel protection equivalent to that provided by Class III cabinets can also be obtained with a personnel suit area and Class I or Class II cabinets. This is one in which the laboratory worker is protected from a potentially contaminated environment by a one-piece positive pressure suit ventilated by a life-support system. This area is entered through an airlock fitted with airtight doors. A chemical shower is provided to decontaminate the surfaces of the suit as the worker leaves the area. The exhaust air from the suit area is filtered by two HEPA filter units installed in series.

Appendix **D**

Proposed Addition to BBPS Enforcement Procedures

The following text is proposed to be added to OSHA Instruction CFL 2–2.44C, Enforcement Procedures for the Occupational Exposure to Bloodborne Pathogens Standard, 29 CF 1910.1030 (add as subparagraph (6) to M.6.b):

(6) Under section (f)(2) of the standard, hepatitis B vaccination must be offered to all employees who have occupational exposure to blood or other potentially infectious materials (OPIM). However, as a matter of policy, violations will be considered *de minimis* and citations will not be issued when designated first aid providers who have occupational exposure are not offered pre-exposure hepatitis B vaccine if the following conditions exist:

(a) The primary job assignment of such designated first aid providers is not the rendering of first aid.

<u>1</u> Any first aid rendered by such person is rendered *only as a collateral duty* responding solely to injuries resulting from workplace incidents, generally at the location where the incident occurred.

<u>2</u> This provision does *not* apply to designated first aid providers who render assistance on a regular basis, for example, at a first aid station, clinic, dispensary or other location where injured employees routinely go for such assistance, nor does it apply to any health care, emergency, or public safety personnel who are expected to render first aid in the course of their work.

(b) The employer's Exposure Control Plan specifically addresses the provision of hepatitis B vaccine to all unvaccinated first aid providers who have rendered assistance in any situation involving the presence of blood or OPIM (regardless of whether an actual "exposure incident" as defined by the standard occurred) and prophylaxis and follow-up for those employees who experience an "exposure incident," including:

1 Provision for a reporting procedure that ensures that all first aid incidents involving the presence of blood or OPIM will be reported to the employer before the end of the work shift during which the first aid incident occurred.

   a The report must include the names of all first aid providers who rendered assistance, regardless of whether personal protective equipment was used and must describe the first aid incident, including time and date.

      The description must include a determination of whether or not, in addition to the presence of blood or other potentially infected materials, and "exposure incident," as defined by the standard, occurred.

      This determination is necessary in order to ensure that the proper post-exposure evaluation, prophylaxis and follow-up procedures required by section (f)(3) of the standard are made available immediately if there has been an "exposure incident" as defined by the standard.

   b The report shall be recorded on a list of such first aid incidents. It shall be readily available to all employees and shall be provided to the Assistant Secretary upon request.

2 Provision for the bloodborne pathogens training program for designated first aiders to include the specifics of this reporting procedure.

3 Provision for the full hepatitis B vaccination series to be made available as soon as possible, but in no event later than 24 hours, to all unvaccinated first aid providers who have rendered assistance in any situation involving the presence of blood or OPIM regardless of whether or not a specific "exposure incident," as defined by the standard, has occurred.

(c) The employer must implement a procedure to ensure that all of the provisions of paragraph b are complied with if pre-exposure hepatitis B vaccine is not to be given to employees meeting the conditions of paragraph a.

NOTE: All other requirements of the standard continue to apply.

Recommendations for Preventing Transmission of Human Immunodeficiency Virus and Hepatitis B Virus to Patients during Exposure-prone Invasive Procedures[1]

T his document has been developed by the Centers for Disease Control (CDC) to update recommendations for prevention of transmission of human immunodeficiency virus (HIV) and hepatitis B virus (HBV) in the health-care setting. Current data suggest that the risk for such transmission from a health-care worker (HCW) to a patient during an invasive procedure is small; a precise assessment of the risk is not yet available. This document contains recommendations to provide guidance for prevention of HIV and HBV transmission during those invasive procedures that are considered exposure-prone.

INTRODUCTION

Recommendations have been made by the Centers for Disease Control (CDC) for the prevention of transmission of the human immunodeficiency virus (HIV) and the hepatitis B virus (HBV) in health-care settings (1–6). These recommendations emphasize adherence to universal precautions that require that blood and other specified body fluids of all patients be handled as if they contain blood-borne pathogens (1,2). Previous guidelines contained precautions to be used during invasive procedures and recommendations for the management of HIV- and HBV-infected health-care workers (HCWs) (1). These guidelines did not include specific recommendations on testing HCWs for HIV or HBV infection,

---

1. Centers for Disease Contol, *MMWR* 1991; 40 (no. RR-8): 1–9.

and they did not provide guidance on which invasive procedures may represent increased risk to the patient.

The recommendations outlined in this document are based on the following considerations:

- Infected HCWs who adhere to universal precautions and who do not perform invasive procedures pose no risk for transmitting HIV or HBV to patients.
- Infected HCWs who adhere to universal precautions and who perform certain exposure-prone procedures pose a small risk for transmitting HBV to patients.
- HIV is transmitted much less readily than HBV.

In the interim, until further data are available, additional precautions are prudent to prevent HIV and HBV transmission during procedures that have been linked to HCW-to-patient HBV transmission or that are considered exposure-prone.

BACKGROUND

Infection-Control Practices

Previous recommendations have specified that infection-control programs should incorporate principles of universal precautions (i.e., appropriate use of hand washing, protective barriers, and care in the use and disposal of needles and other sharp instruments) and should maintain these precautions rigorously in all health-care settings (1,2,5). Proper application of these principles will assist in minimizing the risk of transmission of HIV or HBV from patient to HCW, HCW to patient, or patient to patient.

As part of standard infection-control practice, instruments and other reusable equipment used in performing invasive procedures should be appropriately disinfected and sterilized as follows (7):

- Equipment and devices that enter the patient's vascular system or other normally sterile areas of the body should be sterilized before being used for each patient.
- Equipment and devices that touch intact mucous membranes but do not penetrate the patient's body surfaces should be sterilized when possible or undergo high-level disinfection if they cannot be sterilized before being used for each patient.

- Equipment and devices that do not touch the patient or that only touch intact skin of the patient need only be cleaned with a detergent or as indicated by the manufacturer.

Compliance with universal precautions and recommendations for disinfection and sterilization of medical devices should be scrupulously monitored in all health-care settings (1,7,8). Training of HCWs in proper infection-control technique should begin in professional and vocational schools and continue as an ongoing process. Institutions should provide all HCWs with appropriate inservice education regarding infection control and safety and should establish procedures for monitoring compliance with infection-control policies.

All HCWs who might be exposed to blood in an occupational setting should receive hepatitis B vaccine, preferably during their period of professional training and before any occupational exposures could occur (8,9).

Transmission of HBV during Invasive Procedures

Since the introduction of serologic testing for HBV infection in the early 1970s, there have been published reports of 20 clusters in which a total of over 300 patients were infected with HBV in association with treatment by an HBV-infected HCW. In 12 of these clusters, the implicated HCW did not routinely wear gloves; several HCWs also had skin lesions that may have facilitated HBV transmission (10–22). These 12 clusters included nine linked to dentists or oral surgeons and one cluster each linked to a general practitioner, an inhalation therapist, and a cardiopulmonary-bypass-pump technician. The clusters associated with the inhalation therapist and the cardiopulmonary-bypass-pump technician—and some of the other 10 clusters—could possibly have been prevented if current recommendations on universal precautions, including glove use, had been in effect. In the remaining eight clusters, transmission occurred despite glove use by the HCWs; five clusters were linked to obstetricians or gynecologists, and three were linked to cardiovascular surgeons (6,22–28). In addition, recent unpublished reports strongly suggest HBV transmission from three surgeons to patients in 1989 and 1990 during colorectal (CDC, unpublished data), abdominal, and cardiothoracic surgery (29).

Seven of the HCWs who were linked to published clusters in the United States were allowed to perform invasive procedures following modification of invasive techniques (e.g., double-gloving and restriction of certain high-risk procedures) (6,11,13,15,16,24). For five HCWs, no further transmission to patients was observed. In two instances involving an obstetrician/gynecologist and an oral surgeon, HBV was transmitted to patients after techniques were modified (6,12).

Review of the 20 published studies indicates that a combination of risk factors accounted for transmission of HBV from HCWs to patients. Of the

HCWs whose hepatitis B e antigen (HBeAg) status was determined (17 of 20), all were HBeAg-positive. The presence of HBeAg in serum is associated with higher levels of circulating virus and therefore with greater infectivity of hepatitis-B-surface-antigen (HBsAg)–positive individuals; the risk of HBV transmission to an HCW after a percutaneous exposure to HBeAg-positive blood is approximately 30% (30–32). In addition, each report indicated that the potential existed for contamination of surgical wounds or traumatized tissue, either from a major break in standard infection-control practices (e.g., not wearing gloves during invasive procedures) or from unintentional injury to the infected HCW during invasive procedures (e.g., needlesticks incurred while manipulating needles without being able to see them during suturing).

Most reported clusters in the United States occurred before awareness increased of the risks of transmission of bloodborne pathogens in health-care settings and before emphasis was placed on the use of universal precautions and hepatitis B vaccine among HCWs. The limited number of reports of HBV transmission from HCWs to patients in recent years may reflect the adoption of universal precautions and increased use of HBV vaccine. However, the limited number of recent reports does not preclude the occurrence of undetected or unreported small clusters or individual instances of transmission; routine use of gloves does not prevent most injuries caused by sharp instruments and does not eliminate the potential for exposure of a patient to an HCWs blood and transmission of HBV (6,22–29).

Transmission of HIV during Invasive Procedures

The risk of HIV transmission to an HCW after percutaneous exposure to HIV-infected blood is considerably lower than the risk of HBV transmission after percutaneous exposure to HBeAg-positive blood (0.3% versus approximately 30%) (33–35). Thus, the risk of transmission of HIV from an infected HCW to a patient during an invasive procedure is likely to be proportionately lower than the risk of HBV transmission from an HBeAg-positive HCW to a patient during the same procedure. As with HBV, the relative infectivity of HIV probably varies among individuals and over time for a single individual. Unlike HBV infection, however, there is currently no readily available laboratory test for increased HIV infectivity.

Investigation of a cluster of HIV infections among patients in the practice of one dentist with acquired immunodeficiency syndrome (AIDS) strongly suggested that HIV was transmitted to five of the approximately 850 patients evaluated through June 1991 (36–38). The investigation indicates that HIV transmission occurred during dental care, although the precise mechanisms of transmission have not been determined. In two other studies, when patients cared for by a general surgeon and a surgical resident who had AIDS were tested, all patients tested, 75 and 62, respectively, were negative for HIV infection (39,40). In a fourth study, 143 patients who had been treated by a dental student with HIV infection and were later tested were all negative for HIV infection (41). In another investigation, HIV antibody testing was offered to all patients whose surgical procedures had been performed by a general surgeon within 7 years before the surgeon's diagnosis of AIDS; the date at which the surgeon became infected with HIV is unknown (42). Of 1,340 surgical patients contacted, 616 (46%) were tested for HIV. One patient, a known intravenous drug user, was HIV positive when tested but may already have been infected at the time of surgery. HIV test results for the 615 other surgical patients were negative (95% confidence interval for risk of transmission per operation = 0.0%–0.5%).

The limited number of participants and the differences in procedures associated with these five investigations limit the ability to generalize from them and to define precisely the risk of HIV transmission from HIV-infected HCWs to patients. A precise estimate of the risk of HIV transmission from infected HCWs to patients can be determined only after careful evaluation of a substantially larger number of patients whose exposure-prone procedures have been performed by HIV-infected HCWs.

Exposure-Prone Procedures

Despite adherence to the principles of universal precautions, certain invasive surgical and dental procedures have been implicated in the transmission of HBV from infected HCWs to patients, and should be considered exposure-prone. Reported examples include certain oral, cardiothoracic, colorectal (CDC, unpublished data), and obstetric/gynecologic procedures (6,12,22–29).

Certain other invasive procedures should also be considered exposure-prone. In a prospective study CDC conducted in four hospitals, one or more percutaneous injuries occurred among surgical personnel during 96 (6.9%) of 1,382 operative procedures on the general surgery, gynecology, orthopedic, cardiac, and trauma services (43). Percutaneous exposure of the patient to the HCW's blood may have occurred when the sharp object causing the injury recontacted the patient's open wound in 28 (32%) of the 88 observed injuries to surgeons (range among surgical specialties = 8%–57%; range among hospitals = 24%–42%).

Characteristics of exposure-prone procedures include digital palpation of a needle tip in a body cavity or the simultaneous presence of the HCW's fingers and a needle or other sharp instrument or object in a poorly visualized or highly confined anatomic site. Performance of exposure-prone procedures presents a recognized risk of percutaneous injury to the HCW, and—if such an injury occurs—the HCW's blood is likely to contact the patient's body cavity, subcutaneous tissues, and/or mucous membranes.

Experience with HBV indicates that invasive procedures that do not have the above characteristics would be expected to pose substantially lower risk, if any, of transmission of HIV and other bloodborne pathogens from an infected HCW to patients.

RECOMMENDATIONS

Investigations of HIV and HBV transmission from HCWs to patients indicate that, when HCWs adhere to recommended infection-control procedures, the risk of transmitting HBV from an infected HCW to a patient is small, and the risk of transmitting HIV is likely to be even smaller. However, the likelihood of exposure of the patient to an HCW's blood is greater for certain procedures designated as exposure-prone. To minimize the risk of HIV or HBV transmission, the following measures are recommended:

- **All HCWs should adhere to universal precautions, including the appropriate use of hand washing, protective barriers, and care in the use and disposal of needles and other sharp instruments. HCWs who have exudative lesions or weeping dermatitis should refrain from all direct patient care and from handling patient-care equipment and devices used in performing invasive procedures until the condition resolves. HCWs should also comply with current guidelines for disinfection and sterilization of reusable devices used in invasive procedures.**
- **Currently available data provide no basis for recommendations to restrict the practice of HCWs infected with HIV or HBV who perform invasive procedures not identified as exposure-prone, provided the infected HCWs practice recommended surgical or dental technique and comply with universal precautions and current recommendations for sterilization/disinfection.**
- **Exposure-prone procedures should be identified by medical/surgical/dental organizations and institutions at which the procedures are performed.**
- **HCWs who perform exposure-prone procedures should know their HIV antibody status. HCWs who perform exposure-prone procedures and who do not have serologic evidence of immunity to HBV from vaccination or from previous infection should know their HBsAg status and, if that is positive, should also know their HBeAg status.**
- **HCWs who are infected with HIV or HBV (and are HBeAg-positive) should not perform exposure-prone procedures unless they have sought counsel from an expert review panel and been advised under what**

circumstances, if any, they may continue to perform these procedures.[2] Such circumstances would include notifying prospective patients of the HCW's seropositivity before they undergo exposure-prone invasive procedures.

- Mandatory testing of HCWs for HIV antibody, HBsAg, or HBeAg is not recommended. The current assessment of the risk that infected HCWs will transmit HIV or HBV to patients during exposure-prone procedures does not support the diversion of resources that would be required to implement mandatory testing programs. Compliance by HCWs with recommendations can be increased through education, training, and appropriate confidentiality safeguards.

HCWs WHOSE PRACTICES ARE MODIFIED BECAUSE OF HIV OR HBV STATUS

HCWs whose practices are modified because of their HIV or HBV infection status should, whenever possible, be provided opportunities to continue appropriate patient-care activities. Career counseling and job retraining should be encouraged to promote the continued use of the HCW's talents, knowledge, and skills. HCW's whose practices are modified because of HBV infection should be reevaluated periodically to determine whether their HBeAg status changes due to resolution of infection or as a result of treatment (44).

NOTIFICATION OF PATIENTS AND FOLLOW-UP STUDIES

The public health benefit of notification of patients who have had exposure-prone procedures performed by HCWs infected with HIV or positive for HBeAg should be considered on a case-by-case basis, taking into consideration an assessment of specific risks, confidentiality issues, and available resources. Care-

---

2. The review panel should include experts who represent a balanced perspective. Such experts might include all of the following: (a) the HCW's personal physician(s), (b) an infectious disease specialist with expertise in the procedures performed by the HCW, and (c) state or local public health officials. If the HCW's practice is institutionally based, the expert review panel might also include a member of the infection-control committee, preferably a hospital epidemiologist. HCWs who perform exposure-prone procedures outside the hospital/institutional setting should seek advice from appropriate state and local public health officials regarding the review process. Panels must recognize the importance of confidentiality and the privacy rights of infected HCWs.

fully designed and implemented follow-up studies are necessary to determine more precisely the risk of transmission during such procedures. Decisions regarding notification and follow-up studies should be made in consultation with state and local public health officials.

ADDITIONAL NEEDS

- Clearer definition of the nature, frequency, and circumstances of blood contact between patients and HCWs during invasive procedures.
- Development and evaluation of new devices, protective barriers, and techniques that may prevent such blood contact without adversely affecting the quality of patient care.
- More information on the potential for HIV and HBV transmission through contaminated instruments.
- Improvements in sterilization and disinfection techniques for certain reusable equipment and devices.
- Identification of factors that may influence the likelihood of HIV or HBV transmission after exposure to HIV- or HBV-infected blood.

Definition of Invasive Procedure

An invasive procedure is defined as "surgical entry into tissues, cavities, or organs or repair of major traumatic injuries" associated with any of the following: "1) an operating or delivery room, emergency department, or outpatient setting, including both physicians' and dentists' offices; 2) cardiac catheterization and angiographic procedures; 3) a vaginal or cesarean delivery or other invasive obstetric procedure during which bleeding may occur; or 4) the manipulation, cutting, or removal of any oral or perioral tissues, including tooth structure, during which bleeding occurs or the potential for bleeding exists." *(See Appendix I.)*

REFERENCES

1. CDC. Recommendations for prevention of HIV transmission in health-care settings. *MMWR* 1987;36(suppl 2S):1–18S.
2. CDC. Update: universal precautions for prevention of transmission of

human immunodeficiency virus, hepatitis B virus, and other bloodborne pathogens in health-care settings. *MMWR* 1988,37:377–82, 387–8.

3. CDC. *Hepatitis surveillance report no. 48.* Atlanta: U.S. Department of Health and Human Services, Public Health Service, 1982:2–3.

4. CDC. *CDC guideline for infection control in hospital personnel.* Atlanta: Public Health Service, 1983. 24 pages. (GPO Publication no. 6AR031488305.)

5. CDC. Guidelines for prevention of transmission of human immunodeficiency virus and hepatitis B virus to health-care and public-safety workers. *MMWR* 1989;38;(suppl S–6):1–37.

6. Lettau LA, Smith JD, Williams D, et al. Transmission of hepatitis B with resultant restriction of surgical practice. *JAMA* 1986;255:934–7.

7. CDC. *Guidelines for the prevention and control of nosocomial infections: guideline for handwashing and hospital environmental control.* Atlanta: Public Health Service, 1985. 20 pages. (GPO Publication no. 544–436/24441.)

8. Department of Labor, Occupational Safety and Health Administration. Occupational exposure to bloodborne pathogens: proposed rule and notice of hearing. *Federal Register* 1989;54:23042–139.

9. CDC. Protection against viral hepatitis: recommendations of the immunization practices advisory committee (ACIP). *MMWR* 1990;39(no. RR-2).

10. Levin ML, Maddrey WC, Wands JR, Mendeloff Al. Hepatitis B transmission by dentists. *JAMA* 1974;228:1139–40.

11. Rimland D, Parkin WE, Miller GB, Schrack WD. Hepatitis B outbreak traced to an oral surgeon. *N Engl J Med* 1977;296:953–8.

12. Goodwin D, Fannin SL, McCracken BB. An oral-surgeon related hepatitis-B outbreak. *California Morbidity* 1976;14.

13. Hadler SC, Sorley DL, Acree KH, et al. An outbreak of hepatitis B in a dental practice. *Ann Intern Med* 1981;95:133–8.

14. Reingold AL, Kane MA, Murphy BL, Checko P, Francis DP, Maynard JE. Transmission of hepatitis B by an oral surgeon. *J Infect Dis* 1982;145:262–8.

15. Goodman RA, Ahtone JL, Finton RJ. Hepatitis B transmission from dental personnel to patients: unfinished business [Editorial]. *Ann Intern Med* 1982;96:119.

16. Ahtone J, Goodman RA. Hepatitis B and dental personnel: transmission to patients and prevention issues. *J Am Dent Assoc* 1983;106:219–22.

17. Shaw FE, Jr, Barrett CL, Hamm R, et al. Lethal outbreak of hepatitis B in a dental practice. *JAMA* 1986;255:3260–4.

18. CDC. Outbreak of hepatitis B associated with an oral surgeon, New Hampshire. *MMWR* 1987;36:132–3.

19. Grob PJ, Moeschlin P. Risk to contacts of a medical practitioner carrying HBsAg [Letter]. *N Engl J Med* 1975;293:197.

20. Grob PJ, Bischof B, Naeff F. Cluster of hepatitis B transmitted by a physician. *Lancet* 1981;2:1218–20.
21. Snydman DR, Hindman SH, Wineland MD, Bryan JA, Maynard JE. Nosocomial viral hepatitis B: a cluster among staff with subsequent transmission to patients. *Ann Intern Med* 1976;85:573–7.
22. Coutinho RA, Albrecht-van Lent P, Stoutjesdijk L, et al. Hepatitis B from doctors [Letter]. *Lancet* 1982;1:345–6.
23. Anonymous. Acute hepatitis B associated with gynaecological surgery. *Lancet* 1980;1:1–6.
24. Carl M, Blakey DL, Francis DP, Maynard JE. Interruption of hepatitis B transmission by modification of a gynaecologist's surgical technique. *Lancet* 1982;1:731–3.
25. Anonymous. Acute hepatitis B following gynaecological surgery. *J Hosp Infect* 1987;9:34–8.
26. Welch J, Webster M, Tilzey AJ, Noah ND, Banatvala JE. Hepatitis B infections after gynecological surgery. *Lancet* 1989;1:205–7.
27. Haeram JW, Siebke JC, Ulstrup J, Geiram D, Helle I. HBsAg transmission from a cardiac surgeon incubating hepatitis B resulting in chronic antigenemia in four patients. *Acts Med Scand* 1981;210:389–92.
28. Flower AJE, Prentice M, Morgan G, et al. Hepatitis B infection following cardiothoracic surgery [Abstract]. *1990 International Symposium on Viral Hepatitis and Liver Diseases, Houston.* 1990;94.
29. Heptonstall J. Outbreaks of hepatitis B virus infection associated with infected surgical staff in the United Kingdom. *Communicable Disease Reports* 1991 (in press).
30. Alter HJ, Seef LB, Kaplan PM, et al. Type B hepatitis: the infectivity of blood positive for e antigen and DNA polymerase after accidental needlestick exposure. *N Engl J Med* 1976;295:909–13.
31. Seeff LB, Wright EC, Zimmerman HJ, et al. Type B hepatitis after needlestick exposure: prevention with hepatitis B immunoglobulin: final report of the Veterans Administration Cooperative Study. *Ann Intern Med* 1978;88:285–93.
32. Grady GF, Lee VA, Prince AM, et al. Hepatitis B immune globulin for accidental exposures among medical personnel: final report of a multicenter controlled trial. *J Infect Dis* 1978;138:625–38.
33. Henderson DK, Fahey BJ, Willy M, et al. Risk for occupational transmission of human immunodeficiency virus type 1 (HIV-1) associated with clinical exposures: a prospective evaluation. *Ann Intern Med* 1990;113:740–6.
34. Marcus R, CDC Cooperative Needlestick Study Group. Surveillance of health–care workers exposed to blood from patients infected with the human immunodeficiency virus. *N Engl J Med* 1988;319:1118–23.
35. Gerberding JL, Bryant-LeBlanc CE, Nelson K, et al. Risk of transmitting the

human immunodeficiency virus, cytomegalovirus, and hepatitis B virus to health-care workers exposed to patients with AIDS and AIDS-related conditions. *J Infect Dis* 1987;156:1–8.

36. CDC. Possible transmission of human immunodeficiency virus to a patient during an invasive dental procedure. *MMWR* 1990;39:489–93.

37. CDC. Update: transmission of HIV infection during an invasive dental procedure—Florida. *MMWR* 1991;40:21–27,33.

38. CDC. Update: transmission of HIV infection during invasive dental procedures—Florida. *MMWR* 1991,40:377–81.

39. Porter JD, Cruikshank JG, Gentle PH, Robinson RG, Gill ON. Management of patients treated by a surgeon with HIV infection [Letter]. *Lancet* 1990;335:1134.

40. Armstrong FP, Miner JC, Wolfe WH. Investigation of a health-care worker with symptomatic human immunodeficiency virus infection: an epidemiologic approach. *Milit Med* 1987;152:414–8.

41. Comer RW, Myers DR, Steadman CD, Carter MJ, Rissing JP, Tedesco FJ. Management considerations for an HIV-positive dental student. *J Dent Educ* 1991;55:187–91.

42. Mishu B, Schaffner W, Horan JM, Wood LH, Hutcheson R, McNabb P. A surgeon with AIDS: lack of evidence of transmission to patients. *JAMA* 1990;264:467–70.

43. Tokars J, Bell D, Marcus R, et al. Percutaneous injuries during surgical procedures [Abstract]. *VII International Conference on AIDS.* Vol 2. Florence, Italy, June 16–21, 1991:83.

44. Perrillo RP, Schiff ER, Davis GL, et al. A randomized, controlled trial of interferon alfa–2b alone and after prednisone withdrawal for the treatment of chronic hepatitis B. *N Engl J Med* 1990;323:295–301.

Protection against Viral Hepatitis: Recommendations of the Immunization Practices Advisory Committee (ACIP)[1]

INTRODUCTION

The term "viral hepatitis" is commonly used for several clinically similar diseases that are etiologically and epidemiologically distinct (1). Two of these, hepatitis A (formerly called infectious hepatitis) and hepatitis B (formerly called serum hepatitis), have been recognized as separate entities since the early 1940s and can be diagnosed with specific serologic tests. A third category, currently known as non-A, non-B hepatitis, includes two epidemiologically distinct types of hepatitis: parenterally transmitted and enterically transmitted non-A, non-B hepatitis. Parenterally transmitted non-A, non-B hepatitis is associated with both posttransfusion and sporadic cases of acute hepatitis and may be caused by at least two different agents. Part of the genome for one of these agents has recently been cloned, and a candidate serologic assay for antibody to this virus (proposed as hepatitis C virus) has been developed (2,3). Enterically transmitted non-A, non-B hepatitis, which is spread by the fecal-oral route and is different from the types seen in the United States, has been reported in parts of Asia, Africa, and Mexico (4). Another distinct type of hepatitis, delta hepatitis, is an infection

---

1. Centers for Disease Control, *MMWR* 1990;39(suppl S–2):1–26.

dependent on the hepatitis B virus. It may occur as a coinfection with acute hepatitis B infection or as superinfection of a hepatitis B carrier (5).

HEPATITIS SURVEILLANCE

Approximately 28,500 cases of hepatitis A, 23,200 cases of hepatitis B, 2,620 cases of non-A, non-B hepatitis, and 2,470 cases of hepatitis type unspecified were reported in 1988 in the United States. Most cases of each type occur among young adults. Since reporting from many localities is incomplete, the actual number of hepatitis cases occurring annually is thought to be several times the reported number.

IMMUNE GLOBULINS

Immune globulins are important tools for preventing infection and disease before or after exposure to hepatitis viruses. Immune globulins used in medical practice are sterile solutions of antibodies (immunoglobulins) from human plasma. They are prepared by cold ethanol fractionation of large plasma pools and contain 10–18% protein. In the United States, plasma is primarily obtained from paid donors. Only plasma shown to be free of hepatitis B surface antigen (HBsAg) and antibody to human immunodeficiency virus (HIV) is used to prepare immune globulins.

Immune globulin (IG) (formerly called immune serum globulin, ISG, or gamma globulin) produced in the United States contains antibodies against the hepatitis A virus (anti-HAV) and the HBsAg (anti-HBs). Hepatitis B immune globulin (HBIG) is an IG prepared from plasma containing high titers of anti-HBs.

There is no evidence that hepatitis B virus (HBV), HIV (the causative agent of acquired immunodeficiency syndrome [AIDS]), or other viruses have ever been transmitted by IG or HBIG commercially available in the United States (6). Since late April 1985, all plasma units for preparation of IGs have been screened for antibody to HIV, and reactive units are discarded. No instances of HIV infection or clinical illness have occurred that can be attributed to receiving IG or HBIG, including lots prepared before April 1985. Laboratory studies have shown that the margin of safety based on the removal of HIV infectivity by the fractionation process is extremely high (7). Some HBIG lots prepared before April 1985 have detectable HIV antibody. Shortly after being given HBIG, recipients have occasionally been noted to have low levels of passively acquired HIV antibody, but this reactivity does not persist (8).

Serious adverse effects from IGs administered as recommended have been rare. IGs prepared for intramuscular administration should be used for hepatitis prophylaxis. IGs prepared for intravenous administration to immunodeficient and other selected patients are not intended for hepatitis prophylaxis. IG and HBIG are not contraindicated for pregnant or lactating women

HEPATITIS A

Hepatitis A is caused by the hepatitis A virus (HAV), a 27-nm ribonucleic acid (RNA) agent that is classified as a picornavirus. Patients with illness caused by HAV characteristically have abrupt onsets of symptoms including fever, malaise, anorexia, nausea, abdominal discomfort, dark urine, and jaundice. Severity is related to age. Among children, most infections are asymptomatic, and illness is usually not accompanied by jaundice. Most infected adults become symptomatically ill with jaundice. The case-fatality rate among reported cases is about 0.6%.

Hepatitis A is primarily transmitted by person-to-person contact, generally through fecal contamination and oral ingestion. Transmission is facilitated by poor personal hygiene, poor sanitation, and intimate (intrahousehold or sexual) contact. In recent years, cases of hepatitis A among intravenous drug users, most likely due to person-to-person contact, have been reported with increasing frequency (9). Common-source epidemics from contaminated food and water also occur. Sharing utensils or cigarettes or kissing is not believed to transmit the hepatitis A virus.

The incubation period of hepatitis A is 15–50 days (average 28). High concentrations of HAV (10^8 particles/g) are found in stool specimens from infected persons. Virus in the feces reaches its highest concentration late in the incubation period and early in the prodromal phase of illness, and it diminishes rapidly once jaundice appears. Greatest infectivity is during the 2-week period immediately before the onset of jaundice. Viremia probably occurs during the period that the virus is shed in feces. Virus has not been found in urine. A chronic carrier state with HAV in blood or feces has not been demonstrated. Transmission of HAV by blood transfusion has been reported but is uncommon (10).

The diagnosis of acute hepatitis A is confirmed by finding IgM anti-HAV in serum collected during the acute or early convalescent phase of the disease. IgG anti-HAV, which appears in the convalescent phase of the disease and remains detectable in serum thereafter, confers enduring protection against the disease.

Commercial tests are available to detect IgM anti-HAV and total anti-HAV in serum.

Although the incidence of hepatitis A in the United States in the 1980s was lower than that in the 1970s, a 26% increase in incidence was observed between 1983 and 1988. It is still a common infection among older children and young adults. In 1988, 50% of reported cases of hepatitis in this country were attributable to hepatitis A.

Recommendations for IG Prophylaxis for Hepatitis A

Numerous field studies conducted in the past 4 decades confirm that IG given before exposure or during the incubation period of hepatitis A is protective against clinical illness (11–13). Its prophylactic value is greatest (80–90%) when given early in the incubation period and declines thereafter (13). Recent tests have shown slightly decreased titers of anti-HAV in current IG lots compared with lots tested 8 years previously; however, no differences in IG efficacy have been noted.

Preexposure Prophylaxis

The major group for whom preexposure prophylaxis is recommended is international travelers. The risk of hepatitis A for U.S. citizens traveling abroad varies with living conditions, length of stay, and the incidence of hepatitis A infection in areas visited (14–16). In general, travelers to developed areas of North America, Western Europe, Japan, Australia, and New Zealand are at no greater risk of infection than they would be in the United States. For travelers to developing countries, risk of infection increases with duration of travel and is highest for those who live in or visit rural areas, trek in back country, or frequently eat or drink in settings of poor sanitation. Nevertheless, recent studies have shown that many cases of travel-related hepatitis A occur in travelers with "standard" tourist itineraries, accommodations, and food and beverage consumption behaviors (16 and CDC, unpublished data). In developing countries, travelers should minimize their exposure to hepatitis A and other enteric diseases by avoiding potentially contaminated water or food. Travelers should avoid drinking water (or beverages with ice) of unknown purity and eating uncooked shellfish or uncooked fruits or vegetables that they did not prepare.

IG is recommended for all susceptible travelers to developing countries (17). IG is especially important for persons who will be living in or visiting rural areas, eating or drinking in settings of poor or uncertain sanitation, or who will have close contact with local persons (especially young children) in settings with poor sanitary conditions. Persons who plan to reside in developing areas for long periods should receive IG regularly.

For travelers, a single dose of IG of 0.02 ml/kg of body weight is recommended if travel is for <3 months. For prolonged travel or residence in developing countries, 0.06 ml/kg should be given every 5 months. For persons who require repeated IG prophylaxis, screening for total anti-HAV before travel is useful to define susceptibility and eliminate unnecessary doses of IG for those who are immune. IG produced in developing countries may not meet the standards for purity required in most developed countries. Persons needing repeat doses overseas should use products that meet U.S. license requirements.

Postexposure Prophylaxis

Hepatitis A cannot be reliably diagnosed on clinical presentation alone, and serologic confirmation of index patients is recommended before contacts are treated. Serologic screening of contacts for anti-HAV before they are given IG is not recommended because screening is more costly than IG and would delay its administration.

For postexposure IG prophylaxis, a single intramuscular dose of 0.02 ml/kg is recommended. IG should be given as soon as possible after last exposure; giving IG more than 2 weeks after exposure is not indicated.

Specific recommendations for IG prophylaxis for hepatitis A depend on the nature of the HAV exposure.

1. Close personal contact. IG is recommended for all household and sexual contacts of persons with hepatitis A.
2. Day-care centers. Day-care facilities attended by children in diapers can be important settings for HAV transmission (18–20). IG should be administered to all staff and attendees of day-care centers or homes if (a) one or more children or employee, are diagnosed as having hepatitis A, or (b) cases are recognized in two or more households of center attendees. When an outbreak (hepatitis cases in three or more families) occurs, IG should also be considered for members of households that have children (center attendees) in diapers. In centers not enrolling children in diapers, IG need only be given to classroom contacts of an index patient.
3. Schools. Contact at elementary and secondary schools is usually not an important means of transmitting hepatitis A. Routine administration of IG is not indicated for pupils and teachers in contact with a patient. However, when an epidemiologic investigation clearly shows the existence of a school- or classroom-centered outbreak, IG may be given to persons who have close contact with patients.
4. Institutions for custodial care. Living conditions in some institutions,

such as prisons and facilities for the developmentally disabled, favor transmission of hepatitis A. When outbreaks occur, giving IG to residents and staff who have close contact with patients with hepatitis A may reduce the spread of disease. Depending on the epidemiologic circumstances, prophylaxis can be limited or can involve the entire institution.

5. Hospitals. Routine IG prophylaxis for hospital personnel is not indicated. Rather, sound hygienic practices should be emphasized. Staff education should point out the risk of exposure to hepatitis A and should emphasize precautions regarding direct contact with potentially infective materials (21).

Outbreaks of hepatitis A occur occasionally among hospital staff, usually in association with an unsuspected index patient who is fecally incontinent. Large outbreaks have occurred from contact with infected infants in neonatal intensive care units (10). In outbreaks, prophylaxis of persons exposed to feces of infected patients may be indicated.

6. Offices and factories. Routine IG administration is not indicated under the usual office or factory conditions for persons exposed to a fellow worker with hepatitis A. Experience shows that casual contact in the work setting does not result in virus transmission.

7. Common-source exposure. IG use might be effective in preventing foodborne or waterborne hepatitis A if exposure is recognized in time. However, IG is not recommended for persons exposed to a common source of hepatitis infection after cases have begun to occur, since the 2-week period during which IG is effective will have been exceeded.

If a food handler is diagnosed as having hepatitis A, common-source transmission is possible but uncommon. IG should be administered to other food handlers but is usually not recommended for patrons (22). However, IG administration to patrons may be considered if all of the following conditions exist: (a) the infected person is directly involved in handling, without gloves, foods that will not be cooked before they are eaten, and (b) the hygienic practices of the food handler are deficient or the food handler has had diarrhea, and (c) patrons can be identified and treated within 2 weeks of exposure. Situations in which repeated exposures may have occurred, such as in institutional cafeterias, may warrant stronger consideration of IG use.

HEPATITIS B

Hepatitis B infection is caused by the hepatitis B virus (HBV), a 42-nm, double-shelled deoxyribonucleic acid (DNA) virus of the class hepadnaviridae. Several well-defined antigen-antibody systems are associated with HBV infection (Table F1). HBsAg is found on the surface of the virus and is also produced in excess amounts, circulating in blood as 22-nm spherical and tubular particles. HBsAg can be identified in serum 30–60 days after exposure to HBV and persists for variable periods. Anti-HBs develops after a resolved infection and is responsible for long-term immunity. Antibody to the core antigen (anti-HBc) develops in all HBV infections and persists indefinitely. IgM anti-HBc appears early in infection and persists for 6 months. It is a reliable marker of acute or recent HBV infection A third antigen, hepatitis B e antigen (HBeAg), may be detected in samples from persons with acute or chronic HBV infection. The presence of HBeAg correlates with viral replication and high infectivity. Antibody to HBeAg (anti-HBe) develops in most HBV infections and correlates with the loss of replicating virus and with lower infectivity.

The incubation period of hepatitis B is long (45–160 days; average, 120), and the onset of acute disease is generally insidious. Clinical symptoms and signs include anorexia, malaise, nausea, vomiting, abdominal pain, and jaundice. Extrahepatic manifestations of disease—such as skin rashes, arthralgias, and arthritis—can also occur. The case-fatality rate for reported cases is approximately 1.4%.

A variable proportion of individuals infected with HBV will become chronically infected with the virus. The HBV carrier is central to the epidemiology of HBV transmission. A carrier is defined as a person who is either HBsAg-positive on at least two occasions (at least 6 months apart) or who is HBsAg-positive and IgM anti-HBc negative when a single serum specimen is tested. Although the degree of infectivity is best correlated with HBeAg-positivity, any person positive for HBsAg is potentially infectious. The likelihood of becoming chronically infected with HBV varies inversely with the age at which infection occurs. HBV transmitted from HBsAg-positive mothers to their newborns results in HBV carriage for up to 90% of infants. Between 25% and 50% of children infected before 5 years of age become carriers, whereas only 6–10% of acutely infected adults become carriers.

Carriers and persons with acute infection have the highest concentrations of HBV in blood and serious fluids. A lower concentration is present in other body fluids, such as saliva and semen. Transmission occurs via percutaneous or permucosal routes, and infective blood or body fluids can be introduced at birth, through sexual contact, or by contaminated needles. Infection can also occur in settings of continuous close personal contact (such as in households or among children in institutions for the developmentally disabled), presumably via inapparent or unnoticed contact of infective secretions with skin lesions or mucosal surfaces. Transmission of infection by transfusion of blood or blood products is rare because of routine screening of blood for HBsAg and because of current donor selection procedures. Transmission of HBV from infected health-care workers to patients is uncommon but has been documented during types of

Table F1.   Hepatitis nomenclature

	Abbreviation	Term	Definition/comments
A. Hepatitis A	HAV	Hepatitis A virus	Etiologic agent of "infectious" hepatitis; a picornavirus; single serotype
	Anti-HAV	Antibody to HAV	Detectable at onset of symptoms; lifetime persistence.
	IgM anti-HAV	IgM class antibody to HAV	Indicates recent infection from hepatitis A; detectable for 4–6 months after infection.
B. Hepatitis B	HBV	Hepatitis B virus	Etiologic agent of "serum" hepatitis; also known as Dane particle.
	HBsAg	Hepatitis B surface antigen	Surface antigen(s) of HBV detectable in large quantity in serum; several subtypes identified.
	HBeAg	Hepatitis B e antigen	Soluble antigen; correlates with HBV replication, high titer HBV in serum, and infectivity or serum.
	HBcAg	Hepatitis B core antigen	No commercial test available.
	Anti-HBs	Antibody to HBsAg	Indicates past infection with an immmunity to HBV, passive antibody from HBIG, or immune response from HB vaccine.
	Anti-HBe	Antibody to HBeAg	Presence in serum of HBsAg carrier indicates lower titer of HBV.
	Anti-HBc	Antibody to HBcAg	Indicates prior infection with HBV at some unspecified time.
	IgM anti-HBc	IgM class antibody to HBcAg	Indicates prior infection with HBV; detectable for 4–6 months after infection.
C. Delta hepatitis	HDV	Hepatitis D virus	Etiologic agent of delta hepatitis; can cause infection only in presence of HBV.
	HDAg	Delta antigen	Detectable in early acute delta infection.
	Anti-HDV	Antibody to delta antigen	Indicates present or past infection with delta virus.

D. Non-A, non-B hepatitis	PT-NANB	Parenterally transmitted	Diagnosis by exclusion. At least two candidate viruses, one of which has been proposed as hepatitis C virus; shares epidemiologic features with hepatitis B.
	ET-NANB	Enterically transmitted	Diagnosis by exclusion. Causes large epidemics in Asia, Africa, and Mexico; fecal-oral or waterborne.
E. Immune globulins	IG	Immune globulin	Contains antibodies to HAV, low-titer antibodies to HBV. Previously called ISG, immune serum globulin, or gamma globulin.
	HBIG	Hepatitis B immune globulin	Contains high-titer antibodies to HBV.

invasive procedures (e.g., oral and gynecologic surgery) (23,24). HBsAg-positive health-care workers need not be restricted from patient contact unless they have been epidemiologically associated with HBV transmission. Rather, they should be educated about the potential mechanisms of HBV transmission. Adherence to aseptic techniques minimizes the risk of transmission. HBV is not transmitted via the fecal-oral route.

Worldwide, HBV infection is a major cause of acute and chronic hepatitis, cirrhosis, and primary hepatocellular carcinoma. The frequency of HBV infection and patterns of transmission vary markedly in different parts of the world. In the United States, Western Europe, and Australia, it is a disease of low endemicity, with infection occurring primarily during adulthood and with only 0.2–0.9% of the population being chronically infected. In contrast, HBV infection is highly endemic in China and Southeast Asia, most of Africa, most Pacific Islands, parts of the Middle East, and in the Amazon Basin. In these areas, most persons acquire infection at birth or during childhood, and 8–15% of the population are chronically infected with HBV. In other parts of the world, HBV infection is moderately endemic, with 2–7% of the population being HBV carriers. Prevention strategies for populations in which HBV infection is highly endemic are directed at vaccinating infants with hepatitis B vaccine, usually beginning at birth, to prevent both perinatal and childhood transmission of infection (25). Recommendations for hepatitis B prophylaxis in other areas should be designed to maximize the interruption of HBV transmission in accordance with local patterns of transmission. The recommendations that follow are intended for use in the United States.

Hepatitis B Virus Infection in the United States

Each year, an estimated 300,000 persons, primarily young adults, are infected with HBV. One-quarter become ill with jaundice, more than 10,000 patients require hospitalization, and an average of 250 die of fulminant disease. The United States currently contains an estimated pool of 750,000–1,000,000 infectious carriers. Approximately 25% of carriers develop chronic active hepatitis, which often progresses to cirrhosis. Furthermore, HBV carriers have a risk of developing primary liver cancer that is 12–300 times higher than that of other persons. An estimated 4,000 persons die each year from hepatitis B–related cirrhosis, and more than 800 die from hepatitis B–related liver cancer.

Serologic surveys demonstrate that, although HBV infection is uncommon among adults in the general population, it is highly prevalent in certain groups. Those at risk, based on the prevalence of serologic markers of infection, are described in Table F2. Persons born in areas of high HBV endemicity and their descendants remain at high risk of infection, as do certain populations in which HBV is highly endemic (Alaskan Natives and Pacific Islanders). Certain lifestyles (e.g., homosexual activity, intravenous drug abuse) result in early acquisition of HBV infection and high rates of infection. Persons who have heterosexual activity with multiple partners are at significant risk of infection. Inmates of prisons have a high prevalence of HBV markers, usually because of parenteral drug abuse before or during imprisonment. Patients in custodial institutions for the developmentally disabled are also at increased risk of having HBV infection. Household contacts and sexual partners of HBV carriers are at increased risk, as are hemodialysis patients and recipients of certain plasma-derived products that have not been inactivated (e.g., anti-hemophilic factor).

Those at occupational risk of HBV infection include medical and dental workers, related laboratory and support personnel, and public service employees who have contact with blood, as well as staff in institutions or classrooms for the mentally retarded.

Hepatitis B Prevention Strategies in the United States

The incidence of reported acute hepatitis B cases increased steadily over the past decade and reached a peak in 1985 (11.50 cases/10^5/year), despite the introduction of hepatitis B vaccine 3 years previously. Incidence decreased modestly (18%) by 1988, but still remains higher than a decade ago. This minimal impact of hepatitis B vaccine on disease incidence is attributable to several factors. The sources of infection for most cases include intravenous drug abuse (28%), heterosexual contact with infected persons or multiple partners (22%), and homosexual activity (9%). In addition, 30% of patients with hepatitis B deny any of the recognized risk factors for infection.

Table F2. Prevalence of hepatitis B serologic markers in various population groups

Population group	Prevalence of serologic markers of HBV infection	
	HBsAg (%)	Any marker (%)
Immigrants/refugees from areas of high HBV endemicity	13	70–85
Alaskan Natives/Pacific Islanders	5–15	40–70
Clients in institutions for the developmentally disabled	10–20	35–80
Users of illicit parenteral drugs	7	60–80
Sexually active homosexual men	6	35–80
Household contacts of HBV carriers	3–6	30–60
Patients of hemodialysis units	3–10	20–80
Health care workers—frequent blood contact	1–2	15–30
Prisoners (male)	1–8	10–80
Staff of institutions for the developmentally disabled	1	10–25
Heterosexuals with multiple partners	0.5	5–20
Health care workers—no or infrequent blood contact	0.3	3–10
General population (NHANES II)[a]		
Blacks	0.9	14
Whites	0.2	3

[a]Second National Health and Nutrition Examination Survey.

The present strategy for hepatitis B prevention is to vaccinate those individuals at high risk of infection. Most persons receiving vaccine as a result of this strategy have been persons at risk of acquiring HBV infection through occupational exposure, a group that accounts for approximately 4% of cases. The major deterrents to vaccinating the other high-risk groups include their lack of knowledge about the risk of disease and its consequences, the lack of public-sector programs, the cost of vaccine, and the inability to access most of the high-risk populations.

For vaccine to have an impact on the incidence of hepatitis B, a comprehensive strategy must be developed that will provide hepatitis B vaccination to persons before they engage in behaviors or occupations that place them at risk of infection. Universal HBsAg screening of pregnant women was recently recommended to prevent perinatal HBV transmission. The previous recommendations for selective screening failed to identify most HBsAg-positive pregnant women (22). As an alternative to high-risk group vaccination, universal vaccination of infants and adolescents needs to be examined as a possible strategy to control the transmission of disease.

Hepatitis B Prophylaxis

Two types of products are available for prophylaxis against hepatitis B. Hepatitis B vaccines, first licensed in 1981, provide active immunization against HBV infection, and their use is recommended for both preexposure and postexposure prophylaxis. HBIG provides temporary, passive protection and is indicated only in certain postexposure settings.

HBIG

HBIG is prepared from plasma preselected to contain a high titer of anti-HBs. In the United States, HBIG has an anti-HBs titer of >100,000 by radioimmunoassay (RIA). Human plasma from which HBIG is prepared is screened for antibodies to HIV, in addition, the Cohn fractionation process used to prepare this product inactivates and eliminates HIV from the final product. There is no evidence that the causative agent of AIDS (HIV) has been transmitted by HBIG (6).

Hepatitis B Vaccine

Two types of hepatitis B vaccines are currently licensed in the United States. Plasma-derived vaccine consists of a suspension of inactivated, alum-adsorbed, 22-nm, HBsAg particles that have been purified from human plasma by a combination of biophysical (ultracentrifugation) and biochemical procedures. Inactivation is a threefold process using 8M urea, pepsin at pH 2, and 1:4,000 formalin. These treatment steps have been shown to inactivate representatives of all classes of viruses found in human blood, including HIV (28). Plasma-derived vaccine is no longer being produced in the United States, and use is now limited to hemodialysis patients, other immunocompromised hosts, and persons with known allergy to yeast.

Currently licensed recombinant hepatitis B vaccines are produced by *Saccharomyces cerevisiae* (common baker's yeast), into which a plasmid containing the gene for the HBsAg has been inserted. Purified HBsAg is obtained by lysing the yeast cells and separating HBsAg from yeast components by biochemical and biophysical techniques. These vaccines contain more than 95% HBsAg protein. Yeast-derived protein constitutes no more than 5% of the final product.

Hepatitis B vaccines are packaged to contain 10–40 μg HBsAg protein/ml and are adsorbed with aluminum hydroxide (0.5mg/ml). Thimerosal (1:20,000 concentration) is added as a preservative.

The recommended series of three intramuscular doses of hepatitis B vaccine induces an adequate antibody response[2] in >90% of healthy adults and in 95% of infants, children, and adolescents from birth through 19 years of age (29–31). The deltoid (arm) is the recommended site for hepatitis B vaccination of adults and children; immunogenicity of vaccine for adults is substantially lower when injections are given in the buttock (32). Larger vaccine doses (two to four times normal adult dose) or an increased number of doses (four doses) are required to induce protective antibody in a high proportion of hemodialysis patients and may also be necessary for other immunocompromised persons (such as those on immunosuppressive drugs or with HIV infection) (33,34).

Field trials of the vaccines licensed in the United States have shown 80–95% efficacy in preventing infection or clinical hepatitis among susceptible persons (31,35). Protection against illness is virtually complete for persons who develop an adequate antibody response after vaccination. The duration of protection and need for booster doses are not yet fully defined. Between 30% and 50% of persons who develop adequate antibody after three doses of vaccine will lose detectable antibody within 7 years, but protection against viremic infection and clinical disease appears to persist (36–38). Immunogenicity and efficacy of the licensed vaccines for hemodialysis patients are much lower than in normal adults. Protection in this group may last only as long as adequate antibody levels persist (33).

Vaccine Usage

Primary vaccination comprises three intramuscular doses of vaccine, with the second and third doses given 1 and 6 months, respectively, after the first. Adults and older children should be given a full 1.0 ml/dose, while children <11 years of age should usually receive half (0.5 ml) this dose. See Table F3 for complete information on age-specific dosages of currently available vaccines. An alternative schedule of four doses of vaccine given at 0, 1, 2, and 12 months has been approved for one vaccine for postexposure prophylaxis or for more rapid induction of immunity. However, there is no clear evidence that this regimen provides greater protection than the standard three-dose series. Hepatitis B vaccine should

---

2. An adequate antibody level is 10 milliInternational Units (mIU)/ml, approximately equivalent to 10 sample ratio units (SRU) by RIA or positive by enzyme immunoassay (EIA), measured 1–6 months after completion of the vaccine series.

be given only in the deltoid muscle for adults and children or in the anterolateral thigh muscle for infants and neonates.

For patients undergoing hemodialysis and for other immunosuppressed patients, higher vaccine doses or increased numbers of doses are required. A special formulation of one vaccine is now available for such persons (Table F3). Persons with HIV infection have an impaired response to hepatitis B vaccine. The immunogenicity of higher doses of vaccine is unknown for this group, and firm recommendations on dosage cannot be made at this time (34).

Vaccine doses administered at longer intervals provide equally satisfactory protection, but optimal protection is not conferred until after the third dose. If the vaccine series is interrupted after the first dose, the second and third doses should be given separated by an interval of 3–5 months. Persons who are late for the third dose should be given this dose when convenient. Postvaccination testing is not considered necessary in either situation.

In one study, the response to vaccination by the standard schedule using one or two doses of one vaccine, followed by the remaining doses of a different vaccine, was comparable to the response to vaccination with a single vaccine.

Table F3. Recommended doses and schedules of currently licensed HB vaccines

	Vaccine					
	Heptavax-B[a,b]		Recombivax-HB[a]		Engerix-B[a,c]	
Group	Dose (µg)	(ml)	Dose (µg)	(ml)	Dose (µg)	(ml)
Infants of HBV-carrier mothers	10	(0.5)	5	(0.5)	10	(0.5)
Other infants and children < 11 years	10	(0.5)	2.5	(0.25)	10	(0.5)
Children and adolescents 11–19 years	20	(1.0)	5	(0.5)	20	(1.0)
Adults > 19 years	20	(1.0)	10	(1.0)	20	(1.0)
Dialysis patients and other immunocompromised persons	40	(2.0)[d]	40	(1.0)[e]	40	(2.0)[d,f]

[a]Usual schedule: three doses at 0, 1, 6 months

[b]Available only for hemodialysis and other immunocompromised patients and for persons with known allergy to yeast.

[c]Alternative schedule: four doses at 0, 1, 2, 12 months.

[d]Two 1.0 ml doses given at different sites.

[e]Special formulation for dialysis patients.

[f]Four-dose schedule recommended at 0, 1, 2, 6 months.

Moreover, because the immunogenicities of the available vaccines are similar, it is likely that responses in such situations will be comparable to those induced by any of the vaccines alone.

The immunogenicity of a series of three low doses (0.1 standard dose) of plasma-derived hepatitis B vaccine administered by the intradermal route has been assessed in several studies. The largest studies of adults show lower rates of developing adequate antibody (80–90%) and twofold to fourfold lower antibody titers than with intramuscular vaccination with recommended doses (39 and CDC, unpublished data). Data on immunogenicity of low doses of recombinant vaccines given intradermally are limited. At this time, intradermal vaccination of adults using low doses of vaccine should be done only under research protocol, with appropriate informed consent and with postvaccination testing to identify persons with inadequate response who would be eligible for revaccination. Intradermal vaccination is not recommended for infants or children.

All hepatitis B vaccines are inactivated (noninfective) products, and there is no evidence of interference with other simultaneously administered vaccines.

Data are not available on the safety of hepatitis B vaccines for the developing fetus. Because the vaccines contain only noninfectious HBsAg particles, there should be no risk to the fetus. In contrast, HBV infection of a pregnant woman may result in severe disease for the mother and chronic infection of the newborn. Therefore, pregnancy or lactation should not be considered a contraindication to the use of this vaccine for persons who are otherwise eligible.

Vaccine storage and shipment

Vaccine should be shipped and stored at 2–8°C but not frozen. *Freezing destroys the potency of the vaccine.*

Side effects and adverse reactions

The most common side effect observed following vaccination with each of the available vaccines has been soreness at the injection site. Postvaccination surveillance for 3 years after licensure of the plasma-derived vaccine showed an association of borderline significance between Guillain-Barré syndrome and receipt of the first vaccine dose (40). The rate of this occurrence was very low (0.5/100,000 vaccines) and was more than compensated by disease prevented by the vaccine even if Guillain-Barré syndrome is a true side effect. Such postvaccination surveillance information is not available for the recombinant hepatitis B vaccines. Early concerns about safety of plasma-derived vaccine have proven to be unfounded, particularly the concern that infectious agents such as HIV present in the donor plasma pools might contaminate the final product.

Effect of vaccination on carriers and immune persons

Hepatitis B vaccine produces neither therapeutic nor adverse effects for HBV carriers (41). Vaccination of individuals who possess antibodies against HBV from a previous infection is not necessary but will not cause adverse effects. Such individuals will have a postvaccination increase in their anti-HBs levels. Passively acquired antibody, whether acquired from HBIG or IG administration or from the transplacental route, will not interfere with active immunization (42).

Prevaccination serologic testing for susceptibility

The decision to test potential vaccine recipients for prior infection is primarily a cost-effectiveness issue and should be based on whether the costs of testing balance the costs of vaccine saved by not vaccinating individuals who have already been infected. Estimation of cost-effectiveness of testing depends on three variables: the cost of vaccination, the cost of testing for susceptibility, and the expected prevalence of immune individuals in the group.

Testing in groups with the highest risk of HBV infection (HBV marker prevalence >20%, Table F2) is usually cost-effective unless testing costs are extremely high. Cost-effectiveness of screening may be marginal for groups at intermediate risk. For groups with a low expected prevalence of HBV serologic markers, such as health professionals in their training years, prevaccination testing is not cost-effective.

For routine testing, only one antibody test is necessary (either anti-HBc or anti-HBs). Anti-HBc identifies all previously infected persons, both carriers and those who are not carriers, but does not differentiate members of the two groups. Anti-HBs identifies persons previously infected, except for carriers. Neither test has a particular advantage for groups expected to have carrier rates of <2%, such as health-care workers. Anti-HBc may be preferred to avoid unnecessary vaccination of carriers for groups with higher carrier rates. If RIA is used to test for anti-HBs, a minimum of 10 sample ratio units should be used to designate immunity (2.1 is the usual designation of a positive test). If EIA is used, the positive level recommended by manufacturers is appropriate.

Postvaccination testing for serologic response and revaccination of nonresponders

Hepatitis B vaccine, when given in the deltoid, produces protective antibody (anti-HBs) in >90% of healthy persons. Testing for immunity after vaccination is not recommended routinely but is advised for persons whose subsequent management depends on knowing their immune status (such as dialysis patients and staff). Testing for immunity is also advised for persons for whom a suboptimal response may be anticipated, such as those who have received vaccine in the buttock, persons ≥50 years of age, and persons known to have HIV infection. Postvaccination testing should also be considered for persons at occupational risk who may have needlestick exposures necessitating postexposure prophylaxis. When necessary, postvaccination testing should be done between 1 and 6 months after completion of the vaccine series to provide definitive information on response to the vaccine.

Revaccination of persons who do not respond to the primary series (nonresponders) produces adequate antibody in 15–25% after one additional dose and in 30–50% after three additional doses when the primary vaccination has been given in the deltoid (36). For persons who did not respond to a primary vaccine series given in the buttock, data suggest that revaccination in the arm induces adequate antibody in >75%. Revaccination with one or more additional doses should be considered for persons who fail to respond to vaccination in the deltoid and is recommended for those who have failed to respond to vaccination in the buttock.

Need for vaccine booster doses

Available data show that vaccine-induced antibody levels decline steadily with time and that up to 50% of adult vaccinees who respond adequately to vaccine may have low or undetectable antibody levels by 7 years after vaccination. Nevertheless, both adults and children with declining antibody levels are still protected against hepatitis B disease. Current data also suggest excellent protection against disease for 5 years after vaccination among infants born to hepatitis B–carrier mothers. For adults and children with normal immune status, booster doses are not routinely recommended within 7 years after vaccination, nor is routine serologic testing to assess antibody levels necessary for vaccine recipients during this period. For infants born to hepatitis B–carrier mothers, booster doses are not necessary within 5 years after vaccination. The possible need for booster doses after longer intervals will be assessed as additional information becomes available.

For hemodialysis patients, for whom vaccine-induced protection is less complete and may persist only as long as antibody levels remain above 10 mIU/ml, the need for booster doses should be assessed by annual antibody testing, and booster doses should be given when antibody levels decline to <10 mIU/ml.

Groups recommended for preexposure vaccination

Persons at substantial risk of HBV infection who are demonstrated or judged likely to be susceptible should be vaccinated. They include the following:

  1. Persons with occupational risk. HBV infection is a major infectious occupational hazard for health-care and public-safety workers. The risk

of acquiring HBV infection from occupational exposures is dependent on the frequency of percutaneous and permucosal exposures to blood or blood products. Any health-care or public-safety worker may be at risk for HBV exposure depending on the tasks that he or she performs. If those tasks involve contact with blood or blood-contaminated body fluids, such workers should be vaccinated. Vaccination should be considered for other workers depending on the nature of the task (43).

Risks among health-care professionals vary during the training and working career of each individual but are often highest during the professional training period. For this reason, when possible, vaccination should be completed during training in schools of medicine, dentistry, nursing, laboratory technology, and other allied health professions before workers have their first contact with blood.

2. Clients and staff of institutions for the developmentally disabled. Susceptible clients in institutions for the developmentally disabled should be vaccinated. Staff who work closely with clients should also be vaccinated. The risk in institutional environments is associated not only with blood exposure but may also be consequent to bites and contact with skin lesions and other infective secretions. Susceptible clients and staff who live or work in smaller (group) residential settings with known HBV carriers should also receive hepatitis B vaccine. Clients discharged from residential institutions into community settings should be screened for HBsAg so that the community programs may take appropriate measures to prevent HBV transmission. These measures should include both environmental controls and appropriate use of vaccine

Staff of nonresidential day-care programs (e.g., schools, sheltered workshops for the developmentally disabled) attended by known HBV carriers have a risk of HBV infection comparable to that among health-care workers and therefore should be vaccinated (44). The risk of HBV infection for clients appears to be lower than the risk for staff. Vaccination of clients in day-care programs may be considered. Vaccination of classroom contacts is strongly encouraged if a classmate who is an HBV carrier behaves aggressively or has special medical problems that increase the risk of exposure to his/her blood or serous secretions.

3. Hemodialysis patients. Hepatitis B vaccination is recommended for susceptible hemodialysis patients. Although seroconversion rates and anti-HBs titers are lower than those for healthy persons, for those patients who do respond, hepatitis B vaccine will protect them from HBV infection and reduce the necessity for frequent serologic screening (45). Some studies have shown higher seroconversion rates and antibody titers for patients with uremia who were vaccinated before they required dialysis (46). Identification of patients for vaccination early in the course of their renal disease is encouraged.

4. Sexually active homosexual men. Susceptible sexually active homosexual men should be vaccinated regardless of their age or the duration of their homosexual practices. Persons should be vaccinated as soon as possible after their homosexual activity begins. Homosexual and bisexual men known to have HIV infection should be tested for anti-HBs response after completion of the vaccine series and should be counseled accordingly.

5. Users of illicit injectable drugs. All users of illicit injectable drugs who are susceptible to HBV should be vaccinated as early as possible after their drug abuse begins.

6. Recipients of certain blood products. Patients with clotting disorders who receive clotting-factor concentrates have an increased risk of HBV infection. Vaccination is recommended for these persons, and it should be initiated at the time their specific clotting disorder is identified. Prevaccination testing is recommended for patients who have already received multiple infusions of these products.

7. Household and sexual contacts of HBV carriers. Household contacts of HBV carriers are at high risk of HBV infection. Sexual contacts appear to be at greatest risk. When HBV carriers are identified through routine screening of donated blood, diagnostic testing in hospitals, prenatal screening, screening of refugees from certain areas, or other screening programs, they should be notified of their status. All household and sexual contacts should be tested and susceptible contacts vaccinated.

8. Adoptees from countries of high HBV endemicity. Families accepting orphans or unaccompanied minors from countries of high or intermediate HBV endemicity should have the children screened for HBsAg. If the children are HBsAg-positive, family members should be vaccinated (47).

9. Other contacts of HBV carriers. Persons in casual contact with carriers in settings such as schools and offices are at minimal risk of HBV infection, and vaccine is not routinely recommended for them. At child-care centers, HBV transmission between children or between children and staff has rarely been documented. Unless special circumstances exist, such as behavior problems (biting or scratching) or medical conditions (severe skin disease) that might facilitate transmission, vaccination of contacts of carriers in child care is not indicated.

10. Populations with high endemicity of HBV infection. In certain U.S. populations, including Alaskan Natives, Pacific Islanders, and refugees from HBV-endemic areas, HBV infection is highly endemic, and transmission occurs primarily during childhood. In such groups, universal hepatitis B vaccination of infants is recommended to prevent disease transmission during childhood. In addition, more extensive programs of "catch-up" childhood vaccination should be considered if resources are available.

Immigrants and refugees from areas with highly endemic HBV disease (particularly Africa and eastern Asia) should be screened for HBV markers upon resettlement in the United States. If an HBV carrier is identified, all susceptible household contacts should be vaccinated. Even if no HBV carriers are found within a family, vaccination should be considered for susceptible children <7 years of age because of the high rate of interfamilial HBV infection that occurs among these children (48). Vaccination is recommended for all infants of women who were born in areas in which infection is highly endemic.

11. Inmates of long-term correctional facilities. The prison environment may provide a favorable setting for the transmission of HBV because of the use of illicit injectable drugs and because of male homosexual practices. Moreover, it provides an access point for vaccination of percutaneous drug abusers. Prison officials should consider undertaking screening and vaccination programs directed at inmates with histories of high-risk behaviors.

12. Sexually active heterosexual persons. Sexually active heterosexual persons with multiple sexual partners are at increased risk of HBV infection. Risk increases with increasing numbers of sexual partners. Vaccination is recommended for persons who are diagnosed as having recently acquired other sexually transmitted diseases, for prostitutes, and for persons who have a history of sexual activity with multiple partners in the previous 6 months.

13. International travelers. Vaccination should be considered for persons who plan to reside for more than 6 months in areas with high levels of endemic HBV and who will have close contact with the local population. Vaccination should also be considered for short-term travelers who are likely to have contact with blood from or sexual contact with residents of areas with high levels of endemic disease. Ideally, hepatitis B vaccination of travelers should begin at least 6 months before travel to allow for completion of the full vaccine series. Nevertheless, a partial series will offer some protection from HBV infection. The alternative four-dose schedule may provide better protection during travel if the first three doses can be delivered before travel (second and third doses given 1 and 2 months, respectively, after first).

Postexposure Prophylaxis for Hepatitis B

Prophylactic treatment to prevent hepatitis B infection after exposure to HBV should be considered in the following situations: perinatal exposure of an infant born to an HBsAg-positive mother, accidental percutaneous or permucosal exposure to HBsAg-positive blood, sexual exposure to an HBsAg-positive person, and household exposure of an infant <12 months of age to a primary care giver who has acute hepatitis B.

Various studies have established the relative efficacies of HBIG and/or hepatitis B vaccine in different exposure situations. For an infant with perinatal exposure to an HBsAg-positive and HBeAg-positive mother, a regimen combining one dose of HBIG at birth with the hepatitis B vaccine series started soon after birth is 85–95% effective in preventing development of the HBV carrier state (35,49–51). Regimens involving either multiple doses of HBIG alone, or the vaccine series alone, have 70–85% efficacy (52,53).

For accidental percutaneous exposure, only regimens including HBIG and/or IG have been studied. A regimen of two doses of HBIG, one given after exposure and one a month later, is about 75% effective in preventing hepatitis B in this setting (54,55). For sexual exposure, a single dose of HBIG is 75% effective if given within 2 weeks of last sexual exposure (56). The efficacy of IG for postexposure prophylaxis is uncertain. IG no longer has a role in postexposure prophylaxis of hepatitis B because of the availability of HBIG and the wider use of hepatitis B vaccine.

Recommendations on postexposure prophylaxis are based on available efficacy data and on the likelihood of future HBV exposure of the person requiring treatment. In all exposures, a regimen combining HBIG with hepatitis B vaccine will provide both short- and long-term protection, will be less costly than the two-dose HBIG treatment alone, and is the treatment of choice.

Perinatal Exposure and Recommendations

Transmission of HBV from mother to infant during the perinatal period represents one of the most efficient modes of HBV infection and often leads to severe long-term sequelae. Infants born to HBsAg-positive and HBeAg-positive mothers have a 70–90% chance of acquiring perinatal HBV infection, and 85–90% of infected infants will become chronic HBV carriers. Estimates are that >25% of these carriers will die from primary hepatocellular carcinoma (PHC) or cirrhosis of the liver (57). Infants born to HBsAg-positive and HBeAg-negative mothers have a lower risk of acquiring perinatal infection; however, such infants have had acute disease, and fatal fulminant hepatitis has been reported (58,59). Based on 1987 data in the United States, an estimated 18,000 births occur to HBsAg-positive women each year, resulting in approximately 4,000 infants who become chronic HBV carriers. Prenatal screening of all pregnant women identifies those who are HBsAg-positive and allows treatment of their newborns with HBIG and hepatitis B vaccine, a regimen that is 85–95% effective in preventing the development of the HBV chronic carrier state.

The following are perinatal recommendations:

1. All pregnant women should be routinely tested for HBsAg during an early prenatal visit in each pregnancy. This testing should be done at the same time that other routine prenatal screening tests are ordered. In special situations (e.g., when acute hepatitis is suspected, when a history of exposure to hepatitis has been reported, or when the mother has a particularly high-risk behavior, such as intravenous drug abuse), an additional HBsAg test can be ordered later in the pregnancy. No other HBV marker tests are necessary for the purpose of maternal screening, although HBsAg-positive mothers identified during screening may have HBV-related acute or chronic liver disease and should be evaluated by their physicians.

2. If a woman has not been screened prenatally or if test results are not available at the time of admission for delivery, HBsAg testing should be done at the time of admission, or as soon aş possible thereafter. If the mother is identified as HBsAg-positive 1 month after giving birth, the infant should be tested for HBsAg. If the results are negative, the infant should be given HBIG and hepatitis B vaccine.

3. Following all initial positive tests for HBsAg, a repeat test for HBsAg should be performed on the same specimen, followed by a confirmatory test using a neutralization assay. For women in labor who did not have HBsAg testing during pregnancy and who are found to be HBsAg-positive on first testing, initiation of treatment of their infants should not be delayed by more than 24 hours for repeat or confirmatory testing.

4. Infants born to HBsAg-positive mothers should receive HBIG (0.5 ml) intramuscularly once they are physiologically stable, preferably within 12 hours of birth (Table F4). Hepatitis B vaccine should be administered intramuscularly at the appropriate infant dose. The first dose should be given concurrently with HBIG but at a different site. If vaccine is not immediately available, the first dose should be given as soon as possible. Subsequent doses should be given as recommended for the specific vaccine. Testing infants for HBsAg and anti-HBs is recommended when they are 12–15 months of age to monitor the success or failure of therapy. If HBsAg is not detectable and anti-HBs is present, children can be considered protected. Testing for anti-HBc is not useful, since maternal anti-HBc can persist for >1 year. HBIG and hepatitis B vaccination do not interfere with routine childhood vaccinations. Breast-feeding poses no risk of HBV infection for infants who have begun prophylaxis.

5. Household members and sexual partners of HBV carriers identified through prenatal screening should be tested to determine susceptibility to HBV infection, and, if susceptible, should receive hepatitis B vaccine.

6. Obstetric and pediatric staff should be notified directly about HBsAg-

Table F4.   Hepatitis B virus postexposure recommendations

Exposure	HBIG		Vaccine	
	Dose	Recommended timing	Dose	Recommended timing
Perinatal	0.5 ml IM	Within 12 hours of birth	0.5 ml IM[a]	Within 12 hours of birth[b]
Sexual	0.06 ml/kg IM	Single dose within 14 days of last sexual contact	1.0 ml IM[a]	First dose at time of HBIG treatment[b]

[a]For appropriate age-specific doses of each vaccine, see Table F3.

[b]The first dose can be given the same time as the HBIG dose but in a different site; subsequent doses should be given as recommended for specific vaccine.

positive mothers so that neonates can receive therapy without delay after birth and follow-up doses of vaccine can be given. Programs to coordinate the activities of persons providing prenatal care, hospital-based obstetrical services, and pediatric well-baby care must be established to assure proper follow-up and treatment both of infants born to HBsAg-positive mothers and of other susceptible household and sexual contacts.

7. In those populations under U.S. jurisdiction in which hepatitis B infection is highly endemic (including certain Alaskan Natives, Pacific Island groups, and refugees from highly endemic areas accepted for resettlement in the United States), universal vaccination of newborns with hepatitis B vaccine is the recommended strategy for hepatitis B control. HBsAg screening of mothers and use of HBIG for infants born to HBV-carrier mothers may be added to routine hepatitis B vaccination when practical, but screening and HBIG alone will not adequately protect children from HBV infection in endemic areas. In such areas, hepatitis B vaccine doses should be integrated into the childhood vaccination schedule. More extensive programs of childhood hepatitis B vaccination should be considered if resources are available.

Acute Exposure to Blood That Contains (or Might Contain) HBsAg

For accidental percutaneous (needlestick, laceration, or bite) or permucosal (ocular or mucous membrane) exposure to blood, the decision to provide prophylaxis must include consideration of several factors: (a) whether the source of the blood is available, (b) the HBsAg status of the source, and (c) the hepatitis B vaccination and vaccine-response status of the exposed person. Such exposures usually affect persons for whom hepatitis B vaccine is recommended. For any exposure of a person not previously vaccinated, hepatitis B vaccination is recommended.

Following any such exposure, a blood sample should be obtained from the person who was the source of the exposure and should be tested for HBsAg. The hepatitis B vaccination status and anti-HBs response status (if known) of the exposed person should be reviewed. The outline below and Table F5 summarize prophylaxis for percutaneous or permucosal exposure to blood according to the HBsAg status of the source of exposure and the vaccination status and vaccine response of the exposed person.

Table F5. Recommendations for hepatitis B prophylaxis following percutaneous or permucosal exposure

Exposed person	Treatment when source is found to be:		
	HBsAg-positive	HBsAg-negative	Source not tested or unknown
Unvaccinated	HBIG × 1[a] and initiate HB vaccine[b]	Initiate HB vaccine[b]	Initiate HB vaccine[b]
Previously vaccinated, known responder	Test exposed for anti-HBs 1. If adequate,[c] no treatment 2. If inadequate, HB vaccine booster dose	No treatment	No treatment
Known nonresponder	HBIG × 2 or HBIG × 1 plus 1 dose HB vaccine	No treatment	If known high-risk source, may treat as if source were HBsAg-positive
Response unknown	Test exposed for anti-HBs 1. If inadequate,[c] HBIG × 1 plus HB vaccine booster dose 2. If adequate, no treatment	No treatment	Test exposed for anti-HBs 1. If inadequate,[c] HB vaccine booster dose 2. If adequate, no treatment

[a]HBIG dose 0.06ml/kg IM.

[b]HB vaccine dose—see Table F3.

[c]Adequate anti-HBs is ≥10 SRU by RIA or positive by EIA.

For greatest effectiveness, passive prophylaxis with HBIG, when indicated, should be given as soon as possible after exposure (its value beyond 7 days after exposure is unclear).

1. Source of exposure HBsAg-positive

   a. Exposed person has not been vaccinated or has not completed vaccination. Hepatitis B vaccination should be initiated. A single dose of HBIG (0.06 ml/kg) should be given as soon as possible after exposure and within 24 hours, if possible. The first dose of hepatitis B vaccine (Table F3) should be given intramuscularly at a separate site (deltoid for adults) and can be given simultaneously with HBIG or within 7 days of exposure. Subsequent doses should be given as recommended for the specific vaccine. If the exposed person has begun but not completed vaccination, one dose of HBIG should be given immediately, and vaccination should be completed as scheduled.

   b. Exposed person has already been vaccinated against hepatitis B, and anti-HBs response status is known.

      (1) If the exposed person is known to have had adequate response in the past, the anti-HBs level should be tested unless an adequate level has been demonstrated within the last 24 months. Although current data show that vaccine-induced protection does not decrease as antibody level wanes, most experts consider the following approach to be prudent:

         a) If anti-HBs level is adequate, no treatment is necessary.

         b) If anti-HBs level is inadequate,[3] a booster dose of hepatitis B vaccine should be given.

      (2) If the exposed person is known not to have responded to the primary vaccine series, the exposed person should be given either a single dose of HBIG and a dose of hepatitis B vaccine as soon as possible after exposure, or two doses of HBIG (0.06 ml/kg), one given as soon as possible after exposure and the second 1 month later. The latter treatment is preferred for those who have failed to respond to at least four doses of vaccine.

   c. Exposed person has already been vaccinated against hepatitis B, and the anti-HBs response is unknown. The exposed person should be tested for anti-HBs.

      (1) If the exposed person has adequate antibody, no additional treatment is necessary.

      (2) If the exposed person has inadequate antibody on testing, one

---

3. An adequate antibody response is 10 milliInternational Units (mIU)/ml, approximately equivalent to 10 sample ratio units (SRU) by RIA or positive by EIA.

dose of HBIG (0.06 ml/kg) should be given immediately and a standard booster dose of vaccine (Table F3) given at a different site.

2. Source of exposure known and HBsAg-negative

   a. Exposed person has not been vaccinated or has not completed vaccination. If unvaccinated, the exposed person should be given the first dose of hepatitis B vaccine within 7 days of exposure, and vaccination should be completed as recommended. If the exposed person has not completed vaccination, vaccination should be completed as scheduled.

   b. Exposed person has already been vaccinated against hepatitis B. No treatment is necessary.

3. Source of exposure unknown or not available for testing

   a. Exposed person has not been vaccinated or has not completed vaccination. If unvaccinated, the exposed person should be given the first dose of hepatitis B vaccine within 7 days of exposure and vaccination completed as recommended. If the exposed person has not completed vaccination, vaccination should be completed as scheduled.

   b. Exposed person has already been vaccinated against hepatitis B, and anti-HBs response status is known.

      (1) If the exposed person is known to have had adequate response in the past, no treatment is necessary.

      (2) If the exposed person is known not to have responded to the vaccine, prophylaxis as described earlier in section 1.b.(2) under "Source of exposure HBsAg-positive" may be considered if the source of the exposure is known to be at high risk of HBV infection.

   c. Exposed person has already been vaccinated against hepatitis B, and the anti-HBs response is unknown. The exposed person should be tested for anti-HBs.

      (1) If the exposed person has adequate anti-HBs, no treatment is necessary.

      (2) If the exposed person has inadequate anti-HBs, a standard booster dose of vaccine should be given.

Sexual Partners of Persons with Acute HBV Infection

Sexual partners of HBsAg-positive persons are at increased risk of acquiring HBV infection, and HBIG has been shown to be 75% effective in preventing such infections (56). Because data are limited, the period after sexual exposure during which HBIG is effective is unknown, but extrapolation from other settings makes it unlikely that this period would exceed 14 days. Before treatment, testing of sexual partners for susceptibility is recommended if it does not delay treatment beyond 14 days after last exposure. Testing for anti-HBc is the most efficient prescreening test to use in this population.

All susceptible persons whose sexual partners have acute hepatitis B infection or whose sexual partners are discovered to be hepatitis A carriers should receive a single dose of HBIG (0.06 ml/kg) and should begin the hepatitis B vaccine series if prophylaxis can be started within 14 days of the last sexual contact, or if ongoing sexual contact with the infected person will occur. Giving the vaccine with HBIG may improve the efficacy of postexposure treatment. The vaccine has the added advantage of conferring long-lasting protection.

An alternative treatment for persons who are not from a high-risk group for whom vaccine is routinely recommended and whose regular sexual partners have acute HBV infection is to give one dose of HBIG (without vaccine) and retest the sexual partner for HBsAg 3 months later. No further treatment is necessary if the sexual partner becomes HBsAg-negative. If the sexual partner remains HBsAg-positive, a second dose of HBIG should be given and the hepatitis B vaccine series started.

Household Contacts of Persons with Acute HBV Infection

Since infants have close contact with primary care givers and they have a higher risk of becoming HBV carriers after acute HBV infection, prophylaxis of an infant <12 months of age with HBIG (0.5 ml) and hepatitis B vaccine is indicated if the mother or primary care giver has acute HBV infection. Prophylaxis for other household contacts of persons with acute HBV infection is not indicated unless they have had identifiable blood exposure to the index patient, such as by sharing toothbrushes or razors. Such exposures should be treated similarly to sexual exposures. If the index patient becomes an HBV carrier, all household contacts should be given hepatitis B vaccine.

DELTA HEPATITIS

The delta virus (also known as hepatitis D virus [HDV]) is a defective virus that may cause infection only in the presence of active HBV infection. The HDV is a 35- to 37-nm viral particle, consisting of single-stranded RNA (mw 500,000) and an internal protein antigen (delta antigen [HDAg]), coated with HBsAg as the surface protein (5). Infection may occur as either coinfection with HBV or superinfection of an HBV carrier, each of which usually causes an episode of clinical acute hepatitis. Coinfection usually resolves, whereas superinfection frequently causes chronic HDV infection and chronic active hepatitis. Both types of infection may cause fulminant hepatitis.

HDV infection may be diagnosed by detecting HDAg in serum during early infection and by the appearance of total or IgM-specific delta antibody (anti-HDV) during or after infection. A test for detection of total anti-HDV is commercially available. Other tests (HDAg, IgM anti-HDV) are available only in research laboratories.

Routes of transmission of HDV are similar to those of HBV. In the United States, HDV infection most commonly affects persons at high risk of HBV infection, particularly parenteral drug abusers and persons with hemophilia.

Since HDV is dependent on HBV for replication, prevention of hepatitis B infection, either preexposure or postexposure, will suffice to prevent HDV infection for a person susceptible to hepatitis B. Known episodes of perinatal, sexual, or percutaneous exposure to serum or exposure to persons known to be positive for both HBV and HDV should be treated exactly as such exposures to HBV alone.

Persons who are HBsAg carriers are at risk of HDV infection, especially if they participate in activities that put them at high risk of repeated exposure to HBV (parenteral drug abuse, male homosexual activity). However, at present no products are available that might prevent HDV infection in HBsAg carriers either before or after exposure.

NON-A, NON-B HEPATITIS

Parenterally Transmitted (PT) Non-A, Non-B Hepatitis

Parenterally transmitted non-A, non-B hepatitis accounts for 20–40% of acute viral hepatitis in the United States and has epidemiologic characteristics similar to those of hepatitis B (60). Recently, a portion of the genome of a virus thought to be responsible for PT non-A, non-B hepatitis was cloned (2). A candidate serologic assay for antibody to this virus (proposed as hepatitis C virus) has been developed. This assay appears to detect a substantial number of persons with chronic infection and is being evaluated for screening potential blood donors (3). Although PT non-A, non-B hepatitis has traditionally been considered a transfusion-associated disease, most reported cases have not been associated with blood transfusion (61–64). Groups at high risk of acquiring this disease include transfusion recipients, parenteral drug users, and dialysis patients (62,63). Health-care work that entails frequent contact with blood, personal contact with others who have had hepatitis in the past, and contact with infected persons within households have also been documented in some studies as risk factors for acquiring PT non-A, non-B hepatitis (63–65). However, the role of person-to-person contact in disease transmission has not been well defined, and the importance of sexual activity in the transmission of this type of hepatitis is unclear.

Multiple episodes of non-A, non-B hepatitis have been observed among the same individuals and may be due to different bloodborne agents. An average of 50% of patients who have acute PT non-A, non-B hepatitis infection later develop chronic hepatitis (66). Experimental studies of chimpanzees have confirmed the existence of a carrier state, which may be present in 1–3% of the population (67,68).

The risk and consequences of perinatal transmission of PT non-A, non-B hepatitis are not well defined. Only one small study has been published in which infants born of 12 women who had acute PT non-A, non-B hepatitis during pregnancy were followed. Six infants developed transient alanine aminotransferase (ALT) elevations at 4–8 weeks of age (69).

The results have been equivocal in several studies attempting to assess the value of prophylaxis with IGs against PT non-A, non-B hepatitis (70–72). For persons with percutaneous exposure to blood from a patient with PT non-A, non-B hepatitis, it may be reasonable to administer IG (0.06 ml/kg) as soon as possible after exposure. In other circumstances, no specific recommendations can be made.

Enterically Transmitted (ET) Non-A, Non-B Hepatitis

A distinct type of non-A, non-B hepatitis acquired by the fecal-oral route was first identified through investigations of large waterborne epidemics in developing countries. This ET non-A, non-B hepatitis, which has occurred in epidemics or sporadically in parts of Asia, North and West Africa, and Mexico, is serologically distinct from other known hepatitis viruses (4,73). Young to middle-aged adults are most often affected, with an unusually high mortality among pregnant women. The disease has been transmitted to experimental animals, and candidate viruses have been identified; however, no serologic tests have yet been developed (74).

ET non-A, non-B hepatitis has not been recognized as an endemic disease in the United States or Western Europe, and it is unknown whether the causative agent is present in these areas. Cases have been documented, however, among persons returning from travel to countries in which this disease occurs (75).

Travelers to areas having ET non-A, non-B hepatitis may be at some risk of acquiring this disease by close contact with infected persons or by consuming contaminated food or water. There is no evidence that U.S.-manufactured IG will prevent this infection. As with hepatitis A and other enteric infections, the best

238 THE BLOODBORNE PATHOGENS STANDARD

means of preventing ET non-A, non-B hepatitis is avoiding potentially contaminated food or water.

REFERENCES

1. Francis DP, Maynard JE. The transmission and outcome of hepatitis A, B, and non-A, non-B: a review. *Epidemiol Rev* 1979;1:17–31.
2. Choo Q-L, Kuo G, Weiner AJ, et al. Isolation of a cDNA clone derived from a blood-borne non-A, non-B hepatitis genome. *Science* 1989;244:359–62.
3. Kuo G, Choo Q-L, Alter HJ, et al. An assay for circulating antibodies to a major etiologic virus of human non-A, non-B hepatitis. *Science* 1989;244:362–4.
4. Ramalingaswami V, Purcell RH. Waterborne non-A, non-B hepatitis. *Lancet* 1988;1:571–3.
5. Rizzetto M. The delta agent. *Hematology* 1983;3:729–37.
6. CDC. Safety of therapeutic immune globulin preparations with respect to transmission of human T-lymphotropic virus type III/lymphadenopathy-associated virus infection. *MMWR* 1986;35:231–3.
7. Wells MA, Wittek AE, Epstein JS, et al. Inactivation and partition of human T-cell lymphotropic virus, type III, during ethanol fractionation of plasma. *Transfusion* 1986;26:210–3.
8. Tedder RS, Uttley A, Cheingsong-Popov R. Safety of immunoglobulin preparation containing anti-HTLV-III [Letter]. *Lancet* 1985:1:815.
9. CDC. Hepatitis A among drug abusers. *MMWR* 1988;37:297–300,305.
10. Noble RC, Kane MA, Reeves SA, et al. Posttransfusion hepatitis A in a neonatal intensive care unit. *JAMA* 1984;252:2711–5.
11. Kluge I. Gamma-globulin in the prevention of viral hepatitis a study of the effect of medium-site doses. *Acta Med Scand* 1963;174:469–77.
12. Stokes J Jr, Neefe JR. Prevention and attenuation of infectious hepatitis by gamma globulin: preliminary note. *JAMA* 1945;127:144–5.
13. Mosley JW, Reisler DM, Brachott D, Roth D, Weiser J. Comparison of two lots of immune serum globulin for prophylaxis of infectious hepatitis *Am J Epidemiol* 1968;87:539–50.
14. Woodson RD, Cahill KM. Viral hepatitis abroad. Incidence in Catholic missionaries. *JAMA* 1971;219:1191–3.
15. Woodson RD, Clinton JJ. Hepatitis prophylaxis abroad. Effectiveness of immune serum globulin in protecting Peace Corps volunteers. *JAMA* 1969;209:1053–8.
16. Steffen R, Rickenbach M, Wilhelm U, Helminger A, Schar M. Health problems after travel to developing countries. *J Infect Dis* 1987;156:84–91.
17. CDC. *Health information for international travel 1989.* Atlanta: CDC, 1989; HHS publication no. (CDC) 89–8280.

18. Storch G, McFarland LM, Kelso K, Heilman CJ. Caraway CT. Viral hepatitis associated with day-care centers. *JAMA* 1979;242:1514–8.
19. Hadler SC, Webster HM, Erben JJ, Swanson JE, Maynard JE. Hepatitis A in day-care centers: a community-wide assessment. *N Engl J Med* 1980;302:1222–7.
20. Hadler SC, Erben JJ, Matthews D, Starko K, Francis DP, Maynard JE. Effect of immunoglobulin on hepatitis A in day care centers. *JAMA* 1983;249:48–53.
21. Favero MS, Maynard JE, Leger RT, Graham DR, Dixon RE. Guidelines for the care of patients hospitalized with viral hepatitis. *Ann Intern Med* 1979;91:872–6.
22. Carl M, Francis DP, Maynard JE. Food-borne hepatitis A: recommendations for control. *J Infect Dis* 1983;148:1133–5.
23. Lettau LA, Smith JD, Williams D, et al. Transmission of hepatitis B with resultant restriction of surgical practice. *JAMA* 1986;255:934–7.
24. Kane MA, Lettau L. Transmission of HBV from dental personnel to patients. *J Am Dental Assoc* 1985;110:634–6.
25. Maynard JE, Kane MA, Hadler SC. Global control of hepatitis B through vaccination: role of hepatitis B vaccine in the expanded programme on immunization. *Rev Infect Dis* 1989;11(suppl 3):S574–8.
26. McQuillan GM, Townsend TR, Fields HA, et al. Seroepidemiology of hepatitis B virus infection in the United States: 1976 to 1980. *Am J Med* 1989;87(3A):5S–10S.
27. CDC. Prevention of perinatal transmission of hepatitis B virus: prenatal screening of all pregnant women for hepatitis B surface antigen. *MMWR* 1988;37:341–6,351.
28. Francis DP, Feorino PM, McDougall S, et al. The safety of hepatitis B vaccine: inactivation of the AIDS virus during routine vaccine manufacture. *JAMA* 1986;256:869–72.
29. Zajac BA, West DJ, McAleer WJ, Scolnick EM. Overview of clinical studies with hepatitis B vaccine made by recombinant DNA. *J Infect Dis* 1986;13(suppl A):39–45.
30. Andre FE, Safary A. Clinical experience with a yeast-derived hepatitis B vaccine. In: Zuckerman AJ, ed. *Viral hepatitis and liver disease.* New York: Alan R. Liss, 1988:1023–30.
31. Szmuness W, Stevens CE. Harley EJ, et al. Hepatitis B vaccine: demonstration of efficacy in a controlled clinical trial in a high-risk population in the United States. *N Engl J Med* 1980;303:833–41.
32. CDC. Suboptimal response to hepatitis B vaccine given by injection into the buttock. *MMWR* 1985;34:105–13.
33. Stevens CE, Alter HJ, Taylor PE, et al. Hepatitis B vaccine in patients receiving hemodialysis. Immunogenicity and efficacy. *N Engl J Med* 1984;311:496–501.

34. Collier AC, Corey L, Murphy VL, Handsfield HH. Antibody to human immunodeficiency virus and suboptimal response to hepatitis B vaccination. *Ann Intern Med* 1988;109:101–5.
35. Stevens CE, Taylor PE. Tong MJ, et al. Yeast-recombinant hepatitis B vaccine: efficacy with hepatitis B immune globulin in prevention of perinatal hepatitis B virus transmission. *JAMA* 1987;257:2612–6.
36. Hadler SC, Francis DP, Maynard JE, et al. Long term immunogenicity and efficacy of hepatitis B vaccine in homosexual men. *N Engl J Med* 1986;315:209–14.
37. Wainwright RB, McMahon BJ, Bulkow LR, et al. Duration of immunogenicity and efficacy of hepatitis B vaccine in a Yupik Eskimo population. *JAMA* 1989;261:2362–6.
38. Hadler SC. Are booster doses of hepatitis B vaccine necessary? *Ann Intern Med* 1988;109:457–8.
39. Redfield RR, Innis BL, Scott RM, Cannon HG, Bancroft WH. Clinical evaluation of low-dose intradermally administered hepatitis B vaccine: a cost reduction strategy. *JAMA* 1985;254:3203–6.
40. Shaw FE, Graham DJ, Guess HA, et al. Postmarketing surveillance for necrologic adverse events reported after hepatitis B vaccination. Experience of the first three years. *Am J Epidemiol* 1988;127:337–52.
41. Dienstag JL, Stevens CE, Bhan AK, et al. Hepatitis B vaccine administered to chronic carriers of hepatitis B surface antigen. *Ann Intern Med* 1982;96:575–9.
42. Szmuness W, Stevens CE, Oleszko WR, et al. Passive-active immunization against hepatitis B: immunogenicity studies in adult Americans. *Lancet* 1981;1:575–7.
43. CDC. Guidelines for prevention of transmission of human immunodeficiency virus and hepatitis B virus to health-care and public safety workers. *MMWR* 1989;38(suppl S–6).
44. Beuer B, Friedman SM, Millner ES, et al. Transmission of hepatitis B in school contacts of retarded HBsAg carriers. *JAMA* 1985;254:3190–5.
45. CDC. Routine screening for viral hepatitis in chronic hemodialysis centers. *Hepatitis surveillance report no 49*. Atlanta: CDC, 1985:5–6.
46. Seaworth B, Drucker J, Starling J, Drucker R, Stevens C, Hamilton J. Hepatitis B vaccine in patients with chronic renal failure before dialysis. *J Infect Dis* 1988;157:332–7.
47. Hershow RC, Hadler SC, Kane MA. Adoption of children from countries with endemic hepatitis B transmission risks and medical Issues. *Pediatr Infect Dis J*. 1987;6:431–7.
48. Franks AL, Berg CJ, Kane MA, et al. Hepatitis B virus infection among children born in the United States to Southeast Asian refugees. *N Engl J Med* 1989;321:1301–5.
49. Beasley RP, Hwang L-Y, Lee GC, et al. Prevention of perinatally transmit-

ted hepatitis B virus infections with hepatitis B immune globulin and hepatitis B vaccine. *Lancet* 1983;2:1099–102.

50. Wong VCW, Ip HMH, Reesink HW, et al. Prevention of the HBsAg carrier state in newborn infants of mothers who are chronic carriers of HBsAg and HBeAg by administration of hepatitis-B vaccine and hepatitis-B immunoglobulin: double-blind randomized placebo-controlled study. *Lancet* 1984;1:921–6.

51. Stevens CE, Toy PT, Tong MJ, et al. Perinatal hepatitis B virus transmission in the United States: prevention by passive-active immunization. *JAMA* 1985;253:1740–5.

52. Beasley RP, Hwang LY, Stevens CE, et al. Efficacy of hepatitis B immune globulin for prevention of perinatal transmission of the hepatitis B virus carrier state: final report of a randomized double-blind, placebo-controlled trial. *Hematology* 1983;3:135–41.

53. Xu ZY, Liu CB. Francis DP, et al. Prevention of perinatal acquisition of hepatitis B virus carriage using vaccine: preliminary report of a randomized, double-blind placebo-controlled and comparative trial. *Pediatrics* 1985;76:713–8.

54. Seeff LB, Wright EC, Zimmerman HJ, et al. Type B hepatitis after needlestick exposure: prevention with hepatitis B immune globulin. Final report of the Veterans Administration Cooperative Study. *Ann Intern Med* 1978;88:285–93.

55. Grady GF, Lee VA, Prince AM, et al. Hepatitis B immune globulin for accidental exposures among medical personnel: final report of a multicenter controlled trial. *J Infect Dis* 1978;138:625–38.

56. Redeker AG, Mosley JW, Gocke DJ, McKee AP, Pollack W. Hepatitis B immune globulin as a prophylactic measure for spouses exposed to acute type B hepatitis. *N Engl J Med* 1975;293:1055–9.

57. Beasley RP, Hwang L-Y. Epidemiology of hepatocellular carcinoma. In: Vyas GN, Dienstag JL, Hoofnagle JH, eds. *Viral hepatitis and liver disease.* New York: Grune & Stratton, 1984:209–24.

58. Sinatra FR, Shah P, Weissman JY, Thomas DW, Merritt RJ, Tong MJ. Perinatal transmitted acute icteric hepatitis B in infants born to hepatitis B surface antigen-positive and anti-hepatitis Be–positive carrier mothers. *Pediatrics* 1982;70:557–9.

59. Delaplane D, Yogev R, Crussi F, Schulman ST. Fatal hepatitis B in early infancy: the importance of identifying HBsAg-positive pregnant women and providing immunoprophylaxis to their newborns. *Pediatrics* 1983;72:176–80.

60. Alter MJ, Hadler SC, Francis DP, Maynard JE. The epidemiology of non-A, non-B hepatitis in the United States. In: Dodd RY, Barker LF, eds. *Infection, immunity, and blood transfusion.* New York: Alan R. Liss, 1985:71–9.

61. Alter HJ, Purcell RH, Holland PV, et al. Clinical and serological analysis of transfusion-associated hepatitis. *Lancet* 1975;2:838–41.
62. Dienstag JL. Non-A, non-B hepatitis I. Recognition, epidemiology, and clinical features. *Gastroenterology* 1983;85:439–62.
63. Alter MJ, Gerety RJ, Smallwood LA, et al. Sporadic non-A, non-B hepatitis: frequency and epidemiology in an urban U.S. population. *J Infect Dis* 1982;145:886–93.
64. Alter MJ, Coleman PJ, Alexander WJ, et al. Importance of heterosexual activity in the transmission of hepatitis B and non-A, non-B hepatitis. *JAMA* 1989;262:1201–5.
65. Guyer B, Bradley DW, Bryan JA, Maynard JE. Non-A, non-B hepatitis among participants in a plasmapheresis stimulation program. *J Infect Dis* 1979;139:634–40.
66. Dienstag JL, Alter HJ. Non-A, non-B hepatitis: evolving epidemiologic and clinical perspectives. *Semin Liver Dis* 1986;6:67–81.
67. Tabor E, Seeff LB, Gerety RJ. Chronic non-A, non-B hepatitis carrier state: transmissible agent documented in one patient over a six-year period. *N Engl J Med* 1980;303:140–3.
68. Aach RD, Szmuness W, Mosley JW, et al. Serum alanine aminotransferase of donors in relation to the risk of non-A, non-B hepatitis in recipients: the Transfusion-Transmitted Viruses Study. *N Engl J Med* 1981;304:989–94.
69. Tong MJ, Thursby M, Rakela J, et al. Studies on the maternal-infant transmission of the viruses which cause acute hepatitis. *Gastroenterology* 1981;80:999–1003.

References 70–75 may be obtained by writing to the Hepatitis Branch, Division of Viral and Rickettsial Diseases, Center for Infectious Diseases, Mailstop A33, Centers for Disease Control, Atlanta, GA 30333.

Public Health Service Statement on Management of Occupational Exposure to Human Immunodeficiency Virus, Including Considerations Regarding Zidovudine Postexposure Use[1,2]

INTRODUCTION

CDC has issued guidelines to reduce the risk of human immunodeficiency virus (HIV) infection among health-care workers, emergency-response and public-safety workers, and others who might be exposed to HIV while performing job duties (1–4). The safety practices outlined in these guidelines remain the primary means of preventing occupational acquisition of HIV infection (5). Additionally, some physicians and some institutions have offered the option of using zidovudine (azidothymidine, AZT, ZDV, Retrovir) after occupational exposure to HIV (6). Data collected in an ongoing CDC surveillance project of health-care workers who have been occupationally exposed to blood from HIV-infected patients (7) indicate that during the period April–December 1989, 13 (8.6%) of 151 newly enrolled participants began a postexposure regimen of zidovudine.

This report reviews Public Health Service (PHS) recommendations for postexposure management of workers who have occupational exposures that may place them at risk of acquiring HIV infection, provides background information on zidovudine and experience with zidovudine postexposure prophylaxis, and presents considerations relevant to a decision to offer postexposure prophylaxis.

---

1. Centers for Disease Control, *MMWR* 1990;39(suppl RR-1):1–14.

2. A recently published article by J. L. Gerberding, "Management of Occupational Exposures to Blood-borne Viruses" (*New England Journal of Medicine* [16 February 1995] 332 (7):444–51) gives a more current discussion of postexposure treatment.

Definition of Occupational Exposure

For purposes of this document, an occupational exposure (i.e., exposure that occurs during the performance of job duties) that may place a worker at risk of HIV infection is defined as a percutaneous injury (e.g., a needlestick or cut with a sharp object), contact of mucous membranes, or contact of skin (especially when the exposed skin is chapped, abraded, or afflicted with dermatitis or the contact is prolonged or involving an extensive area) with blood, tissues, or other body fluids to which universal precautions apply, including: (a) semen, vaginal secretions, or other body fluids contaminated with visible blood, because these substances have been implicated in the transmission of HIV infection (2); (b) cerebrospinal fluid, synovial fluid, pleural fluid, peritoneal fluid, pericardial fluid, and amniotic fluid, because the risk of transmission of HIV from these fluids has not yet been determined (2); and (c) laboratory specimens that contain HIV (e.g., suspensions of concentrated virus).

PHS Recommendations for Management of Persons after Occupational Exposures That May Place Them at Risk of Acquiring HIV Infection

Employers should make available to workers a system for promptly initiating evaluation, counseling, and follow-up after a reported occupational exposure that may place the worker at risk of acquiring HIV infection. Workers should be educated to report exposures immediately after they occur, because certain interventions that may be appropriate, e.g., prophylaxis against hepatitis B, must be initiated promptly to be effective (3,8,9). Workers who might reasonably be considered at risk of occupational exposure to HIV should be familiarized with the principles of postexposure management as part of job orientation and ongoing job training.

If an exposure occurs, the circumstances should be recorded in the workers confidential medical record. Relevant information includes the following:

- date and time of exposure
- job duty being performed by worker at time of exposure
- details of exposure, including amount of fluid or material, type of fluid or material, and severity of exposure (e.g., for a percutaneous exposure, depth of injury and whether fluid was injected; for a skin or mucous membrane exposure, the extent and duration of contact and the condition of the skin, e.g., chapped, abraded, intact)

- description of source of exposure—including, if known, whether the source material contained HIV or HBV
- details about counseling, postexposure management, and follow-up

After an occupational exposure, both the exposed worker and the source individual should be evaluated to determine the possible need for the exposed worker to receive prophylaxis against hepatitis B according to previously published CDC recommendations (3,8,9). Because of the potentially severe consequences of hepatitis B virus infection, hepatitis B vaccine, which is both safe and highly effective (10), should be offered to any susceptible health-care worker who has an occupational exposure and has not previously been vaccinated with hepatitis B vaccine. Hepatitis B immune globulin may also be indicated, particularly if the source patient or material is found to be positive for hepatitis B surface antigen (HBsAg) (3,8,9).

In addition, the source individual should be informed of the incident and, if consent is obtained, tested for serologic evidence of HIV infection. If consent cannot be obtained (e.g., patient is unconscious), policies should be developed for testing source individuals in compliance with applicable state and local laws. **Confidentiality of the source individual should be maintained at all times.**

If the source individual has AIDS, is known to be HIV-seropositive, or refuses testing, the worker should be evaluated clinically and serologically for evidence of HIV infection as soon as possible after the exposure (baseline) and if seronegative, should be retested periodically for a minimum of 6 months after exposure (e.g., 6 weeks, 12 weeks, and 6 months after exposure) to determine whether HIV infection has occurred. The worker should be advised to report and seek medical evaluation for any acute illness that occurs during the follow-up period. Such illness, particularly if characterized by fever, rash, myalgia, fatigue, malaise, or lymphadenopathy, may be indicative of acute HIV infection, drug reaction, or another medical condition. During the follow-up period, especially the first 6–12 weeks after the exposure when most infected persons are expected to seroconvert, exposed workers should follow PHS recommendations for preventing transmission of HIV. These recommendations include refraining from blood, semen, or organ donation and abstaining from or using measures to prevent HIV transmission during sexual intercourse (11–14). In addition, in countries such as the United States where safe and effective alternatives to breast-feeding are available, exposed women should not breast-feed infants during the follow-up period in order to prevent the infant's possible exposure to HIV in breast milk. **During all phases of follow-up, confidentiality of the worker should be protected.**

If the source individual is HIV-seronegative and has no clinical manifestations of AIDS or HIV infection, no further HIV follow-up of the exposed worker is necessary unless epidemiologic evidence suggests that the source individual may have recently been exposed to HIV or if testing is desired by the worker or recommended by the health-care provider. In these instances, the guidelines may be followed as described above.

If the source individual cannot be identified, decisions regarding appropriate follow-up should be individualized, based on factors such as whether potential sources are likely to include a person at increased risk of HIV infection.

The employer should make serologic testing available to all workers who are concerned about possible infection with HIV through an occupational exposure. Appropriate psychological counseling may be indicated as well.

ZIDOVUDINE

Background

Zidovudine is a thymidine analogue that has been shown in vitro to inhibit replication of some retroviruses, including HIV, by interfering with the action of viral ribonucleic acid (RNA)–dependent deoxyribonucleic acid (DNA) polymerase (reverse transcriptase) and possibly also by other mechanisms (15).

In a double-blind, placebo-controlled trial, zidovudine was shown to increase the length and quality of life of patients with advanced HIV infection and AIDS (16). Largely on the basis of the results of this trial, zidovudine was approved for marketing by the Food and Drug Administration (FDA) and is indicated for treatment of adults with symptomatic HIV infection, including AIDS, who have a history of cytologically confirmed *Pneumocystis carinii* pneumonia or an absolute CD4, lymphocyte count of $<200/mm^3$. The dose of zidovudine originally approved for oral use by patients who have AIDS and advanced symptomatic HIV infection was 200 mg every 4 hours. On January 16, 1990, FDA approved a change in the labeling that now recommends administering the drug at 600 mg/day (100 mg every 4 hours) after a patient has received 1 month of zidovudine therapy at a dose of 1,200 mg/day (200 mg every 4 hours).

Later studies (National Institute of Allergy and Infectious Diseases [NIAID] AIDS Clinical Trial Group Protocols no. 016 and no. 019) have indicated that zidovudine can delay disease progression in patients with less advanced HIV infection (patients with an absolute CD4, count of $<500/mm^3$, whether symptomatic or asymptomatic) (NIAID Administrative Report: "AIDS Clinical Trials Alert," August 29, 1989).

Toxicity

Among patients who have AIDS or symptomatic HIV infection and who are treated with zidovudine, the most frequently reported adverse events are granulocytopenia and anemia. Other adverse events that affect ≥5% of zidovudine recipients include one or more of the following: headache, nausea, insomnia, myalgia, diaphoresis, fever, malaise, anorexia, diarrhea, dyspepsia, vomiting, dyspnea, rash, and taste abnormalities (17). Occurrences less commonly reported in the published literature include polymyositis, peripheral neuropathy, and seizures.

Among 3,200 patients with asymptomatic HIV infection treated in NIAID protocol no. 019 with placebo or with zidovudine doses of either 1,500 mg or 500 mg daily (either 300 mg or 100 mg given every 4 hours, five times daily), investigators have reported the following toxicity after a median of 44 weeks of therapy: in the 1,500-mg/day group, approximately 12% of the subjects developed moderate to severe hematologic toxicity, defined as hemoglobin of <8 g/dl, granulocytes of <750/mm^3, or platelets of <50,000/mm^3. In the 500-mg/day group, this toxicity occurred at a rate of about 3%, compared with approximately 2% in the placebo group. Nausea was rarely reported in the placebo group; however, 3–5% of zidovudine recipients, irrespective of dose group, experienced moderate to severe nausea. No statistically significant difference was observed between zidovudine dose and placebo for any other moderate to severe clinical adverse experiences (NIAID Administrative Report: "AIDS Clinical Trials Alert," August 29, 1989).

Preliminary data from a study sponsored by the Burroughs-Wellcome Company of health-care workers who received 200 mg of zidovudine or placebo every 4 hours for 6 weeks after occupational exposure to HIV indicate that adverse effects most frequently consisted of nausea and vomiting. In no instance did the prescribing physician discontinue a participant's study drug or placebo because of hematologic or other serious toxicity; however, during the therapy period, 14 (28.6%) of 49 participants who received zidovudine had a hemoglobin concentration between 9.5 and 12 g/dl, compared with one (2.9%) of 35 participants in the placebo group. Seven (14.3%) of the 49 participants who received zidovudine, compared with one (2.9%) of the 35 placebo recipients, elected to discontinue therapy because of subjective, reversible symptoms, including nausea, vomiting, fatigue, headache, myalgia, or cough.

Several anecdotal reports of short-term toxicity among health-care workers receiving zidovudine have been received by PHS. Symptoms include fever, myalgia, fatigue, nausea, and vomiting. Single reports have been received of severe anemia, reversible peripheral neuropathy, and transient clinical hepatitis.

Although the risk of acute zidovudine toxicity for exposed health-care workers cannot be determined from this limited information, data from the NIAID protocol no. 019 trial and from the Burroughs-Wellcome study of exposed health-care workers suggest that the risk of acute toxicity associated with short-term use of the drug is lower than the risk observed during long-term therapy of symptomatic HIV-infected individuals.

For healthy persons not infected with HIV, the risk of long-term toxicity, including teratogenic and carcinogenic effects, related to a course of zidovudine is not known. It is not known whether zidovudine can cause fetal harm when administered to a pregnant woman or whether it can affect reproductive capacity

(17). To assess the safety of zidovudine use during pregnancy, the Burroughs-Wellcome Company has developed a registry to evaluate pregnancy outcomes of women who took zidovudine during pregnancy. Physicians are encouraged to register such persons by telephoning the pregnancy registry, (919) 248-8465 (collect) or (800) 722-9292. It is also not known whether zidovudine is excreted in human milk. However, because of the potential for adverse side effects among breast-fed infants, as well as the potential for transmission of HIV if the mother is infected, mothers should be instructed to discontinue breast-feeding whether or not they are receiving zidovudine (17).

In other studies conducted by the Burroughs-Wellcome Company (*see Appendix G1*), vaginal tumors, including carcinomas, were observed in mice and rats receiving zidovudine at doses that the FDA has determined resulted in plasma levels in mice approximately equal to human plasma levels at the dose originally approved for treatment of persons with symptomatic HIV infection (200 mg every 4 hours). In rats, the plasma levels were determined by the FDA to be about 10 times higher than human plasma levels achieved with the originally approved dose. The results of these rodent carcinogenicity studies are of uncertain predictive value for humans.

Studies of Zidovudine Postexposure Prophylaxis Involving Animals

Data involving studies of laboratory animals (*see Appendix G2*) are limited and must be interpreted with caution, as they have most often been derived by using nonhuman retroviruses having pathogenic mechanisms different from the pathogenesis of HIV infection in humans. In one study using HIV in a mouse model, zidovudine prophylaxis was begun 24 hours before intrathymic injection of a large inoculum of HIV and continued for 2 weeks thereafter. HIV infection was not prevented in any of the animals studied, although the course of infection was modified. It is not known whether prophylaxis would be effective in conditions that more closely resemble occupational exposures, i.e., zidovudine begun after exposure, with the exposure consisting of a percutaneous injection of a lower inoculum of HIV. **Data from animal studies are inadequate to support or reject the hypothesis that zidovudine may be effective prophylaxis for persons who have been occupationally exposed to HIV.**

Studies of Zidovudine Postexposure Prophylaxis Involving Humans

The efficacy of zidovudine prophylaxis for humans after exposure to HIV cannot be assessed because of insufficient data. The Burroughs-Wellcome

Company recently sponsored a double-blind, placebo-controlled study to evaluate 6 weeks of zidovudine prophylaxis (200mg orally every 4 hours) involving health-care workers who had experienced occupational percutaneous, mucous membrane, or nonintactskin exposures to HIV-infected blood. Of 84 workers who initially enrolled in the study (49 of whom were given zidovudine), none developed HIV infection after at least 6 months of follow-up. The risk of transmission of HIV per episode of percutaneous exposure to HIV-infected blood is, on the average, approximately 0.4% (7). Thus, the absence of seroconversions in this small group of participants is not unexpected, regardless of whether they took zidovudine. Enrollment in this study was terminated in June 1989.

NIAID has enrolled three persons in an ongoing open trial of zidovudine prophylaxis after a "massive exposure" to HIV. The first person received a blood transfusion from an HIV-infected donor, was started on zidovudine 7 days after exposure, and was culture-positive for HIV 4 months after completing 6 weeks of chemotherapy. The second person was exposed to a high concentration of HIV on abraded skin in a research laboratory, was started on zidovudine within 24 hours postexposure, and remains HIV-seronegative after 11 months. The risk of seroconversion after this type of laboratory exposure is unknown. The third person was exposed to a high concentration of HIV on broken skin in a research laboratory, was started on zidovudine within 24 hours after the exposure, and is HIV-seronegative 3 months after the exposure. The risk of seroconversion after this type of laboratory exposure also is unknown. All individuals were able to complete a 6-week course of therapy (200 mg orally every 4 hours) without clinically significant adverse effects. Information regarding enrollment in this study can be obtained by calling the NIAID study coordinator at (800) 537-9978.

Prophylaxis Schedules Currently Used after Occupational Exposure

Various regimens have been prescribed for zidovudine prophylaxis after occupational exposure. No data are available to enable investigators to determine the efficacy or compare the toxicity of these or other regimens. At the National Institutes of Health Clinical Center, workers who elect to receive zidovudine are treated with 200 mg every 4 hours (six times daily) for 6 weeks (6). At San Francisco General Hospital, workers who elect to receive zidovudine are treated with 200 mg every 4 hours (five times daily; no dose is given at 4:00 a.m.) for 4 weeks (6). Some clinicians have used an initial dose of 400 mg, and others have prescribed treatment courses ranging from 4 days to 4 months. At several institutions, attempts are made to begin prophylaxis within 1 hour after exposure for workers who elect to receive the drug.

DISCUSSION

Data from animal and human studies are inadequate to establish the efficacy or safety of zidovudine for prophylaxis after occupational exposure to HIV. However, some physicians believe that zidovudine should be offered as prophylaxis to persons after certain occupational exposures for the following reasons: the severity of the illness that may result from HIV infection, the documented antiviral effect of zidovudine in the treatment of persons with established HIV infection, the apparent reversibility of acute toxicity in persons taking zidovudine for a brief period, and the suggestion that in some animal studies, zidovudine postexposure may modify the course of some retroviral infections. Other physicians believe that zidovudine should not be recommended for uninfected persons after occupational exposures because of the lack of data demonstrating efficacy in postexposure prophylaxis, the limited data on toxicity in uninfected individuals, and the fact that zidovudine has been shown to be carcinogenic in rats and mice.

At this time, prophylaxis with zidovudine cannot be considered a necessary component of postexposure management. However, workers who might be at risk of occupational exposure to HIV should be informed, as part of job orientation and ongoing job training, of the considerations pertaining to the use of zidovudine for postexposure prophylaxis. The PHS recommends that if a physician decides to offer zidovudine to a worker after an exposure incident, that decision by the physician and the decision by the worker to take zidovudine should take into account the following considerations.

Considerations Regarding Use of Zidovudine after an Occupational Exposure

Risk of HIV infection after exposure

Evaluation of the risk of HIV infection after exposure should take into account existing knowledge from prospective studies of exposed workers, which demonstrate that on the average the risk of transmission of HIV per episode of percutaneous exposure (e.g., a needlestick or cut with a sharp object) to HIV-infected blood is approximately 0.4%. These studies also suggest that the risk of HIV transmission per episode of mucous membrane or skin exposure to HIV-infected blood is less than that after a percutaneous exposure (7,18–21). The risk of HIV transmission after occupational exposure to body fluids other than blood, for which universal precautions are recommended, is unknown. The risk of HIV infection for persons who take zidovudine postexposure prophylaxis cannot be determined at present because of the small number of persons studied.

Risk evaluation should also include an assessment of factors that may increase or decrease the probability of HIV transmission after an individual occupational exposure. These factors are not well understood, but include the likelihood that the source fluid contained HIV and probably also the concentration of HIV in the source fluid, the route of exposure, and the volume of fluid involved. For example, a percutaneous exposure to concentrated HIV in a research laboratory is probably more likely to result in transmission of infection than a similar exposure to HIV-infected blood in a clinical setting. A percutaneous exposure to HIV-infected blood is probably more likely to result in transmission than a mucous membrane exposure to the same blood. Finally, an exposure to a larger quantity of HIV-infected blood, such as injection of several milliliters, is probably more likely to result in HIV transmission than an exposure to a smaller quantity of the same blood, such as in a needlestick exposure.

Interval between exposure and initiation of prophylaxis, if given

Data from animal studies suggest that prophylaxis against certain retroviral infections other than HIV may be more effective when started within hours after exposure (22,23). Because in vitro studies indicate that human HIV infection may be established in human lymphocytes within hours after exposure (24), and epidemiologic studies of exposed health-care workers indicate that acute retroviral illness may occur as early as 2 weeks after exposure (7), it appears that if the decision is made to use postexposure prophylaxis, prophylaxis should be initiated promptly.

Counseling and informed consent

If zidovudine prophylaxis is being considered, the worker should be counseled regarding (a) the theoretical rationale for postexposure prophylaxis, (b) the risk of occupationally acquired HIV infection due to the exposure, (c) the limitations of current knowledge of the efficacy of zidovudine when used as postexposure prophylaxis, (d) current knowledge of the toxicity of zidovudine (including the data from animal and human studies) and the limitations of this knowledge in predicting toxicity in uninfected individuals who take the drug after occupational exposures, and (e) the need for postexposure follow-up (including HIV serologic testing), regardless of whether zidovudine is taken. **The worker should also be informed that there are diverse opinions among physicians regarding the use of zidovudine for postexposure prophylaxis, and the PHS cannot make a**

recommendation for or against the use of zidovudine for this purpose because of the limitations of current knowledge.

The duration of follow-up needed to detect evidence of HIV transmission or delayed toxicity among workers who take zidovudine is presently unknown. Workers taking zidovudine postexposure may require follow-up to detect HIV seroconversion for a longer period than that recommended for workers who do not take zidovudine. Regardless of the length of follow-up, mechanisms should be developed to permit workers taking zidovudine to be contacted if future information indicates the need for additional evaluation.

If a physician offers zidovudine as prophylaxis after an occupational exposure and the exposed worker elects to take the drug, the physician or other appropriate health-care provider should obtain written informed consent from the worker for this use of this drug. The consent document should reflect the information presented in the counseling session, as outlined above, emphasizing the need for follow-up medical evaluations and for precautions to prevent the transmission of HIV infection during the follow-up period, including refraining from blood, semen, or organ donation, refraining from breast-feeding, and either abstaining from sexual intercourse or using latex condoms during sexual intercourse, as discussed below.

Considerations regarding sexual intercourse for exposed workers taking zidovudine include (a) the possible risk of teratogenesis associated with zidovudine use, and (b) the risk of transmission of HIV to a sexual partner. The risk of teratogenesis among offspring of either men or women taking zidovudine is unknown. Therefore, men and women of reproductive age who are receiving zidovudine should abstain from, or use effective contraception during, sexual intercourse throughout the time zidovudine is being taken. In addition, to prevent HIV transmission to sexual partners, all exposed workers, including pregnant women, should abstain from, or use latex condoms during, sexual intercourse throughout the follow-up period.

Research Needs

Further data are needed to determine risk factors for occupational exposure to HIV, to evaluate measures for preventing these exposures, and to identify risk factors for HIV transmission after occupational exposure. Appropriate animal models of HIV infection are needed, and animal studies should be conducted under experimental conditions that mimic the circumstances of occupational exposure affecting humans. Studies involving humans should be conducted to determine whether postexposure prophylaxis with zidovudine or other agents is effective, and, if effective, should define the optimal time that postexposure prophylaxis should be initiated and the optimal duration of prophylaxis. Studies should also assess the toxicity of candidate prophylactic agents, establish the optimal dosage for healthy individuals and for persons with preexisting hepatic or renal dysfunction, and define the duration of follow-up needed to detect evidence of HIV infection in persons receiving prophylaxis. Strains of HIV isolated from treated workers should be monitored to detect development of drug resistance.

Expanded Surveillance of Workers with Occupational Exposures to HIV

CDC has expanded its ongoing surveillance of workers with occupational exposures to HIV (7) to collect additional information on postexposure chemoprophylaxis. No names or other personal identifiers of workers are collected.
Information is collected on the following:

- circumstances associated with exposures
- extent to which zidovudine and other antiretroviral agents are prescribed for postexposure chemoprophylaxis, including dosage and timing
- incidence of associated toxicity
- rate of HIV seroconversion among workers who do and do not receive postexposure chemoprophylaxis

All physicians who provide care to a worker within 1 month after an occupational exposure to HIV, regardless of whether an antiretroviral agent is prescribed, are encouraged to enroll the worker in the CDC surveillance system. Enrollment and follow-up requirements have been simplified; in particular, it is no longer necessary to send blood specimens to CDC for HIV serologic testing unless the enzyme immunoassay (EIA) performed by a licensed local laboratory is reactive or equivocal. CDC will continue, however, to offer EIA testing at no charge on specimens from surveillance participants on request. Additional information and enrollment materials can be obtained from the Hospital Infections Program, Center for Infectious Diseases, Centers for Disease Control, Mail Stop C-10, Atlanta, GA 30333; telephone (404) 639-1644.

CONTACTS FOR PHYSICIANS AND FOR INFECTION CONTROL AND OCCUPATIONAL HEALTH PROFESSIONALS

- To enroll persons who have had a "massive exposure" to HIV in NIAID study of zidovudine prophylaxis, telephone (800) 537-9978.

- To report adverse effects associated with zidovudine to FDA, use "Adverse Reaction Report" forms (FDA no. 1639), obtainable from:

    Food and Drug Administration Office of
    Epidemiology and Biostatistics
    HFD-730
    Rockville, MD 20857
    (301) 443-4580

- To enroll an exposed worker in the CDC prospective surveillance system, telephone (404) 639-1644
- To enroll pregnant women who receive zidovudine during pregnancy, contact:

    Zidovudine in Pregnancy Registry
    Epidemiology, Information, and Surveillance Division
    Burroughs-Wellcome Company
    3030 Cornwallis Road
    Research Triangle Park, NC 27709
    (919) 248-8465 (collect) or (800) 722-9292

REFERENCES

1. CDC. Recommendations for prevention of HIV transmission in health-care settings. *MMWR* 1987;36(no. 2S).
2. CDC. Update: universal precautions for prevention of transmission of human immunodeficiency virus, hepatitis B virus, and other bloodborne pathogens in health-care settings. *MMWR* 1988;37:377–88.
3. CDC. Guidelines for prevention of transmission of human immunodeficiency virus and hepatitis B virus to health-care and public-safety workers. *MMWR* 1989;38(no. S-6).
4. CDC. 1988 Agent summary statement for human immunodeficiency virus and report on laboratory-acquired infection with human immunodeficiency virus. *MMWR* 1988;37 (no. S-4).
5. U.S. Department of Labor, U.S. Department of Health and Human Services. *Joint advisory notice: protection against occupational exposure to hepatitis B virus (HBV) and human immunodeficiency virus (HIV).* Washington, DC: U.S. Department of Labor, US Department of Health and Human Services, 1987.

6. Henderson DK, Gerberding JL. Prophylactic zidovudine after occupational exposure to the human immunodeficiency virus: an interim analysis. *J Infect Dis* 1989;160:321–7.
7. Marcus R, CDC Cooperative Needlestick Study Group. Surveillance of health-care workers exposed to blood from patients infected with the human immunodeficiency virus. *N Engl J Med* 1988;319:1118–23.
8. CDC. Recommendations for protection against viral hepatitis: recommendations of the Immunization Practices Advisory Committee (ACIP). *MMWR* 1985;34:313–35.
9. CDC. Protection against viral hepatitis: recommendations of the Immunization Practices Advisory Committee (ACIP). *MMWR* 1990 (in press).
10. CDC. Update on hepatitis B prevention. MMWR 1987;36:353–66.
11. CDC. Public Health Service guidelines for counseling and antibody testing to prevent HIV infection and AIDS. *MMWR* 1987;36:509–15.
12. CDC. Additional recommendations to reduce sexual and drug abuse-related transmission of human T-lymphotropic virus type III/lymphadenopathy-associated virus. *MMWR* 1986; 35:152–5.
13. CDC. Prevention of acquired immune deficiency syndrome (AIDS): report of inter-agency recommendations. *MMWR* 1983;32:101-3.
14. CDC. Provisional Public Health Service inter-agency recommendations for screening donated blood and plasma for antibody to the virus causing acquired immunodeficiency syndrome. *MMWR* 1985;34:1–5.
15. Yarchoan R, Mitsuya H, Myers C, Broder S. Clinical pharmacology of 3-azido-2, 3dideoxythymidine (zidovudine) and related dideoxynucleosides. *N Engl J Med* 1989; 321: 726–38.
16. Fischl MA, Richman DD, Grieco MH, et al. The efficacy of azidothymidine (AZT) in the treatment of patients with AIDS and AIDS-related complex. *N Engl J Med* 1987;317:185–91.
17. Huff BB, ed. *1989 Physicians desk reference.* 43rd ed. Oradell, NJ: Edward R. Barnhart, 1989:793–5.
18. Henderson DK, Fahey BJ, Saah AJ, Schmitt JM, Lane HC. Longitudinal assessment of risk for occupational/nosocomial transmission of human immunodeficiency virus, type 1 in health care workers [Abstract]. In: *Program and abstracts of the twenty-eighth Interscience Conference on Antimicrobial Agents and Chemotherapy (Los Angeles).* Washington, DC: American Society for Microbiology, 1988:221.
19. Gerberding JL, Littell CG, Chambers HF, et al. Risk of occupational HIV transmission in intensively exposed health-care workers: follow-up [Abstract]. In: *Program and abstracts of the twenty-eighth Interscience Conference on Antimicrobial Agents and Chemotherapy (Los Angeles).* Washington, DC: American Society for Microbiology, 1988:169.
20. Elmslie K, Mulligan L, O'Shaughnessy M. National surveillance program:

256 THE BLOODBORNE PATHOGENS STANDARD

occupational exposure to human immunodeficiency virus (HIV-1) infection in Canada. *V International Conference on AIDS.* Montreal, June 4–9, 1989:148.

21. McEvoy M, Porter K, Mortimer P, Simmons N, Shanson D. Prospective study of clinical, laboratory, and ancillary staff with accidental exposures to blood or body fluids from patients infected with HIV. *Br Med J* 1987;294:595–7.
22. Ruprecht RM, OBrien LG, Rossoni LD, Nusinoff-Lehrman S. Suppression of mouse viraemia and retroviral disease by 3-azido-3-deoxythymidine. *Nature* 1986;323:467–9.
23. Tavares L, Roneker C, Johnston K, Nusmoff-Lehrman S, de Noronha F. 3-Azido-3deoxythymidine in feline leukemia virus-infected cats: a model for therapy and prophylaxis of AIDS. *Cancer Res* 1987;47:3190–4.
24. Sunyoung K, Byrn R, Groopman J, Baltimore D. Kinetics of HIV gene expression during the one-step multiplication of HIV [Abstract]. *IV International Conference on AIDS.* Book 1. Stockholm, June 12–16, 1988:119.

APPENDIX G1
RESULTS OF STUDIES CONDUCTED BY THE
BURROUGHS-WELLCOME COMPANY OF ZIDOVUDINE
CARCINOGENICITY INVOLVING ANIMALS

In lifetime carcinogenicity bioassay, mice and rats were given various doses of zidovudine, up to the maximum tolerated doses, for most of their lifespans. Dose reductions were necessary for both species during the study because of the onset and persistence of drug-related anemia. Mice were treated initially with 30, 60, or 120 mg/kg/day; after 90 days, these doses were reduced to 20, 30, or 40 mg/kg/day, respectively. Rats were treated initially with 80, 220, or 600 mg/kg/day; after 90 days, the 600-mg/kg/day group was reduced to 450 mg/kg/day; and after 280 days, this group was further reduced to 300 mg/kg/day. Although anemia persisted at the reduced doses, drug treatment did not adversely affect survival in either species.

Among mice dosed for approximately 22 months, seven vaginal neoplasms occurred in 60 female animals at the highest dose. The earliest a tumor was discovered was after 19 months of continuous dosing; most tumors were discovered after 21 months of treatment. The tumors consisted of five nonmetastasizing squamous cell carcinomas and two benign tumors (one squamous cell papilloma and one squamous cell polyp). One benign vaginal tumor (squamous cell papilloma) was discovered in the middle-dose group after 22 months of treatment. In all instances, these lesions were discovered during histologic examination of tissues from animals that either died or were sacrificed, late in life from nontreat-ment-related causes, or sacrificed upon completion of lifetime dosing.

Among rats dosed for approximately 22 months, two nonmetastasizing vagi-nal squamous cell carcinomas were diagnosed on the basis of histologic exami-nation of tissues from animals receiving the highest dose. These carcinomas were discovered after 20–22 months of dosing. No vaginal tumors occurred among rats given the middle or low dose. No other drug-related tumors were observed among animals of either sex or of either species (Burroughs-Wellcome Company [letter to physicians], December 5, 1989).

APPENDIX G2
STUDIES OF ZIDOVUDINE PROPHYLAXIS INVOLVING ANIMALS

Studies of retrovirus infections other than HIV in mice and cats suggest that zidovudine may alter the course of some retroviral infections when given before or shortly after exposure to the virus. In one study, mice were injected with a large challenge inoculum (1×10^4 plaque-forming units) of Rauscher murine leukemia virus (RMLV) and were given a 20-day course of zidovudine, at vari-ous doses, beginning 4 hours after inoculation. By day 69, all untreated mice had died of RMLV infection, whereas those treated with high doses of zidovudine had no clinical signs of infection and were not viremic. Both the protective effect of zidovudine and the incidence of zidovudine-induced bone marrow depression were greater with increasing doses (1).

In another study, cats were injected with a large challenge dose (2×10^3 focus-inducing units) of Rickard feline leukemia virus (RFLV) and were given zidovudine at various doses and various intervals after inoculation. Of eight cats injected with RFLV and treated with a 6-week course of zidovudine beginning 1 hour after inoculation, none developed clinical evidence of RFLV disease, none had virus isolated from serum, and one had evidence of infection manifested by the development of neutralizing antibody within 3 months after treatment with zidovudine was stopped. In contrast, 11 of 12 untreated cats either became viremic or died of infection in the same period. When zidovudine prophylaxis was initiated 3 or 7 days after inoculation, a substantial proportion of animals in different dosage groups became viremic, developed neutralizing antibody, or both. All animals treated beginning 28 days after inoculation were viremic when zidovudine treatment was initiated (2).

Limited studies involving primates have not shown success in postexposure prophylaxis against simian immunodeficiency virus (SIV). In one study, macaque monkeys were inoculated with a small dose (10 TCID$_{50}$) of a rapidly lethal variant of SIV (SMM/PBj-14) and later treated with zidovudine for 14 days. Of three animals whose treatment was begun 1 hour after inoculation, two developed infection, and one died. Of three animals treated within 24 hours, all developed infection, and two died. Of three animals treated within 72 hours, all developed infection, and two died. Of three control animals that were inoculated with the virus but not given zidovudine treatment, all developed infection, and two died (3). In another study of macaque monkeys, a 1-week course of zidovudine begun 8 hours before the animals were inoculated with SIV did not prevent viremia, but delayed its onset until 1-2 days after the zidovudine treatment was completed (4).

Finally, studies have been conducted by using the SCID-hu mouse model, an immunodeficient mouse with an immune system that has been reconstituted with transplanted human hematolymphoid organs susceptible to infection with HIV (5). Seventeen mice were treated with zidovudine for 24 hours before and for 2 weeks after intrathymic injection of a standard challenge dose of HIV (400-4,000 IU), the smallest dose causing infection in all animals. At 2 weeks after injection, none of the mice tested positive for HIV DNA by the polymerase chain reaction (PCR), although the presence of HIV RNA in some cells was detected by in situ hybridization. Four weeks after zidovudine was stopped, HIV DNA was detected by PCR in all 17 mice. In comparison, all of 40 mice not receiving zidovudine tested positive for HIV DNA by PCR 2 weeks after injection (6).

REFERENCES

1. Ruprecht RM, O'Brien LG, Rossoni LD, Nusinoff-Lehrman S. Suppression of mouse viraemia and retroviral disease by 3'-azido-3'-deoxythymidine. Nature 1986;323:467-9.
2. Tavares L, Roneker C, Johnston K, Nusinoff-Lehrman S, de Noronha F. 3'-Azido-3'deoxythvmidine in feline leukemia virus-infected cats: a model for therapy and prophylaxis of AIDS. Cancer Res 1987;47:3190-4.
3. McClure HM, Anderson DC, Fultz P, Ansari A, Brodie A, Lehrman A. Prophylactic effects of AZT following exposure of macaques to an acutely lethal variant of SIV (SIV/SMM/PBj-14) [Abstracts]. V International Conference on AIDS. Montreal June 4-9, 1989;522.
4. Lundgren B, Hedstrom KG, Norrby E, Oberq B, Wahren B. Inhibition of early occurrence of antigen in SIV-infected macaques as a measurement of

antiviral efficacy [Abstract]. Symposium on Nonhuman Primate Models for AIDS. November 1988.

5. Namikawa R, Kaneshima H, Lieberman M, Weissman IL, McCune JM. Infection of the SCID-hu mouse by HIV-1. Science 1988;242:1684-6.

6. McCune JM, Namikawa R, Shih CC, Rabin L, Kaneshima H. 3′-Azido-3′ deoxythymidine suppresses HIV infection in SCID-hu mouse. Science 1990 (in press).

Guidelines for Prevention of Transmission of Human Immunodeficiency Virus and Hepatitis B Virus to Health Care and Public Safety Workers[1]

I. Introduction

A. Background

This document is a response to recently enacted legislation, Public Law 100-607, The Health Omnibus Programs Extension Act of 1988, Title II, Programs with Respect to Acquired Immune Deficiency Syndrome ("AIDS Amendments of 1988"). Subtitle E, General Provisions, Section 253(a) of Title II specifies that "the Secretary of Health and Human Services, acting through the Director of the Centers for Disease Control, shall develop, issue, and disseminate guidelines to all health workers, public safety workers (including emergency response employees) in the United States concerning—

(1) methods to reduce the risk in the workplace of becoming infected with the etiologic agent for acquired immune deficiency syndrome; and
(2) circumstances under which exposure to such etiologic agent may occur."

It is further noted that "The Secretary [of Health and Human Services] shall transmit the guidelines issued under subsection (a) to the Secretary of Labor for use by the Secretary of Labor in the development of standards to be issued under the Occupational Safety and Health Act of 1970," and that "the Secretary, acting through the Director of the Centers for Disease Control, shall develop a model

---

1. Centers for Disease Control, *MMWR* 1989; 38(no. S-6): 1–37.

curriculum for emergency response employees with respect to the prevention of exposure to the etiologic agent for acquired immune deficiency syndrome during the process of responding to emergencies."

Following development of these guidelines and curriculum, "[t]he Secretary shall—

(A) transmit to State public health officers copies of the guidelines and the model curriculum developed under paragraph (1) with the request that such officers disseminate such copies as appropriate throughout the State; and

(B) make such copies available to the public."

B. Purpose and Organization of Document

The purpose of this document is to provide an overview of the modes of transmission of human immunodeficiency virus (HIV) in the workplace, an assessment of the risk of transmission under various assumptions, principles underlying the control of risk, and specific risk-control recommendations for employers and workers. This document also includes information on medical management of persons who have sustained an exposure at the workplace to these viruses (e.g., emergency medical technicians who incur a needlestick injury while performing professional duties). These guidelines are intended for use by a technically informed audience. As noted above, a separate model curriculum based on the principles and practices discussed in this document is being developed for use in training workers and will contain less technical wording.

Information concerning the protection of workers against acquisition of the human immunodeficiency virus (HIV) while performing job duties, the virus that causes AIDS, is presented here. Information on hepatitis B virus (HBV) is also presented in this document on the basis of the following assumptions:

- the modes of transmission for hepatitis B virus (HBV) are similar to those of HIV,
- the potential for HBV transmission in the occupational setting is greater than for HIV,
- there is a larger body of experience relating to controlling transmission of HBV in the workplace, and
- general practices to prevent the transmission of HBV will also minimize the risk of transmission of HIV.

Bloodborne transmission of other pathogens not specifically addressed here will be interrupted by adherence to the precautions noted below. It is important to note that the implementation of control measures for HIV and HBV does not obviate the need for continued adherence to general infection-control principles and general hygiene measures (e.g., hand washing) for preventing transmission of other infectious diseases to both worker and client. General guidelines for control of these diseases have been published (1–3).

This document was developed primarily to provide guidelines for fire-service personnel, emergency medical technicians, paramedics (see section IV), and law-enforcement and correctional-facility personnel (see section V). Throughout the report, paramedics and emergency medical technicians are called "emergency medical workers" and fire-service, law-enforcement, and correctional-facility personnel, "public-safety workers." Previously issued guidelines address the needs of hospital-, laboratory-, and clinic-based health-care workers (4,5). A condensation of general guidelines for protection of workers from transmission of bloodborne pathogens, derived from the Joint Advisory Notice of the Departments of Labor and Health and Human Services (6), is provided in section III.

C. Modes and Risk of Virus Transmission in the Workplace

Although the potential for HBV transmission in the workplace setting is greater than for HIV, the modes of transmission for these two viruses are similar. Both have been transmitted in occupational settings **only** by percutaneous inoculation or contact with an open wound, nonintact (e.g., chapped, abraded, weeping, or dermatitis) skin, or mucous membranes to blood, blood-contaminated body fluids, or concentrated virus. **Blood is the single most important source of HIV and HBV in the workplace setting.** Protection measures against HIV and HBV for workers should focus primarily on preventing these types of exposures to blood as well as on delivery of HBV vaccination.

The risk of hepatitis B infection following a parenteral (i.e., needlestick or cut) exposure to blood is directly proportional to the probability that the blood contains hepatitis B surface antigen (HBsAg), the immunity status of the recipient, and on the efficiency of transmission (7). The probability of the source of the blood being HBsAg positive varies from 1 to 3 per thousand in the general population to 5–15% in groups at high risk for HBV infection, such as immigrants from areas of high endemicity (China and Southeast Asia, sub-Saharan Africa, most Pacific islands, and the Amazon Basin); clients in institutions for the mentally retarded; intravenous drug users; homosexually active males; and household (sexual and nonsexual) contacts of HBV carriers. Of persons who have not had prior hepatitis B vaccination or postexposure prophylaxis, 6–30% of persons who receive a needlestick exposure from an HBsAg-positive individual will become infected (7).

The risk of infection with HIV following one needlestick exposure to blood from a patient known to be infected with HIV is approximately 0.5% (4,5). This rate of transmission is considerably lower than that for HBV, probably as a result of the significantly lower concentrations of virus in the blood of HIV-infected persons. Table H1 presents theoretical data concerning the likelihood of infection given repeated needlestick injuries involving patients whose HIV serostatus is unknown. Though inadequately quantified, the risk from exposure of nonintact skin or mucous membranes is likely to be far less than that from percutaneous inoculation.

D. Transmission of Hepatitis B Virus to Workers

1. Health-care workers

In 1987, the CDC estimated the total number of HBV infections in the United

Table H1.   The risk of HIV infection following needlestick injury: hypothetical model

Prevelence of HIV infection (A)	Probability of infection given needlestick injury with blood containing HIV (B)	Probability of infection given random needlestick (unknown serostatus) A*B = (C)	Probability of infection given 10 random needlesticks $1-(1-C)^{10}$	Probability of infection given 100 random needlesticks $1-(1-C)^{100}$
0.0001	0.001	0.0000001	0.000001	0.00001
0.0001	0.005	0.0000005	0.000005	0.00005
0.001	0.001	0.000001	0.00001	0.0001
0.001	0.005	0.000005	0.00005	0.0005
0.01	0.001	0.00001	0.0001	0.001
0.01[a]	0.005	0.00005	0.0005	0.005
0.05	0.001	0.00005	0.0005	0.005
0.05	0.005	0.00025	0.0025	0.025

[a]For example, if the prevelence of infection in the population is 0.01 (i.e., 1 per 100) and the risk of a seroconversion following a needlestick with blood know to contain HIV is 0.005 (i.e., 1 in 200), then the probability of HIV infection given a random needlestick is 0.00005 (i.e., 5 in 100,000). If an individual sustains 10 needlestick injuries, the probability of acquiring HIV infection in 0.0005 (i.e., 1 in 2,000); if the individual sustains 100 needlestick injuries, the probability a acquiring HIV infection is 0.005 (i.e., 1 in 200).

States to be 300,000 per year, with approximately 75,000 (25%) of infected persons developing acute hepatitis. Of these infected individuals, 18,000–30,000 (6–10%) will become HBV carriers, at risk of developing chronic liver disease (chronic active hepatitis, cirrhosis, and primary liver cancer), and infectious to others.

CDC has estimated that 12,000 health-care workers whose jobs entail exposure to blood become infected with HBV each year, that 500–600 of them are hospitalized as a result of that infection, and that 700–1,200 of those infected become HBV carriers. Of the infected workers, approximately 250 will die (12–15 from fulminant hepatitis, 170–200 from cirrhosis, and 40–50 from liver cancer). Studies indicate that 10–30% of health-care or dental workers show serologic evidence of past or present HBV infection.

2. Emergency medical and public-safety workers

Emergency medical workers have an increased risk for hepatitis B infection (8–10). The degree of risk correlates with the frequency and extent of blood exposure during the conduct of work activities. A few studies are available concerning risk of HBV infection for other groups of public-safety workers (law-enforcement personnel and correctional-facility workers), but reports that have been published do not document any increased risk for HBV infection (11–13). Nevertheless, in occupational settings in which workers may be routinely exposed to blood or other body fluids as described below, an increased risk for occupational acquisition of HBV infection must be assumed to be present.

3. Vaccination for hepatitis B virus

A safe and effective vaccine to prevent hepatitis B has been available since 1982. Vaccination has been recommended for health-care workers regularly exposed to blood and other body fluids potentially contaminated with HBV (7,14,15). In 1987, the Department of Health and Human Services and the Department of Labor stated that hepatitis B vaccine should be provided to all such workers at no charge to the worker (6).

Available vaccines stimulate active immunity against HBV infection and provide over 90% protection against hepatitis B for 7 or more years following vaccination (7). Hepatitis B vaccines also are 70–88% effective when given within 1 week after HBV exposure. Hepatitis B immune globulin (HBIG), a preparation of immunoglobulin with high levels of antibody to HBV (anti-HBs), provides temporary passive protection following exposure to HBV. Combination treatment with hepatitis B vaccine and HBIG is over 90% effective in preventing hepatitis B following a documented exposure (7).

E. Transmission of Human Immunodeficiency Virus to Workers

1. Health-care workers with AIDS

As of September 19, 1988, a total of 3,182 (5.1%) of 61,929 adults with AIDS who had been reported to the CDC national surveillance system and for whom occupational information was available, reported being employed in a health-care setting. Of the health-care workers with AIDS, 95% reported high-risk behavior; for the remaining 5% (169 workers), the means of HIV acquisition was undetermined.

Of these 169 health-care workers with AIDS with undetermined risk, information is incomplete for 28 (17%) because of death or refusal to be interviewed; 97 (57%) are still being investigated. The remaining 44 (26%) health-care workers were interviewed directly or had other follow-up information available. The occupations of these 44 were nine nursing assistants (20%); eight physicians (18%), four of whom were surgeons; eight housekeeping or maintenance workers (18%); six nurses (14%); four clinical laboratory technicians (9%); two respiratory therapists (5%); one dentist (2%); one paramedic (2%); one embalmer (2%); and four others who did not have contact with patients (9%). Eighteen of these 44 health-care workers reported parenteral and/or other nonneedlestick exposure to blood or other body fluids from patients in the 10 years preceding their diagnosis of AIDS. None of these exposures involved a patient with AIDS or known HIV infection, and HIV seroconversion of the health-care worker was not documented following a specific exposure.

2. Human immunodeficiency virus transmission in the workplace

As of July 31, 1988, 1,201 health-care workers had been enrolled and tested for HIV antibody in ongoing CDC surveillance of health-care workers exposed via needlestick or splashes to skin or mucous membranes to blood from patients known to be HIV-infected (16). Of 860 workers who had received needlestick injuries or cuts with sharp objects (i.e., parenteral exposures) and whose serum had been tested for HIV antibody at least 180 days after exposure, four were positive, yielding a seroprevalence rate of 0.47%. Three of these individuals experienced an acute retroviral syndrome associated with documented seroconversion. Investigation revealed no nonoccupational risk factors for these three workers. Serum collected within 30 days of exposure was not available from the fourth person. This worker had an HIV-seropositive sexual partner, and heterosexual acquisition of infection cannot be excluded. None of the 103 workers who had contamination of mucous membranes or nonintact skin and whose serum had been tested at least 180 days after exposure developed serologic evidence of HIV infection.

Two other ongoing prospective studies assess the risk of nosocomial acquisition of HIV infection among health-care workers in the United States. As of April 1988, the National Institutes of Health had tested 983 health-care workers, 137 with documented needlestick injuries and 345 health-care workers who had sustained mucous membrane exposures to blood or other body fluids of HIV-infected patients; none had seroconverted (17) (one health-care worker who subsequently experienced an occupational HIV seroconversion has since been reported from NIH [18]). As of March 15, 1988, a similar study at the University of California of 212 health-care workers with 625 documented accidental parenteral exposures involving HIV-infected patients had identified one seroconversion following a needlestick (19). Prospective studies in the United Kingdom and Canada show no evidence of HIV transmission among 220 health-care workers with parenteral, mucous-membrane, or cutaneous exposures (20,21).

In addition to the health-care workers enrolled in these longitudinal surveillance studies, case histories have been published in the scientific literature for 19 HIV infected health-care workers (13 with documented seroconversion and six without documented seroconversion). None of these workers reported nonoccupational risk factors (see Table H2).

3. Emergency medical service and public-safety workers

In addition to the one paramedic with undetermined risk discussed above, three public-safety workers (law-enforcement officers) are classified in the undetermined risk group. Follow-up investigations of these workers could not determine conclusively if HIV infection was acquired during the performance of job duties.

II. PRINCIPLES OF INFECTION CONTROL AND THEIR APPLICATION TO EMERGENCY AND PUBLIC-SAFETY WORKERS

A. General Infection Control

Within the health-care setting, general infection control procedures have been developed to minimize the risk of patient acquisition of infection from contact with contaminated devices, objects, or surfaces or of transmission of an infectious agent from health-care workers to patients (1–3). Such procedures also protect workers from the risk of becoming infected. General infection-control

Table H2. HIV-infected health care workers with no reported nonoccupational risk factors and for whom case histories have been published in the scientific literature

Case	Occupation	Country	Type of exposure	Source
Cases with documented seroconversion				
1[a]	NS[b]	United States	Needlestick	AIDS patient
2	NS	United States	Needlestick	AIDS patient
3	NS	United States	Needlestick	AIDS patient
4	NS	United States	2 Needlesticks	AIDS and HIV-infected patients
5	NS	United States	Needlestick	AIDS patient
6	Nurse	England	Needlestick	AIDS patient
7	Nurse	France	Needlestick	HIV-infected patient
8	Nurse	Martinique	Needlestick	AIDS patient
9	Research lab worker	United States	Cut with sharp object	Concentrated virus
10	Home health care worker	United States	Cutaneous[c]	AIDS patient
11	NS	United States	Nonintact skin	AIDS patient
12	Phlebotomist	United States	Mucous membrane	HIV-infected patient
13	Technologist	United States	Nonintact skin	HIV-infected patient
14	NS	United States	Needlestick	AIDS patient
15	Nurse	Italy	Mucous membrane	HIV-infected patient
16	Nurse	France	Needlestick	AIDS patient
17	Navy medic	United States	Needlestick	AIDS patient
18	Clinical lab worker	United States	Cut with sharp object	AIDS patient
Case without documented seroconversion				
19	NS	United States	Puncture wound	AIDS patient
20	NS	United States	2 Needlesticks	2 AIDS patients
21	Research lab worker	United States	Nonintact skin	Concentrated virus
22	Home health care provider	England	Nonintact skin	AIDS patient
23	Dentist	United States	Multiple needlesticks	Unknown
24	Technician	Mexico	Multiple needlesticks and mucous membrane	Unknown
25	Lab worker	United States	Needlestick, puncture wound	Unknown

[a]AIDS case.
[b]Not specified.
[c]Mother who provided nursing care for her child with HIV infection; extensive contact with the child's blood and body secretions and excretions occurred; the mother did not wear gloves and often did not wash her hands immediately after exposure.

procedures are designed to prevent transmission of a wide range of microbiological agents and to provide a wide margin of safety in the varied situations encountered in the health-care environment.

General infection-control principles are applicable to other work environments where workers contact other individuals and where transmission of infectious agents may occur. The modes of transmission noted in the hospital and
medical office environment are observed in the work situations of emergency and
public-safety workers, as well. Therefore, the principles of infection control developed for hospital and other health-care settings are also applicable to these
work situations. Use of general infection control measures, as adapted to the
work environments of emergency and public-safety workers, is important to protect both workers and individuals with whom they work from a variety of infection agents, not just HIV and HBV.

Because emergency and public-safety workers work in environments that
provide inherently unpredictable risks of exposures, general infection-control
procedures should be adapted to these work situations. Exposures are unpredictable, and protective measures may often be used in situations that do not appear
to present risk. Emergency and public-safety workers perform their duties in the
community under extremely variable conditions; thus, control measures that are
simple and uniform across all situations have the greatest likelihood of worker
compliance. Administrative procedures to ensure compliance also can be more
readily developed than when procedures are complex and highly variable.

B. Universal Blood and Body Fluid Precautions to Prevent Occupational HIV and HBV Transmission

In 1985, CDC developed the strategy of "universal blood and body fluid
precautions" to address concerns regarding transmission of HIV in the health-
care setting (4). The concept, now referred to simply as "universal precautions"
stresses that **all patients should be assumed to be infectious for HIV and other
bloodborne pathogens.** In the hospital and other health-care setting, "universal
precautions" should be followed when workers are exposed to blood, certain
other body fluids (amniotic fluid, pericardial fluid, peritoneal fluid, pleural fluid,
synovial fluid, cerebrospinal fluid, semen, and vaginal secretions), or any body
fluid visibly contaminated with blood. Since HIV and HBV transmission has not
been documented from exposure to other body fluids (feces, nasal secretions,
sputum, sweat, tears, urine, and vomitus), "universal precautions" do not apply to
these fluids. Universal precautions also do not apply to saliva, except in the
dental setting, where saliva is likely to be contaminated with blood (7).

For the purpose of this document, human "exposure" is defined as contact
with blood or other body fluids to which universal precautions apply through
percutaneous inoculation or contact with an open wound, nonintact skin, or mu-

cous membrane during the performance of normal job duties. An "exposed worker" is defined, for the purposes of this document, as an individual exposed, as described above, while performing normal job duties.

The unpredictable and emergent nature of exposures encountered by emergency and public-safety workers may make differentiation between hazardous body fluids and those which are not hazardous very difficult and often impossible. For example, poor lighting may limit the worker's ability to detect visible blood in vomitus or feces. Therefore, **when emergency medical and public-safety workers encounter body fluids under uncontrolled, emergency circumstances in which differentiation between fluid types is difficult, if not impossible, they should treat all body fluids as potentially hazardous.**

The application of the principles of universal precautions to the situations encountered by these workers results in the development of guidelines (listed below) for work practices, use of personal protective equipment, and other protective measures. To minimize the risks of acquiring HIV and HBV during performance of job duties, emergency and public-safety workers should be protected from exposure to blood and other body fluids as circumstances dictate. Protection can be achieved through adherence to work practices designed to minimize or eliminate exposure and through use of personal protective equipment (i.e., gloves, masks, and protective clothing), which provide a barrier between the worker and the exposure source. In some situations, redesign of selected aspects of the job through equipment modifications or environmental control can further reduce risk. These approaches to primary prevention should be used together to achieve maximal reduction of the risk of exposure.

If exposure of an individual worker occurs, medical management, consisting of collection of pertinent medical and occupational history, provision of treatment, and counseling regarding future work and personal behaviors, may reduce risk of developing disease as a result of the exposure episode (22). Following episodic (or continuous) exposure, decontamination and disinfection of the work environment, devices, equipment, and clothing or other forms of personal protective equipment can reduce subsequent risk of exposures. Proper disposal of contaminated waste has similar benefits.

III. EMPLOYER RESPONSIBILITIES

A. General

Detailed recommendations for employer responsibilities in protecting workers from acquisition of bloodborne diseases in the workplace have been published in the Department of Labor and Department of Health and Human Services Joint Advisory Notice and are summarized here (6). In developing programs to protect workers, employers should follow a series of steps: 1) classification of work activity, 2) development of standard operating procedures, 3) provision of training and education, 4) development of procedures to ensure and monitor compliance, and 5) workplace redesign. As a first step every employer should classify work activities into one of three categories of potential exposure (see Table H3). Employers should make protective equipment available to all workers when they are engaged in Category I or II activities. Employers should ensure that the appropriate protective equipment is used by workers when they perform Category I activities.

As a second step, employers should establish a detailed work practices program that includes standard operating procedures (SOPS) for all activities having the potential for exposure. Once these SOPs are developed, an initial and periodic worker education program to assure familiarity with work practices should be provided to potentially exposed workers. No worker should engage in such tasks or activities before receiving training pertaining to the SOPs, work practices, and protective equipment required for that task. Examples of personal protective equipment for the prehospital setting (defined as a setting where delivery of emergency health care takes place away from a hospital or other health-care setting) are provided in Table H4. (A curriculum for such training programs is being developed in conjunction with these guidelines and should be consulted for further information concerning such training programs.)

To facilitate and monitor compliance with SOPs, administrative procedures

Table H3. Summary of task categorization and implications for personal protective equipment

Joint advisory notice category[a]	Nature of task/activity	*Personal protective equipment should be:*	
		Available?	Worn?
I	Direct contact with blood or other body fluids to which universal precautions apply	Yes	Yes
II	Activity performed without blood exposure but exposure may occur in emergency	Yes	No
III	Task/activity does not entail predictable or unpredictable exposure to blood	No	No

[a]U.S. Department of Labor, U.S. Department of Health and Human Services. *Joint advisory notice: protection against occupational exposure to hepatitis B virus (HBV) and human immunodeficiency virus (HIV).* Washington, DC: U.S. Department of Labor, U.S. Department of Health and Human Services, 1987.

Table H4. Examples of recommended personal preotective equipment for worker protection against HIV and HBV transmission[a] in prehospital[b] settings

Task or activity	Disposable gloves	Gown	Mask[c]	Protective eyewear
Bleeding control with spurting blood	Yes	Yes	Yes	Yes
Bleeding control with minimal bleeding	Yes	No	No	No
Emergency childbirth	Yes	Yes	Yes, if splashing is likely	Yes, if splashing is likely
Blood drawing	At certain times	No	No	No
Starting an intravenous (IV) line	Yes	No	No	No
Endotrachael intubation, esophageal obturator use	Yes	No	No, unless splashing is likely	No, unless splashing is likely
Oral/nasal suctioning, manually cleaning airway	Yes[d]	No	No, unless splashing is likely	No, unless splashing is likely
Handling and cleaning instruments with microbial contamination	Yes	No, unless soiling is likely	No	No
Measuring blood pressure	No	No	No	No
Measuring temperature	No	No	No	No
Giving an injection	No	No	No	No

[a]The examples provided in this table are based on application of Universal Precautions. Universal Precautions are intended to supplement rather than replace recommendations for routine infection control, such as hand washing and using gloves to prevent gross microbial contamination of hands (e.g., contact with urine or feces).

[b]Defined as setting where delivery of emergency health care takes place away from a hospital or other health care facility.

[c]Refers to protective masks to prevent exposure of mucous membranes to blood or other potentially contaminated body fluids. Some resuscitative devices are referred to as "masks."

[d]While not clearly necessary to prevent HIV or HBV transmission unless blood is present, gloves are recommended to prevent transmission of other agents (e.g., *Herpes simplex*).

should be developed and records kept as described in the Joint Advisory Notice (6). Employers should monitor the workplace to ensure that required work practices are observed and that protective clothing and equipment are provided and properly used. The employer should maintain records documenting the administrative procedures used to classify job activities and copies of all SOPs for tasks or activities involving predictable or unpredictable exposure to blood or other body fluids to which universal precautions apply. In addition, training records, indicating the dates of training sessions, the content of those training sessions along with the names of all persons conducting the training, and the names of all those receiving training should also be maintained.

Whenever possible, the employer should identify devices and other approaches to modifying the work environment which will reduce exposure risk. Such approaches are desirable, since they don't require individual worker action or management activity. For example, jails and correctional facilities should have classification procedures that require the segregation of offenders who indicate through their actions or words that they intend to attack correctional-facility staff with the intent of transmitting HIV or HBV.

B. Medical

In addition to the general responsibilities noted above, the employer has the specific responsibility to make available to the worker a program of medical management. This program is designed to provide for the reduction of risk of infection by HBV and for counseling workers concerning issues regarding HIV and HBV. These services should be provided by a licensed health professional. All phases of medical management and counseling should ensure that the confidentiality of the worker's and client's medical data is protected.

1. Hepatitis B vaccination

All workers whose jobs involve participation in tasks or activities with exposure to blood or other body fluids to which universal precautions should be vaccinated with hepatitis B vaccine.

2. Management of percutaneous exposure to blood and other infectious body fluids

Once an exposure has occurred, a blood sample should be drawn after consent is obtained from the individual from whom exposure occurred and tested for hepatitis B surface antigen (HBsAg) and antibody to human immunodeficiency virus (HIV antibody). Local laws regarding consent for testing source individuals should be followed. Policies should be available for testing source individuals in situations where consent cannot be obtained (e.g., an unconscious patient). Testing of the source individual should be done at a location where appropriate pretest counseling is available; posttest counseling and referral for treatment should be provided. It is extremely important that all individuals who seek consultation for any HIV-related concerns receive counseling as outlined in the "Public Health Service Guidelines for Counseling and Antibody Testing to Prevent HIV Infection and AIDS" (22).

a. Hepatitis B virus postexposure management   For an exposure to a source individual found to be positive for HBsAg, the worker who has not previously been given hepatitis B vaccine should receive the vaccine series. A single dose of hepatitis B immune globulin (HBIG) is also recommended, if this can be given within 7 days of exposure. For exposures from an HBsAg-positive source to workers who have previously received vaccine, the exposed worker should be tested for antibody to hepatitis B surface antigen (anti-HBs), and given one dose of vaccine and one dose of HBIG if the antibody level in the worker's blood samples is inadequate (i.e., <10 SRU by RIA, negative by EIA) (7).

If the source individual is negative for HBsAg and the worker has not been vaccinated, this opportunity should be taken to provide hepatitis B vaccination.

If the source individual refuses testing or he/she cannot be identified, the unvaccinated worker should receive the hepatitis B vaccine series. HBIG administration should be considered on an individual basis when the source individual is known or suspected to be at high risk of HBV infection. Management and treatment, if any, of previously vaccinated workers who receive an exposure from a source who refuses testing or is not identifiable should be individualized (7).

b. Human immunodeficiency virus postexposure management   For any exposure to a source individual who has AIDS, who is found to be positive for HIV infection (4), or who refuses testing, the worker should be counseled regarding the risk of infection and evaluated clinically and serologically for evidence of HIV infection as soon as possible after the exposure. In view of the evolving nature of HIV postexposure management, the health-care provider should be well informed of current PHS guidelines on this subject. The worker should be advised to report and seek medical evaluation for any acute febrile illness that occurs within 12 weeks after the exposure. Such an illness, particularly one characterized by fever, rash, or lymphadenopathy, may be indicative of recent HIV infection. Following the initial test at the time of exposure, seronegative workers should be retested 6 weeks, 12 weeks, and 6 months after exposure to determine whether transmission has occurred. During this follow-up period (especially the first 6–12 weeks after exposure, when most infected persons are expected to seroconvert), exposed workers should follow U.S. Public Health

Service (PHS) recommendations for preventing transmission of HIV (22). These include refraining from blood donation and using appropriate protection during sexual intercourse (23). During all phases of follow-up, it is vital that worker confidentiality be protected.

If the source individual was tested and found to be seronegative, baseline testing of the exposed worker with follow-up testing 12 weeks later may be performed if desired by the worker or recommended by the health-care provider.

If the source individual cannot be identified, decisions regarding appropriate follow-up should be individualized. Serologic testing should be made available by the employer to all workers who may be concerned they have been infected with HIV through an occupational exposure as defined above.

3. Management of human bites

On occasion, police and correctional-facility officers are intentionally bitten by suspects or prisoners. When such bites occur, routine medical and surgical therapy (including an assessment of tetanus vaccination status) should be implemented as soon as possible, since such bites frequently result in infection with organisms other than HIV and HBV. Victims of bites should be evaluated as described above for exposure to blood or other infectious body fluids.

Saliva of some persons infected with HBV has been shown to contain HBV-DNA at concentrations 1/1,000 to 1/10,000 of that found in the infected person's serum (5,24). HbsAg-positive saliva has been shown to be infectious when injected into experimental animals and in human bite exposures (25–27). However, HBsAg-positive saliva has not been shown to be infectious when applied to oral mucous membranes in experimental primate studies (27) or through contamination of musical instruments or cardiopulmonary resuscitation dummies used by HBV carriers (28,29). Epidemiologic studies of nonsexual household contacts of HIV-infected patients, including several small series in which HIV transmission failed to occur after bites or after percutaneous inoculation or contamination of cuts and open wounds with saliva from HIV-infected patients, suggest that the potential for salivary transmission of HIV is remote (5,30–33). One case report from Germany has suggested the possibility of transmission of HIV in a household setting from an infected child to a sibling through a human bite (34). The bite did not break the skin or result in bleeding. Since the date of seroconversion to HIV was not known for either child in this case, evidence for the role of saliva in the transmission of virus is unclear (34).

4. Documentation of exposure and reporting

As part of the confidential medical record, the circumstances of exposure should be recorded. Relevant information includes the activity in which the worker was engaged at the time of exposure, the extent to which appropriate work practices and protective equipment were used, and a description of the source of exposure.

Employers have a responsibility under various federal and state laws and regulations to report occupational illnesses and injuries. Existing programs in the National Institute for Occupational Safety and Health (NIOSH), Department of Health and Human Services; the Bureau of Labor Statistics, Department of Labor (DOL); and the Occupational Safety and Health Administration (OSHA) receive such information for the purposes of surveillance and other objectives. Cases of infectious disease, including AIDS and HBV infection, are reported to the Centers for Disease Control through State health departments.

5. Management of HBV- or HIV-infected workers

Transmission of HBV from health-care workers to patients has been documented. Such transmission has occurred during certain types of invasive procedures (e.g., oral and gynecologic surgery) in which health-care workers, when tested, had very high concentrations of HBV in their blood (at least 100 million infectious virus particles per milliliter, a concentration much higher than occurs with HIV infection), and the health-care workers sustained a puncture wound while performing invasive procedures or had exudative or weeping lesions or microlacerations that allowed virus to contaminate instruments or open wounds of patients (35,36). A worker who is HBsAg-positive and who has transmitted hepatitis B virus to another individual during the performance of his or her job duties should be excluded from the performance of those job duties which place other individuals at risk for acquisition of hepatitis B infection.

Workers with impaired immune systems resulting from HIV infection or other causes are at increased risk of acquiring or experiencing serious complications of infectious disease. Of particular concern is the risk of severe infection following exposure to other persons with infectious diseases that are easily transmitted if appropriate precautions are not taken (e.g., measles, varicella). Any worker with an impaired immune system should be counseled about the potential risk associated with providing health care to persons with any transmissible infection and should continue to follow existing recommendations for infection control to minimize risk of exposure to other infectious agents (2,3). Recommendations of the Immunization Practices Advisory Committee (ACIP) and institutional policies concerning requirements for vaccinating workers with live-virus vaccines (e.g., measles, rubella) should also be considered.

The question of whether workers infected with HIV can adequately and safely be allowed to perform patient-care duties or whether their work assignments should be changed must be determined on an individual basis. These decisions should be made by the worker's personal physician(s) in conjunction with the employer's medical advisors.

C. Disinfection, Decontamination, and Disposal

As described in Section I.C., the only documented occupational risks of HIV and HBV infection are associated with parenteral (including open wound) and mucous membrane exposure to blood and other potentially infectious body fluids. Nevertheless, the precautions described below should be routinely followed.

1. Needle and sharps disposal

All workers should take precautions to prevent injuries caused by needles, scalpel blades, and other sharp instruments or devices during procedures; when cleaning used instruments; during disposal of used needles; and when handling sharp instruments after procedures. To prevent needlestick injuries, needles should not be recapped, purposely bent or broken by hand, removed from disposable syringes, or otherwise manipulated by hand. After they are used, disposable syringes and needles, scalpel blades, and other sharp items should be placed in puncture-resistant containers for disposal; the puncture-resistant containers should be located as close as practical to the use area (e.g., in the ambulance or, if sharps are carried to the scene of victim assistance from the ambulance, a small puncture-resistant container should be carried to the scene, as well). Reusable needles should be left on the syringe body and should be placed in a puncture-resistant container for transport to the reprocessing area.

2. Hand washing

Hands and other skin surfaces should be washed immediately and thoroughly if contaminated with blood, other body fluids to which universal precautions apply, or potentially contaminated articles. Hands should always be washed after gloves are removed, even if the gloves appear to be intact. Hand washing should be completed using the appropriate facilities, such as utility or restroom sinks. Waterless antiseptic hand cleanser should be provided on responding units to use when hand-washing facilities are not available. When hand-washing facilities are available, wash hands with warm water and soap. When hand-washing facilities are not available, use a waterless antiseptic hand cleanser. The manufacturer's recommendations for the product should be followed.

3. Cleaning, disinfecting, and sterilizing

Table H5 presents the methods and applications for cleaning, disinfecting, and sterilizing equipment and surfaces in the prehospital setting. These methods also apply to housekeeping and other cleaning tasks. Previously issued guidelines for health-care workers contain more detailed descriptions (4).

Table H5. Reprocessing methods for equipment used in the prehospital[a] health care setting

Sterilization:	Destroys:	All forms of microbial life including high numbers of bacterial spores.
	Methods:	Steam under pressure (autoclave), gas (ethylene oxide), dry heat, or immersion in EPA-approved chemical "sterilant" for prolonged period of time, e.g., 6–10 hours or according to manufacturers' instructions. Note: liquid chemical "sterilants" should be used only on those instruments that are impossible to sterilize or disinfect with heat.
	Use:	For those instruments or devices that penetrate skin or contact normally sterile areas of the body, e.g., scalpels, needles, etc. Disposable invasive equipment eliminates the need to reprocess these types of items. When indicated, however, arrangements should be made with a health care facility for reprocessing of reusable invasive instruments.
High-level disinfection:	Destroys:	All forms of microbial life *except* high numbers of bacterial spores.
	Methods:	Hot water pasteurization (80–100° C, 30 minutes) or exposure to an EPA-registered "sterilant" chemical as above, except for a short exposure time (10–45 minutes or as directed by the manufacturer).
	Use:	For reusable instruments or devices that come into contact with mucous membranes (e.g., laryngoscope blades, endotracheal tubes, etc.).
Intermediate-level disinfection	Destroys:	*Mycobacterium tuberculosis*, vegetative bacteria, most viruses, and most fungi, but does *not* kill bacterial spores.
	Methods:	EPA-registered "hospital disinfectant" chemical germicides that have a label claim for tuberculocidal activity; commercially available hard-surface germicides or solutions containing at least 500 ppm free available chlorine (a 1:100 dilution of common household bleach—approximately 1/4 cup bleach per gallon of tap water).
	Use:	For those surfaces that come into contact only with intact skin, e.g., stethoscopes, blood pressure cuffs, splints, etc., *and* have been visibly contaminated with blood or bloody body fluids. Surfaces *must* be precleaned of visible material before the germicidal chemical is applied for disinfection.
Low-level disinfection	Destroys:	Most bacteria, some viruses, some fungi, but not *Mycobaterium tuberculosis* or bacterial spores.
	Methods:	EPA-registered "hospital disinfectants" (*no* label claim for tuberculocidal activity).
	Use	These agents are excellent cleaners and can be used for routine housecleaning or removal of soiling in the *absence* of visible blood contamination.

| Environmental disinfection: | Environmental surfaces which have become soiled should be cleaned and disinfected using any cleaner or disinfectant agent which is intended for environmental use. Such surfaces include floors, woodwork, ambulance seats, countertops, etc. |
| IMPORTANT: | To assure the effectiveness of any sterilization or disinfection process, equipment and instruments must first be thoroughly cleaned of all visible soil. |

[a]Defined as setting where delivery of emergency health care takes place prior to arrival at hospital or other health care facility.

4. Cleaning and decontaminating spills of blood

All spills of blood and blood-contaminated fluids should be promptly cleaned up using an EPA-approved germicide or a 1:100 solution of household bleach in the following manner **while wearing gloves.** Visible material should first be removed with disposable towels or other appropriate means that will ensure against direct contact with blood. If splashing is anticipated, protective eyewear should be worn along with an impervious gown or apron which provides an effective barrier to splashes. The area should then be decontaminated with an appropriate germicide. Hands should be washed following removal of gloves. Soiled cleaning equipment should be cleaned and decontaminated or placed in an appropriate container and disposed of according to agency policy. Plastic bags should be available for removal of contaminated items from the site of the spill.

Shoes and boots can become contaminated with blood in certain instances. Where there is massive blood contamination on floors, the use of disposable impervious shoe coverings should be considered. Protective gloves should be worn to remove contaminated shoe coverings. The coverings and gloves should be disposed of in plastic bags. A plastic bag should be included in the crime scene kit or the car which is to be used for the disposal of contaminated items. Extra plastic bags should be stored in the police cruiser or emergency vehicle.

5. Laundry

Although soiled linen may be contaminated with pathogenic microorganisms, the risk of actual disease transmission is negligible. Rather than rigid procedures and specifications, hygienic storage and processing of clean and soiled linen are recommended. Laundry facilities and/or services should be made routinely available by the employer. Soiled linen should be handled as little as possible and with minimum agitation to prevent gross microbial contamination of the air and of persons handling the linen. All soiled linen should be bagged at the location where it was used. Linen soiled with blood should be placed and transported in bags that prevent leakage. Normal laundry cycles should be used according to the washer and detergent manufacturer's recommendations.

6. Decontamination and laundering of protective clothing

Protective work clothing contaminated with blood or other body fluids to which universal precautions apply should be placed and transported in bags or containers that prevent leakage. Personnel involved in the bagging, transport, and laundering of contaminated clothing should wear gloves. Protective clothing and station and work uniforms should be washed and dried according to the manufacturer's instructions. Boots and leather goods may be brush-scrubbed with soap and hot water to remove contamination.

7. Infective waste

The selection of procedures for disposal of infective waste is determined by the relative risk of disease transmission and application of local regulations, which vary widely. **In all cases, local regulations should be consulted prior to disposal procedures and followed.** Infective waste, in general, should either be incinerated or should be decontaminated before disposal in a sanitary landfill. Bulk blood, suctioned fluids, excretions, and secretions may be carefully poured down a drain connected to a sanitary sewer, where permitted. Sanitary sewers may also be used to dispose of other infectious wastes capable of being ground and flushed into the sewer, where permitted. Sharp items should be placed in puncture-proof containers and other blood-contaminated items should be placed in leakproof plastic bags for transport to an appropriate disposal location.

Prior to the removal of protective equipment, personnel remaining on the scene after the patient has been cared for should carefully search for and remove contaminated materials. Debris should be disposed of as noted above.

IV. Fire and Emergency Medical Services

The guidelines that appear in this section apply to fire and emergency medical services. This includes structural firefighters, paramedics, emergency medical technicians, and advanced life support personnel. Firefighters often provide emergency medical services and therefore encounter the exposures common to paramedics and emergency medical technicians. Job duties are often performed in uncontrolled environments, which, due to a lack of time and other factors, do not allow for application of a complex decision-making process to the emergency at hand.

The general principles presented here have been developed from existing principles of occupational safety and health in conjunction with data from studies of health-care workers in hospital settings. The basic premise is that workers must be protected from exposure to blood and other potentially infectious body fluids in the course of their work activities. There is a paucity of data concerning the risks these worker groups face, however, which complicates development of control principles. Thus, the guidelines presented below are based on principles of prudent public health practice.

Fire and emergency medical service personnel are engaged in delivery of medical care in the prehospital setting. The following guidelines are intended to assist these personnel in making decisions concerning use of personal protective equipment and resuscitation equipment, as well as for decontamination, disinfection, and disposal procedures.

A. Personal Protective Equipment

Appropriate personal protective equipment should be made available routinely by the employer to reduce the risk of exposure as defined above. For many situations, the chance that the rescuer will be exposed to blood and other body fluids to which universal precautions apply can be determined in advance. Therefore, if the chances of being exposed to blood is high (e.g., CPR, IV insertion, trauma, delivering babies), the worker should put on protective attire before beginning patient care. Table H4 sets forth examples of recommendations for personal protective equipment in the prehospital setting; the list is not intended to be all-inclusive.

1. Gloves

Disposable gloves should be a standard component of emergency response equipment, and should be donned by all personnel prior to initiating any emergency patient care tasks involving exposure to blood or other body fluids to which universal precautions apply. Extra pairs should always be available. Considerations in the choice of disposable gloves should include dexterity, durability, fit, and the task being performed. Thus, there is no single type or thickness of glove appropriate for protection in all situations. For situations where large amounts of blood are likely to be encountered, it is important that gloves fit tightly at the wrist to prevent blood contamination of hands around the cuff. For multiple trauma victims, gloves should be changed between patient contacts, if the emergency situation allows.

Greater personal protective equipment measures are indicated for situations where broken glass and sharp edges are likely to be encountered, such as extricating a person from an automobile wreck. Structural fire-fighting gloves that meet the Federal OSHA requirements for fire-fighters gloves (as contained in 29 CFR 1910.156 or National Fire Protection Association Standard 1973, Gloves for Structural Fire Fighters) should be worn in any situation where sharp or rough surfaces are likely to be encountered (37).

While wearing gloves, avoid handling personal items, such as combs and pens, that could become soiled or contaminated. Gloves that have become contaminated with blood or other body fluids to which universal precautions apply should be removed as soon as possible, taking care to avoid skin contact with the exterior surface. Contaminated gloves should be placed and transported in bags that prevent leakage and should be disposed of or, in the case of reusable gloves, cleaned and disinfected properly.

2. Masks, eyewear, and gowns

Masks, eyewear, and gowns should be present on all emergency vehicles that respond or potentially respond to medical emergencies or victim rescues. These protective barriers should be used in accordance with the level of exposure encountered. Minor lacerations or small amounts of blood do not merit the same extent of barrier use as required for exsanguinating victims or massive arterial bleeding. Management of the patient who is not bleeding, and who has no bloody body fluids present, should not routinely require use of barrier precautions. Masks and eyewear (e.g., safety glasses) should be worn together, or a face shield should be used by all personnel prior to any situation where splashes of blood or other body fluids to which universal precautions apply are likely to occur. Gowns or aprons should be worn to protect clothing from splashes with blood. If large splashes or quantities of blood are present or anticipated, impervious gowns or aprons should be worn. An extra change of work clothing should be available at all times.

3. Resuscitation equipment

No transmission of HBV or HIV infection during mouth-to-mouth resuscitation has been documented. However, because of the risk of salivary transmission of other infectious diseases (e.g., herpes simplex and *Neisseria meningitidis*) and the theoretical risk of HIV and HBV transmission during artificial ventilation of trauma victims, disposable airway equipment or resuscitation bags should be used. Disposable resuscitation equipment and devices should be used once and disposed of or, if reusable, thoroughly cleaned and disinfected after each use according to the manufacturer's recommendations.

Mechanical respiratory assist devices (e.g., bag-valve masks, oxygen demand valve resuscitators) should be available on all emergency vehicles and to all emergency response personnel that respond or potentially respond to medical emergencies or victim rescues.

Pocket mouth-to-mouth resuscitation masks designed to isolate emergency response personnel (i.e., double lumen systems) from contact with victims' blood and blood contaminated saliva, respiratory secretions, and vomitus should be provided to all personnel who provide or potentially provide emergency treatment.

V. Law-Enforcement and Correctional-Facility Officers

Law-enforcement and correctional-facility officers may face the risk of exposure to blood during the conduct of their duties. For example, at the crime scene or during processing of suspects, law-enforcement officers may encounter blood-contaminated hypodermic needles or weapons, or be called upon to assist with body removal. Correctional-facility officers may similarly be required to search prisoners or their cells for hypodermic needles or weapons, or subdue violent and combative inmates.

The following section presents information for reducing the risk of acquiring HIV and HBV infection by law-enforcement and correctional-facility officers as a consequence of carrying out their duties. However, there is an extremely diverse range of potential situations which may occur in the control of persons with unpredictable violent, or psychotic behavior. Therefore, informed judgment of the individual officer is paramount when unusual circumstances or events arise. These recommendations should serve as an adjunct to rational decision making in those situations where specific guidelines do not exist, particularly where immediate action is required to preserve life or prevent significant injury.

The following guidelines are arranged into three sections: a section addressing concerns shared by both law-enforcement and correctional-facility officers, and two sections dealing separately with law-enforcement officers and correctional-facility officers, respectively. Table H4 contains selected examples of personal protective equipment that may be employed by law-enforcement and correctional-facility officers.

A. Law-Enforcement and Correctional-Facilities Considerations

1. Fights and assaults

Law-enforcement and correctional-facility officers are exposed to a range of assaultive and disruptive behavior through which they may potentially become exposed to blood or other body fluids containing blood. Behaviors of particular concern are biting, attacks resulting in blood exposure, and attacks with sharp objects. Such behaviors may occur in a range of law-enforcement situations including arrests, routine interrogations, domestic disputes, and lockup operations, as well as in correctional-facility activities. Hand-to-hand combat may result in bleeding and may thus incur a greater chance for blood-to-blood exposure, which increases the chances for bloodborne disease transmission.

Whenever the possibility for exposure to blood or blood-contaminated body fluids exists, the appropriate protection should be worn, if feasible under the circumstances. In all cases, extreme caution must be used in dealing with the suspect or prisoner if there is any indication of assaultive or combative behavior. When blood is present and a suspect or an inmate is combative or threatening to staff, gloves should always be put on as soon as conditions permit. In case of blood contamination of clothing, an extra change of clothing should be available at all times.

2. Cardiopulmonary resuscitation

Law-enforcement and correctional personnel are also concerned about infection with HIV and HBV through administration of cardiopulmonary resuscitation (CPR). Although there have been no documented cases of HIV transmission through this mechanism, the possibility of transmission of other infectious diseases exists. Therefore, agencies should make protective masks or airways available to officers and provide training in their proper use. Devices with one-way valves to prevent the patients' saliva or vomitus from entering the caregiver's mouth are preferable.

B. Law-Enforcement Considerations

1. Searches and evidence handling

Criminal justice personnel have potential risks of acquiring HBV or HIV infection through exposures which occur during searches and evidence handling. Penetrating injuries are known to occur, and puncture wounds or needlesticks in particular pose a hazard during searches of persons, vehicles, or cells, and during evidence handling. The following precautionary measures will help to reduce the risk of infection:

- An officer should use great caution in searching the clothing of suspects. Individual discretion, based on the circumstances at hand, should determine if a suspect or prisoner should empty his own pockets or if the officer should use his own skills in determining the contents of a suspect's clothing.
- A safe distance should always be maintained between the officer and the suspect.
- Wear protective gloves if exposure to blood is likely to be encountered.

- Wear protective gloves for all body cavity searches.
- If cotton gloves are to be worn when working with evidence of potential latent fingerprint value at the crime scene, they can be worn over protective disposable gloves when exposure to blood may occur.
- Always carry a flashlight, even during daylight shifts, to search hidden areas. Whenever possible, use long-handled mirrors and flashlights to search such areas (e.g., under car seats).
- If searching a purse, carefully empty contents directly from purse, by turning it upside down over a table.
- Use puncture-proof containers to store sharp instruments and clearly marked plastic bags to store other possibly contaminated items.
- To avoid tearing gloves, use evidence tape instead of metal staples to seal evidence.
- Local procedures for evidence handling should be followed. In general, items should be air-dried before sealing in plastic.

Not all types of gloves are suitable for conducting searches. Vinyl or latex rubber gloves provide little protection against sharp instruments, and they are not puncture-proof. There is a direct tradeoff between level of protection and manipulability. In other words, the thicker the gloves, the more protection they provide, but the less effective they are in locating objects. Thus, there is no single type or thickness of glove appropriate for protection in all situations. Officers should select the type and thickness of glove which provides the best balance of protection and search efficiency.

Officers and crime scene technicians may confront unusual hazards, especially when the crime scene involves violent behavior, such as a homicide where large amounts of blood are present. Protective gloves should be available and worn in this setting. In addition, for very large spills, consideration should be given to other protective clothing, such as overalls, aprons, boots, or protective shoe covers. They should be changed if torn or soiled, and always removed prior to leaving the scene. While wearing gloves, avoid handling personal items, such as combs and pens, that could become soiled or contaminated.

Face masks and eye protection or a face shield are required for laboratory and evidence technicians whose jobs entail potential exposures to blood via a splash to the face, mouth, nose, or eyes.

Airborne particles of dried blood may be generated when a stain is scraped. It is recommended that protective masks and eyewear or face shields be worn by laboratory or evidence technicians when removing the blood stain for laboratory analyses.

While processing the crime scene, personnel should be alert for the presence of sharp objects such as hypodermic needles, knives, razors, broken glass, nails, or other sharp objects.

2. Handling deceased persons and body removal

For detectives, investigators, evidence technicians, and others who may have to touch or remove a body, the response should be the same as for situations requiring CPR or first aid: wear gloves and cover all cuts and abrasions to create a barrier and carefully wash all exposed areas after any contact with blood. The precautions to be used with blood and deceased persons should also be used when handling amputated limbs, hands, or other body parts. Such procedures should be followed after contact with the blood of anyone, regardless of whether they are known or suspected to be infected with HIV or HBV.

3. Autopsies

Protective masks and eyewear (or face shields), laboratory coats, gloves, and waterproof aprons should be worn when performing or attending all autopsies. All autopsy material should be considered infectious for both HIV and HBV. Onlookers with an opportunity for exposure to blood splashes should be similarly protected. Instruments and surfaces contaminated during postmortem procedures should be decontaminated with an appropriate chemical germicide (4). Many laboratories have more detailed standard operating procedures for conducting autopsies; where available, these should be followed. More detailed recommendations for health-care workers in this setting have been published (4).

4. Forensic laboratories

Blood from **all** individuals should be considered infective. To supplement other work site precautions, the following precautions are recommended for workers in forensic laboratories.

  a. All specimens of blood should be put in a well-constructed, appropriately labeled container with a secure lid to prevent leaking during transport. Care should be taken when collecting each specimen to avoid contaminating the outside of the container and of the laboratory form accompanying the specimen.
  b. All persons processing blood specimens should wear gloves. Masks and protective eyewear or face shields should be worn if mucous membrane contact with blood is anticipated (e.g., removing tops from vacuum tubes). Hands should be washed after completion of specimen processing.
  c. For routine procedures, such as histologic and pathologic studies or microbiological culturing, a biological safety cabinet is not necessary. However, biological safety cabinets (Class I or II) should be used whenever procedures are conducted that have a high potential for gener-

ating droplets. These include activities such as blending, sonicating, and vigorous mixing.

d. Mechanical pipetting devices should be used for manipulating all liquids in the laboratory. Mouth pipetting must not be done.

e. Use of needles and syringes should be limited to situations in which there is no alternative, and the recommendations for preventing injuries with needles outlined under universal precautions should be followed.

f. Laboratory work surfaces should be cleaned of visible materials and then decontaminated with an appropriate chemical germicide after a spill of blood, semen, or blood-contaminated body fluid and when work activities are completed.

g. Contaminated materials used in laboratory tests should be decontaminated before reprocessing or be placed in bags and disposed of in accordance with institutional and local regulatory policies for disposal of infective waste.

h. Scientific equipment that has been contaminated with blood should be cleaned and then decontaminated before being repaired in the laboratory or transported to the manufacturer.

i. All persons should wash their hands after completing laboratory activities and should remove protective clothing before leaving the laboratory.

j. Area posting of warning signs should be considered to remind employees of continuing hazard of infectious disease transmission in the laboratory setting.

C. Correctional-Facility Considerations

1. Searches

Penetrating injuries are known to occur in the correctional-facility setting, and puncture wounds or needlesticks in particular pose a hazard during searches of prisoners or their cells. The following precautionary measures will help to reduce the risk of infection:

- A correctional-facility officer should use great caution in searching the clothing of prisoners. Individual discretion, based on the circumstances at hand, should determine if a prisoner should empty his own pockets or if the officer should use his own skills in determining the contents of a prisoner's clothing.
- A safe distance should always be maintained between the officer and the prisoner.
- Always carry a flashlight, even during daylight shifts, to search hidden areas.

Whenever possible, use long-handled mirrors and flashlights to search such areas (e.g., under commodes, bunks, and in vents in jail cells).

- Wear protective gloves if exposure to blood is likely to be encountered.
- Wear protective gloves for all body cavity searches.

Not all types of gloves are suitable for conducting searches. Vinyl or latex rubber gloves can provide little, if any, protection against sharp instruments, and they are not puncture-proof. There is a direct trade-off between level of protection and manipulability. In other words, the thicker the gloves, the more protection they provide, but the less effective they are in locating objects. Thus, there is no single type or thickness of glove appropriate for protection in all situations. Officers should select the type and thickness of glove which provides the best balance of protection and search efficiency.

2. Decontamination and disposal

Prisoners may spit at officers and throw feces; sometimes these substances have been purposefully contaminated with blood. Although there are no documented cases of HIV or HBV transmission in this manner and transmission by this route would not be expected to occur, other diseases could be transmitted. These materials should be removed with a paper towel after donning gloves, and the area then decontaminated with an appropriate germicide. Following cleanup, soiled towels and gloves should be disposed of properly.

REFERENCES

1. Garner JS, Favero MS. *Guideline for handwashing and hospital environmental control, 1985.* Atlanta: Public Health Service, Centers for Disease Control, 1985. HHS publication no. 99–1117.
2. Garner JS, Simmons BP. Guideline for isolation precautions in hospitals. *Infect Control* 1983;4(suppl):245–25.
3. Williams WW. Guideline for infection control in hospital personnel. *Infect Control* 1983;4(suppl):326–49.
4. Centers for Disease Control. Recommendations for prevention of HIV transmission in health-care settings. *MMWR* 1987;36(suppl 2S).
5. Centers for Disease Control. Update: Universal precautions for prevention of transmission of human immunodeficiency virus, hepatitis B virus, and other bloodborne pathogens in health-care settings. *MMWR* 1988; 37:377–82,387–88.
6. U.S. Department of Labor, U.S. Department of Health and Human Services. Joint advisory notice: protection against occupational exposure to hepatitis

B virus (HBV) and human immunodeficiency virus (HIV). *Federal Register* 1987;52:41818–24

7. Centers for Disease Control. Recommendations for protection against viral hepatitis. *MMWR* 1985;34:313–324, 329–35.

8. Kunches LM, Craven DE, Werner BG, Jacobs LM. Hepatitis B exposure in emergency medical personnel: prevalence of serologic markers and need for immunization. *Am J Med* 1983; 75:269–72.

9. Pepe PE, Hollinger FB, Troisi CL, Heiberg D. Viral hepatitis risk in urban emergency medical services personnel. *Ann Emerg Med* 1986; 5:454–7.

10. Valenzuela TD, Hook EW, Copass MK, Corey L. Occupational exposure to hepatitis B in paramedics. *Arch Intern Med* 1985;145:1976–77.

11. Morgan-Capner P, Hudson P. Hepatitis B markers in Lancashire police officers. *Epidemiol Inf* 1988; 100:145–51.

12. Peterkin M, Crawford RJ. Hepatitis B vaccine for police forces [Letter] ? Lancet 1986;2:1458–9.

13. Radvan GH, Hewson EG, Berenger S, Brookman DJ. The Newcastle hepatitis B outbreak: observations on cause, management, and prevention. *Med J Aust* 1986;144:461–4.

14. Centers for Disease Control. Inactivated hepatitis B virus vaccine. *MMWR* 1982; 26:317–22, 327–8.

15. Centers for Disease Control. Update on hepatitis B prevention. *MMWR* 1987; 36:353–60, 366.

16. Marcus R, CDC Cooperative Needlestick Surveillance Group. Surveillance of health care workers exposed to blood from patients infected with the human immunodeficiency virus. *N Engl J Med* 1988; 319:1118–23.

17. Henderson DK, Fahey BJ, Saah AJ, Schmitt JM, Lane HC. Longitudinal assessment of risk for occupational/nosocomial transmission of human immunodeficiency virus, type 1 in health care workers [Abstract]. *1988 ICAAC Conference, New Orleans.*

18. Barnes DM. Health workers and AIDS: Questions persist. *Science* 1988; 241:161–2.

19. Gerberding JL, Littell CG, Chambers HF, Moss AR, Carlson J, Drew W, Levy J, Sande MA. Risk of occupational HIV transmission in intensively exposed health-care workers: follow-up [Abstract]. *1988 ICAAC Conference, New Orleans.*

20. Health and Welfare Canada. National surveillance program on occupational exposures to HIV among health-care workers in Canada. *Canada Dis Weekly Rep* 1987;13–37:163–6.

21. McEvoy M, Porter K, Mortimer P, Simmons N, Shanson D. Prospective study of clinical, laboratory, and ancillary staff with accidental exposures to blood or body fluids from patients infected with HIV. *Br Med J* 1987; 294:1595–7.

22. Centers for Disease Control. Public Health Service guidelines for counseling

and antibody testing to prevent HIV infection and AIDS. *MMWR* 1987; 36:509–15.

23. Centers for Disease Control. Additional recommendations to reduce sexual and drug abuse-related transmission of human T-lymphotropic virus type III/lymphadenopathy-associated virus. *MMWR* 1986; 35:152–5.

24. Jenison SA, Lemon SM, Baker LN, Newbold JE. Quantitative analysis of hepatitis B virus DNA in saliva and semen of chronically infected homosexual men. *J Infect Dis* 1987;156:299–306.

25. Cancio-Bello TP, de Medina M, Shorey J, Valledor MD, Schiff ER. An institutional outbreak of hepatitis B related to a human biting carrier. *J Infect Dis* 1982;146:652–6.

26. MacQuarrie MB, Forghani B, Wolochow DA. Hepatitis B transmitted by a human bite. *JAMA* 1974; 230:723-4.

27. Scott RM, Snitbhan R, Bancroft WH, Alter HJ, Tingpalapong M. Experimental transmission of hepatitis B virus by semen and saliva. *J Infect Dis* 1980;142:67-71.

28. Glaser JB, Nadler JP. Hepatitis B virus in a cardiopulmonary resuscitation training course: risk of transmission from a surface antigen-positive participant. *Arch Intern Med* 1985; 145:1653–5.

29. Osterholm MT, Bravo ER, Crosson JT , et al. Lack of transmission of viral hepatitis type B after oral exposure to HBsAg-positive saliva. *Br Med J* 1979; 2:1263–4.

30. Lifson AR. Do alternate modes for transmission of human immunodeficiency virus exists? A review. *JAMA* 1988;259:1353–6.

31. Friedland GH, Saltzman BR, Rogers MF, et al. Lack of transmission of HTLV-III/LAV infection to household contacts of patients with AIDS or AIDS-related complex with oral candidiasis. *N Engl J Med* 1986; 314:344–9.

32. Curran JW, Jaffe HW, Hardy AM, et al. Epidemiology of HIV infection and AIDS in the United States. *Science* 1988; 239:610–6.

33. Jason JM, McDougall JS, Dixon G, et al. HTLV-III/LAV antibody and immune status of household contacts and sexual partners of persons with hemophilia. *JAMA* 1986; 255:212–5.

34. Wahn V, Kramer HH, Voit T, Bruster HT, Scrampical B, Scheid A. Horizontal transmission of HIV infection between two siblings [Letter]. *Lancet* 1986; 2:694.

35. Kane MA, Lettau LA. Transmission of HBV from dental personnel to patients. *J Am Dent Assoc* 1985;110:634–6.

36. Lettau LA, Smith JD, Williams D, et al. Transmission of hepatitis B virus with resultant restriction of surgical practice. *JAMA* 1986; 255:934–7.

37. International Association of Fire Fighters. *Guidelines to prevent transmission of communicable disease during emergency care for fire fighters, paramedics, and emergency medical technicians.* New York: International Association of Fire Fighters, 1988.

Recommendations for Prevention of HIV Transmission in Health Care Settings[1]

INTRODUCTION

Human immunodeficiency virus (HIV), the virus that causes acquired immunodeficiency syndrome (AIDS), is transmitted through sexual contact and exposure to infected blood or blood components and perinatally from mother to neonate. HIV has been isolated from blood, semen, vaginal secretions, saliva, tears, breast milk, cerebrospinal fluid, amniotic fluid, and urine and is likely to be isolated from other body fluids, secretions, and excretions. However, epidemiologic evidence has implicated only blood, semen, vaginal secretions, and possibly breast milk in transmission.

The increasing prevalence of HIV increases the risk that health-care workers will be exposed to blood from patients infected with HIV, especially when blood and body-fluid precautions are not followed for all patients. Thus, this document emphasizes the need for health-care workers to consider all patients as potentially infected with HIV and/or other bloodborne pathogens and to adhere rigorously to infection-control precautions for minimizing the risk of exposure to blood and body fluids of all patients.

The recommendations contained in this document consolidate and update CDC recommendations published earlier for preventing HIV transmission in health-care settings: precautions for clinical and laboratory staffs (1) and precautions for health-care workers and allied professionals (2); recommendations for preventing HIV transmission in the workplaces (3) and during invasive procedures (4); recommendations for preventing possible transmission of HIV from tears (5); and recommendations for providing dialysis treatment for HIV-infected patients (6). These recommendations also update portions of the "Guideline for Isolation Precautions in Hospitals" (7) and reemphasize some of the recommendations

---

1. Centers for Disease Control, *MMWR* 1987;36(no. 2S):1–18.

contained in "Infection Control Practices for Dentistry" (8). The recommendations contained in this document have been developed for use in health-care settings and emphasize the need to treat blood and other body fluids from all patients as potentially infective. These same prudent precautions also should be taken in other settings in which persons may be exposed to blood or other body fluids.

Definition of Health-Care Workers

Health-care workers are defined as persons, including students and trainees, whose activities involve contact with patients or with blood or other body fluids from patients in a health-care setting.

Health-Care Workers with AIDS

As of July 10, 1987, a total of 1,875 (5.8%) of 32,395 adults with AIDS, who had been reported to the CDC national surveillance system and for whom occupational information was available, reported being employed in a health-care or clinical laboratory setting. In comparison, 6.8 million persons—representing 5.6% of the U.S. labor force—were employed in health services. Of the health-care workers with AIDS, 95% have been reported to exhibit high-risk behavior; for the remaining 5%, the means of HIV acquisition was undetermined. Health-care workers with AIDS were significantly more likely than other workers to have an undetermined risk (5% versus 3%, respectively). For both health-care workers and non–health-care workers with AIDS, the proportion with an undetermined risk has not increased since 1982.

AIDS patients initially reported as not belonging to recognized risk groups are investigated by state and local health departments to determine whether possible risk factors exist. Of all health-care workers with AIDS reported to CDC who were initially characterized as not having an identified risk and for whom follow-up information was available, 66% have been reclassified because risk factors were identified or because the patient was found not to meet the surveillance case definition for AIDS. Of the 87 health-care workers currently categorized as having no identifiable risk, information is incomplete on 16 (18%) because of death or refusal to be interviewed; 38 (44%) are still being investigated. The remaining 33 (38%) health-care workers were interviewed or had other follow-up information available. The occupations of these 33 were as follows: five physicians (15%), three of whom were surgeons; one dentist (3%); three nurses (9%); nine nursing assistants (27%); seven housekeeping or maintenance workers (21%); three clinical laboratory technicians (9%); one therapist (3%); and four others who did not have contact with patients (12%). Although 15 of these 33 health-care workers reported parenteral and/or other nonneedlestick exposure to blood or body fluids from patients in the 10 years preceding their diagnosis of AIDS, none of these exposures involved a patient with AIDS or known HIV infection.

Risk to Health-Care Workers of Acquiring HIV in Health-Care Settings

Health-care workers with documented percutaneous or mucous membrane exposures to blood or body fluids of HIV-infected patients have been prospectively evaluated to determine the risk of infection after such exposures. As of June 30, 1987, 883 health-care workers have been tested for antibody to HIV in an ongoing surveillance project conducted by CDC (9). Of these, 708 (80%) had percutaneous exposures to blood, and 175 (20%) had a mucous membrane or an open wound contaminated by blood or body fluid. Of 396 health-care workers, each of whom had only a convalescent-phase serum sample obtained and tested greater than or equal to 90 days post-exposure, one—for whom heterosexual transmission could not be ruled out—was seropositive for HIV antibody. For 425 additional health-care workers, both acute- and convalescent-phase serum samples were obtained and tested; none of 74 health-care workers with nonpercutaneous exposures seroconverted, and three (0.9%) of 351 with percutaneous exposures seroconverted. None of these three health-care workers had other documented risk factors for infection.

Two other prospective studies to assess the risk of nosocomial acquisition of HIV infection for health-care workers are ongoing in the United States. As of April 30, 1987, 332 health-care workers with a total of 453 needlestick or mucous membrane exposures to the blood or other body fluids of HIV-infected patients were tested for HIV antibody at the National Institutes of Health (10). These exposed workers included 103 with needlestick injuries and 229 with mucous membrane exposures; none had seroconverted. A similar study at the University of California of 129 health-care workers with documented needlestick injuries or mucous membrane exposures to blood or other body fluids from patients with HIV infection has not identified any seroconversions (11). Results of a prospective study in the United Kingdom identified no evidence of transmission among 150 health-care workers with parenteral or mucous membrane exposures to blood or other body fluids, secretions, or excretions from patients with HIV infection (12).

In addition to health-care workers enrolled in prospective studies, eight persons who provided care to infected patients and denied other risk factors have been reported to have acquired HIV infection. Three of these health-care workers had needlestick exposures to blood from infected patients (13–15). Two were persons who provided nursing care to infected persons; although neither sustained a needlestick, both had extensive contact with blood or other body fluids, and neither observed recommended barrier precautions (16,17). The other three were health-care workers with nonneedlestick exposures to blood from infected patients (18). Although the exact route of transmission for these last three infections is not known, all three persons had direct contact of their skin with blood from infected patients, all had skin lesions that may have been contaminated by blood, and one also had a mucous membrane exposure.

A total of 1,231 dentists and hygienists, many of whom practiced in areas with many AIDS cases, participated in a study to determine the prevalence of antibody to HIV; one dentist (0.1%) had HIV antibody. Although no exposure to a known HIV-infected person could be documented, epidemiologic investigation did not identify any other risk factor for infection. The infected dentist, who also had a history of sustaining needlestick injuries and trauma to his hands, did not routinely wear gloves when providing dental care (19).

PRECAUTIONS TO PREVENT TRANSMISSION OF HIV

Universal Precautions

Since medical history and examination cannot reliably identify all patients infected with HIV or other bloodborne pathogens, blood and body-fluid precautions should be consistently used for all patients. This approach, previously recommended by CDC (3,4), and referred to as "universal blood and body-fluid precautions" or "universal precautions," should be used in the care of all patients, especially including those in emergency-care settings in which the risk of blood exposure is increased and the infection status of the patient is usually unknown (20).

1. All health-care workers should routinely use appropriate barrier precautions to prevent skin and mucous membrane exposure when contact with blood or other body fluids of any patient is anticipated. Gloves should be worn for touching blood and body fluids, mucous membranes, or non-intact skin of all patients, for handling items or surfaces soiled with blood or body fluids, and for performing venipuncture and other vascular access procedures. Gloves should be changed after contact with each patient. Masks and protective eyewear or face shields should be worn during procedures that are likely to generate droplets of blood or other body fluids to prevent exposure of mucous membranes of the mouth, nose, and eyes. Gowns or aprons should be worn during procedures that are likely to generate splashes of blood or other body fluids.
2. Hands and other skin surfaces should be washed immediately and thor-

oughly if contaminated with blood or other body fluids. Hands should be washed immediately after gloves are removed.

3. All health-care workers should take precautions to prevent injuries caused by needles, scalpels, and other sharp instruments or devices during procedures; when cleaning used instruments; during disposal of used needles; and when handling sharp instruments after procedures. To prevent needlestick injuries, needles should not be recapped, purposely bent or broken by hand, removed from disposable syringes, or otherwise manipulated by hand. After they are used, disposable syringes and needles, scalpel blades, and other sharp items should be placed in puncture-resistant containers for disposal; the puncture-resistant containers should be located as close as practical to the use area. Large-bore reusable needles should be placed in a puncture-resistant container for transport to the reprocessing area.

4. Although saliva has not been implicated in HIV transmission, to minimize the need for emergency mouth-to-mouth resuscitation, mouthpieces, resuscitation bags, or other ventilation devices should be available for use in areas in which the need for resuscitation is predictable.

5. Health-care workers who have exudative lesions or weeping dermatitis should refrain from all direct patient care and from handling patient-care equipment until the condition resolves.

6. Pregnant health-care workers are not known to be at greater risk of contracting HIV infection than health-care workers who are not pregnant; however, if a health-care worker develops HIV infection during pregnancy, the infant is at risk of infection resulting from perinatal transmission. Because of this risk, pregnant health-care workers should be especially familiar with and strictly adhere to precautions to minimize the risk of HIV transmission.

Implementation of universal blood and body-fluid precautions for all patients eliminates the need for use of the isolation category of "Blood and Body Fluid Precautions" previously recommended by CDC (7) for patients known or suspected to be infected with bloodborne pathogens. Isolation precautions [e.g., enteric, AFB (7)] should be used as necessary if associated conditions, such as infectious diarrhea or tuberculosis, are diagnosed or suspected.

Precautions for Invasive Procedures

In this document, an invasive procedure is defined as surgical entry into tissues, cavities, or organs or repair of major traumatic injuries (a) in an operating or delivery room, emergency department, or outpatient setting, including both physicians' and dentists' offices; (b) cardiac catheterization and angiographic procedures; (c) a vaginal or caesarean delivery or other invasive obstetric procedure during which bleeding may occur; or (d) the manipulation, cutting, or removal of any oral or perioral tissues, including tooth structure, during which bleeding occurs or the potential for bleeding exists. The universal blood and body-fluid precautions listed above, combined with the precautions listed below, should be the minimum precautions for all such invasive procedures.

1. All health-care workers who participate in invasive procedures must routinely use appropriate barrier precautions to prevent skin and mucous membrane contact with blood and other body fluids of all patients. Gloves and surgical masks must be worn for all invasive procedures. Protective eyewear or face shields should be worn for procedures that commonly result in the generation of droplets, splashing of blood or other body fluids, or the generation of bone chips. Gowns or aprons made of materials that provide an effective barrier should be worn during invasive procedures that are likely to result in the splashing of blood or other body fluids. All health-care workers who perform or assist in vaginal or caesarean deliveries should wear gloves and gowns when handling the placenta or the infant until blood and amniotic fluid have been removed from the infant's skin and should wear gloves during postdelivery care of the umbilical cord.
2. If a glove is torn or a needlestick or other injury occurs, the glove should be removed and a new glove used as promptly as patient safety permits; the needle or instrument involved in the incident should also be removed from the sterile field.

Precautions for Dentistry[2]

Blood, saliva, and gingival fluid from all dental patients should be considered infective. Special emphasis should be placed on the following precautions for preventing transmission of bloodborne pathogens in dental practice in both institutional and noninstitutional settings.

1. In addition to wearing gloves for contact with oral mucous membranes of all patients, all dental workers should wear surgical masks and protective eyewear or chin-length plastic face shields during dental procedures in which splashing or spattering of blood, saliva, or gingival fluids is likely. Rubber dams, high-speed evacuation, and proper patient position-

---

2. General infection-control precautions are more specifically addressed in previous recommendations for infection-control practices for dentistry (8).

ing, when appropriate, should be utilized to minimize generation of droplets and spatter.

2. Handpieces should be sterilized after use with each patient, since blood, saliva, or gingival fluid of patients may be aspirated into the handpiece or waterline. Handpieces that cannot be sterilized should at least be flushed, the outside surface cleaned and wiped with a suitable chemical germicide, and then rinsed. Handpieces should be flushed at the beginning of the day and after use with each patient. Manufacturers' recommendations should be followed for use and maintenance of waterlines and check valves and for flushing of handpieces. The same precautions should be used for ultrasonic scalers and air/water syringes.

3. Blood and saliva should be thoroughly and carefully cleaned from material that has been used in the mouth (e.g., impression materials, bite registration), especially before polishing and grinding intraoral devices. Contaminated materials, impressions, and intraoral devices should also be cleaned and disinfected before being handled in the dental laboratory and before they are placed in the patient's mouth. Because of the increasing variety of dental materials used intraorally, dental workers should consult with manufacturers as to the stability of specific materials when using disinfection procedures.

4. Dental equipment and surfaces that are difficult to disinfect (e.g., light handles or X-ray–unit heads) and that may become contaminated should be wrapped with impervious-backed paper, aluminum foil, or clear plastic wrap. The coverings should be removed and discarded, and clean coverings should be put in place after use with each patient.

Precautions for Autopsies or Morticians' Services

In addition to the universal blood and body-fluid precautions listed above, the following precautions should be used by persons performing postmortem procedures:

1. All persons performing or assisting in postmortem procedures should wear gloves, masks, protective eyewear, gowns, and waterproof aprons.
2. Instruments and surfaces contaminated during postmortem procedures should be decontaminated with an appropriate chemical germicide.

Precautions for Dialysis

Patients with end-stage renal disease who are undergoing maintenance dialysis and who have HIV infection can be dialyzed in hospital-based or freestanding dialysis units using conventional infection-control precautions (21). Universal blood and body-fluid precautions should be used when dialyzing all patients.

Strategies for disinfecting the dialysis fluid pathways of the hemodialysis machine are targeted to control bacterial contamination and generally consist of using 500–750 parts per million (ppm) of sodium hypochlorite (household bleach) for 30–40 minutes or 1.5–2.0% formaldehyde overnight. In addition, several chemical germicides formulated to disinfect dialysis machines are commercially available. None of these protocols or procedures need to be changed for dialyzing patients infected with HIV.

Patients infected with HIV can be dialyzed by either hemodialysis or peritoneal dialysis and do not need to be isolated from other patients. The type of dialysis treatment (i.e., hemodialysis or peritoneal dialysis) should be based on the needs of the patient. The dialyzer may be discarded after each use. Alternatively, centers that reuse dialyzes—i.e., a specific single-use dialyzer is issued to a specific patient, removed, cleaned, disinfected, and reused several times on the same patient only—may include HIV-infected patients in the dialyzer reuse program. An individual dialyzer must never be used on more than one patient.

Precautions for Laboratories[3]

Blood and other body fluids from all patients should be considered infective. To supplement the universal blood and body-fluid precautions listed above, the following precautions are recommended for health-care workers in clinical laboratories.

1. All specimens of blood and body fluids should be put in a well-constructed container with a secure lid to prevent leaking during transport. Care should be taken when collecting each specimen to avoid contaminating the outside of the container and of the laboratory form accompanying the specimen.
2. All persons processing blood and body fluid specimens (e.g., removing tops from vacuum tubes) should wear gloves. Masks and protective eyewear should be worn if mucous membrane contact with blood or body fluids is anticipated. Gloves should be changed and hands washed after completion of specimen processing.
3. For routine procedures, such as histologic and pathologic studies or microbiologic culturing, a biological safety cabinet is not necessary. However, biological safety cabinets (Class I or II) should be used

---

3. Additional precautions for research and industrial laboratories are addressed elsewhere (22,23).

whenever procedures are conducted that have a high potential for generating droplets. These include activities such as blending, sonicating, and vigorous mixing.

4. Mechanical pipetting devices should be used for manipulating all liquids in the laboratory. Mouth pipetting must not be done.

5. Use of needles and syringes should be limited to situations in which there is no alternative, and the recommendations for preventing injuries with needles outlined under universal precautions should be followed.

6. Laboratory work surfaces should be decontaminated with an appropriate chemical germicide after a spill of blood or other body fluids and when work activities are completed.

7. Contaminated materials used in laboratory tests should be decontaminated before reprocessing or be placed in bags and disposed of in accordance with institutional policies for disposal of infective waste (24).

8. Scientific equipment that has been contaminated with blood or other body fluids should be decontaminated and cleaned before being repaired in the laboratory or transported to the manufacturer.

9. All persons should wash their hands after completing laboratory activities and should remove protective clothing before leaving the laboratory.

Implementation of universal blood and body fluid precautions for all patients eliminates the need for warning labels on specimens since blood and other body fluids from all patients should be considered infective.

ENVIRONMENTAL CONSIDERATIONS FOR HIV TRANSMISSION

No environmentally mediated mode of HIV transmission has been documented. Nevertheless, the precautions described below should be taken routinely in the care of all patients.

Sterilization and Disinfection

Standard sterilization and disinfection procedures for patient-care equipment currently recommended for use (25,26) in a variety of health-care settings—including hospitals, medical and dental clinics and offices, hemodialysis centers, emergency-care facilities, and long-term nursing-care facilities—are adequate to sterilize or disinfect instruments, devices, or other items contaminated with blood or other body fluids from persons infected with bloodborne pathogens including HIV (21,23).

Instruments or devices that enter sterile tissue or the vascular system of any patient or through which blood flows should be sterilized before reuse. Devices or items that contact intact mucous membranes should be sterilized or receive high-level disinfection, a procedure that kills vegetative organisms and viruses but not necessarily large numbers of bacterial spores. Chemical germicides that are registered with the U.S. Environmental Protection Agency (EPA) as "sterilants" may be used either for sterilization or for high-level disinfection depending on contact time.

Contact lenses used in trial fittings should be disinfected after each fitting by using a hydrogen peroxide contact lens disinfecting system or, if compatible, with heat (78–80° C (172.4–176.0° F)) for 10 minutes.

Medical devices or instruments that require sterilization or disinfection should be thoroughly cleaned before being exposed to the germicide, and the manufacturer's instructions for the use of the germicide should be followed. Further, it is important that the manufacturer's specifications for compatibility of the medical device with chemical germicides be closely followed. Information on specific label claims of commercial germicides can be obtained by writing to the Disinfectants Branch, Office of Pesticides, Environmental Protection Agency, 401 M Street, SW, Washington, DC 20460.

Studies have shown that HIV is inactivated rapidly after being exposed to commonly used chemical germicides at concentrations that are much lower than used in practice (27–30). Embalming fluids are similar to the types of chemical germicides that have been tested and found to completely inactivate HIV. In addition to commercially available chemical germicides, a solution of sodium hypochlorite (household bleach) prepared daily is an inexpensive and effective germicide. Concentrations ranging from approximately 500 ppm (1:100 dilution of household bleach) sodium hypochlorite to 5,000 ppm (1:10 dilution of household bleach) are effective depending on the amount of organic material (e.g., blood, mucus) present on the surface to be cleaned and disinfected. Commercially available chemical germicides may be more compatible with certain medical devices that might be corroded by repeated exposure to sodium hypochlorite, especially to the 1:10 dilution.

Survival of HIV in the Environment

The most extensive study on the survival of HIV after drying involved greatly concentrated HIV samples, i.e., 10 million tissue culture infectious doses per milliliter (31). This concentration is at least 100,000 times greater than that typically found in the blood or serum of patients with HIV infection. HIV was detectable by tissue-culture techniques 1–3 days after drying, but the rate of inactivation was rapid. Studies performed at CDC have also shown that drying HIV causes a rapid (within several hours) 1–2 log (90–99%) reduction in HIV concentration. In tissue culture fluid, cell-free HIV could be detected up to 15 days at room temperature, up to 11 days at 37° C (98.6° F), and up to 1 day if the HIV was cell-associated.

When considered in the context of environmental conditions in health-care facilities, these results do not require any changes in currently recommended sterilization, disinfection, or housekeeping strategies. When medical devices are contaminated with blood or other body fluids, existing recommendations include the cleaning of these instruments, followed by disinfection or sterilization, depending on the type of medical device. These protocols assume "worst-case" conditions of extreme virologic and microbiologic contamination, and whether viruses have been inactivated after drying plays no role in formulating these strategies. Consequently, no changes in published procedures for cleaning, disinfecting, or sterilizing need to be made.

Housekeeping

Environmental surfaces such as walls, floors, and other surfaces are not associated with transmission of infections to patients or health-care workers. Therefore, extraordinary attempts to disinfect or sterilize these environmental surfaces are not necessary. However, cleaning and removal of soil should be done routinely. Cleaning schedules and methods vary according to the area of the hospital or institution, type of surface to be cleaned, and the amount and type of soil present. Horizontal surfaces (e.g., bedside tables and hard-surfaced flooring) in patient-care areas are usually cleaned on a regular basis, when soiling or spills occur, and when a patient is discharged. Cleaning of walls, blinds, and curtains is recommended only if they are visibly soiled. Disinfectant fogging is an unsatisfactory method of decontaminating air and surfaces and is not recommended.

Disinfectant-detergent formulations registered by EPA can be used for cleaning environmental surfaces, but the actual physical removal of microorganisms by scrubbing is probably at least as important as any antimicrobial effect of the cleaning agent used. Therefore, cost, safety, and acceptability by housekeepers can be the main criteria for selecting any such registered agent. The manufacturer's instructions for appropriate use should be followed.

Cleaning and Decontaminating Spills of Blood or Other Body Fluids

Chemical germicides that are approved for use as "hospital disinfectants" and are tuberculocidal when used at recommended dilutions can be used to decontaminate spills of blood and other body fluids. Strategies for decontaminating spills of blood and other body fluids in a patient-care setting are different than for spills of cultures or other materials in clinical, public health, or research laboratories. In patient-care areas, visible material should first be removed and then the area should be decontaminated with large spills of cultured or concentrated infectious agents in the laboratory, the contaminated area should be flooded with a liquid germicide before cleaning, then decontaminated with fresh germicidal chemicals. In both settings, gloves should be worn during the cleaning and decontaminating procedures.

Laundry

Although soiled linen has been identified as a source of large numbers of certain pathogenic microorganisms, the risk of actual disease transmission is negligible. Rather than rigid procedures and specifications, hygienic and common-sense storage and processing of clean and soiled linen are recommended (26). Soiled linen should be handled as little as possible and with minimum agitation to prevent gross microbial contamination of the air and of persons handling the linen. All soiled linen should be bagged at the location where it was used; it should not be sorted or rinsed in patient-care areas. Linen soiled with blood or body fluids should be placed and transported in bags that prevent leakage. If hot water is used, linen should be washed with detergent in water at least 71° C (160° F) for 25 minutes. If low-temperature (less than or equal to 70° C (158° F) laundry cycles are used, chemicals suitable for low-temperature washing at proper use concentration should be used.

Infective Waste

There is no epidemiologic evidence to suggest that most hospital waste is any more infective than residential waste. Moreover, there is no epidemiologic evidence that hospital waste has caused disease in the community as a result of improper disposal. Therefore, identifying wastes for which special precautions are indicated is largely a matter of judgment about the relative risk of disease transmission. The most practical approach to the management of infective waste is to identify those wastes with the potential for causing infection during handling and disposal and for which some special precautions appear prudent. Hospital wastes for which special precautions appear prudent include microbiology laboratory waste, pathology waste, and blood specimens or blood products. While any item that has had contact with blood, exudates, or secretions may be potentially infective, it is not usually considered practical or necessary to treat all such waste as infective (23,26). Infective waste, in general, should either be incinerated or should be autoclaved before disposal in a sanitary landfill. Bulk blood, suctioned fluids, excretions, and secretions may be carefully poured down a drain connected to a sanitary sewer. Sanitary sewers may also be used to dispose of other infectious wastes capable of being ground and flushed into the sewer.

Implementation of Recommended Precautions

Employers of health-care workers should ensure that policies exist for:

1. Initial orientation and continuing education and training of all health-care workers—including students and trainees—on the epidemiology, modes of transmission, and prevention of HIV and other bloodborne infections and the need for routine use of universal blood and body fluid precautions for all patients.
2. Provision of equipment and supplies necessary to minimize the risk of infection with HIV and other bloodborne pathogens.
3. Monitoring adherence to recommended protective measures. When monitoring reveals a failure to follow recommended precautions, counseling, education, and/or retraining should be provided, and, if necessary, appropriate disciplinary action should be considered.

Professional associations and labor organizations, through continuing education efforts, should emphasize the need for health-care workers to follow recommended precautions.

SEROLOGIC TESTING FOR HIV INFECTION

Background

A person is identified as infected with HIV when a sequence of tests, starting with repeated enzyme immunoassays (EIA) and including a Western blot or similar, more specific assay, are repeatedly reactive. Persons infected with HIV usually develop antibody against the virus within 6–12 weeks after infection.

The sensitivity of the currently licensed EIA tests is at least 99% when they are performed under optimal laboratory conditions on serum specimens from persons infected for greater than or equal to 12 weeks. Optimal laboratory conditions include the use of reliable reagents, provision of continuing education of personnel, quality control of procedures, and participation in performance-evaluation programs. Given this performance, the probability of a false-negative test is remote except during the first several weeks after infection, before detectable antibody is present. The proportion of infected persons with a false-negative test attributed to absence of antibody in the early stages of infection is dependent on both the incidence and prevalence of HIV infection in a population (Table I1).

The specificity of the currently licensed EIA tests is approximately 99% when repeatedly reactive tests are considered. Repeat testing of initially reactive specimens by EIA is required to reduce the likelihood of laboratory error. To increase further the specificity of serologic tests, laboratories must use a supplemental test, most often the Western blot, to validate repeatedly reactive EIA results. Under optimal laboratory conditions, the sensitivity of the Western blot test is comparable to or greater than that of a repeatedly reactive EIA, and the Western blot is highly specific when strict criteria are used to interpret the test results. The testing sequence of a repeatedly reactive EIA and a positive Western blot test is highly predictive of HIV infection, even in a population with a low prevalence of infection (Table I2). If the Western blot test result is indeterminant, the testing sequence is considered equivocal for HIV infection. When this occurs, the Western blot test should be repeated on the same serum sample, and, if still indeterminant, the testing sequence should be repeated on a sample collected 3–6 months later. Use of other

Table I1 Estimated annual number of patients infected with HIV not detected by HIV-antibody testing in a hypothetical hospital with 10,000 admissions/year[a]

Beginning prevalence of HIV infection	Annual incidence of HIV infection	Approximate no. of HIV-infected patients	Approximate no. of HIV-infected patients not detected
5.0%	1.0%	550	17–18
5.0%	0.5%	525	11–12
1.0%	0.2%	110	3–4
1.0%	0.1%	105	2–3
0.1%	0.02%	11	0–1
0.1%	0.01%	11	0–1

[a]The estimates are based on the following assumptions: (1) the sensitivity of the screening test is 99% (i.e., 99% of HIV-infected persons with antibody will be detected); (2) persons infected with HIV will not develop detectable antibody (seroconvert) until 6 weeks (1.5 months) after infection; (3) new infections occur at an equal rate throughout the year; (4) calculations of the number of HIV-infected persons in the patient population are based on the mid-year prevalence, which is the beginning prevalence plus half the annual incidence of infections.

Table I2 Predictive value of positive HIV-antibody tests in hypothetical populations
with different prevalences of infection

	Prevalence of infection	Predictive value of positive tests[a]
Repeatedly reactive enzyme	0.2%	28.41%
immunoassay (EIA)[b]	2.0%	80.16%
	20.0%	98.02%
Repeatedly reactive EIA	0.2%	99.75%
followed by positive Western	2.0%	99.97%
blot (WB)[c]	20.0%	99.99%

[a]Proportion of person with positive test results who are actually infected with HIV.

[b]Assumes EIA sensitivity of 99.0% and specificity of 99.5%.

[c]Assumes WB sensitivity of 99.0% and specificity of 99.9%.

supplemental tests may aid in interpreting results on samples that are persistently
indeterminant by Western blot.

Testing of Patients

Previous CDC recommendations have emphasized the value of HIV serologic
testing of patients for: (a) management of parenteral or mucous membrane exposures of health-care workers, (b) patient diagnosis and management, and (c)
counseling and serologic testing to prevent and control HIV transmission in the
community. In addition, more recent recommendations have stated that hospitals,
in conjunction with state and local health departments, should periodically determine the prevalence of HIV infection among patients from age groups at highest
risk of infection (32).

Adherence to universal blood and body fluid precautions recommended for
the care of all patients will minimize the risk of transmission of HIV and other
bloodborne pathogens from patients to health-care workers. The utility of routine
HIV serologic testing of patients as an adjunct to universal precautions is unknown.
Results of such testing may not be available in emergency or outpatient settings.
In addition, some recently infected patients will not have detectable antibody to
HIV (Table I1).

Personnel in some hospitals have advocated serologic testing of patients in
settings in which exposure of health-care workers to large amounts of patients'
blood may be anticipated. Specific patients for whom serologic testing has been

advocated include those undergoing major operative procedures and those undergoing treatment in critical care units, especially if they have conditions involving uncontrolled bleeding. Decisions regarding the need to establish testing programs for patients should be made by physicians or individual institutions.

In addition, when deemed appropriate, testing of individual patients may be performed on agreement between the patient and the physician providing care. In addition to the universal precautions recommended for all patients, certain additional precautions for the care of HIV-infected patients undergoing major surgical operations have been proposed by personnel in some hospitals. For example, surgical procedures on an HIV-infected patient might be altered so that hand-to-hand passing of sharp instruments would be eliminated; stapling instruments rather than hand-suturing equipment might be used to perform tissue approximation; electrocautery devices rather than scalpels might be used as cutting instruments; and, even though uncomfortable, gowns that totally prevent seepage of blood onto the skin of members of the operative team might be worn. While such modifications might further minimize the risk of HIV infection for members of the operative team, some of these techniques could result in prolongation of operative time and could potentially have an adverse effect on the patient.

Testing programs, if developed, should include the following principles:

- Obtaining consent for testing.
- Informing patients of test results, and providing counseling for seropositive patients by properly trained persons.
- Assuring that confidentiality safeguards are in place to limit knowledge of test results to those directly involved in the care of infected patients or as required by law.
- Assuring that identification of infected patients will not result in denial of needed care or provision of suboptimal care.
- Evaluating prospectively (a) the efficacy of the program in reducing the incidence of parenteral, mucous membrane, or significant cutaneous exposures of health-care workers to the blood or other body fluids of HIV-infected patients and (b) the effect of modified procedures on patients.

Testing of Health-Care Workers

Although transmission of HIV from infected health-care workers to patients has not been reported, transmission during invasive procedures remains a possibility. Transmission of hepatitis B virus (HBV)—a bloodborne agent with a considerably greater potential for nosocomial spread—from health-care workers to patients has been documented. Such transmission has occurred in situations (e.g., oral and gynecologic surgery) in which health-care workers, when tested, had very high concentrations of HBV in their blood (at least 100 million infectious virus particles per milliliter, a concentration much higher than occurs with HIV infection), and the health-care workers sustained a puncture wound while performing invasive procedures or had exudative or weeping lesions or microlacerations that allowed virus to contaminate instruments or open wounds of patients (33,34).

The hepatitis B experience indicates that only those health-care workers who perform certain types of invasive procedures have transmitted HBV to patients. Adherence to recommendations in this document will minimize the risk of transmission of HIV and other bloodborne pathogens from health-care workers to patients during invasive procedures. Since transmission of HIV from infected health-care workers performing invasive procedures to their patients has not been reported and would be expected to occur only very rarely, if at all, the utility of routine testing of such health-care workers to prevent transmission of HIV cannot be assessed. If consideration is given to developing a serologic testing program for health-care workers who perform invasive procedures, the frequency of testing, as well as the issues of consent, confidentiality, and consequences of test results—as previously outlined for testing programs for patients—must be addressed.

Management of Infected Health-Care Workers

Health-care workers with impaired immune systems resulting from HIV infection or other causes are at increased risk of acquiring or experiencing serious complications of infectious disease. Of particular concern is the risk of severe infection following exposure to patients with infectious diseases that are easily transmitted if appropriate precautions are not taken (e.g., measles, varicella). Any health-care worker with an impaired immune system should be counseled about the potential risk associated with taking care of patients with any transmissible infection and should continue to follow existing recommendations for infection control to minimize risk of exposure to other infectious agents (7,35). Recommendations of the Immunization Practices Advisory Committee (ACIP) and institutional policies concerning requirements for vaccinating health-care workers with live virus vaccines (e.g., measles, rubella) should also be considered.

The question of whether workers infected with HIV—especially those who perform invasive procedures—can adequately and safely be allowed to perform patient-care duties or whether their work assignments should be changed must be determined on an individual basis. These decisions should be made by the health-care worker's personal physician(s) in conjunction with the medical directors and personnel health service staff of the employing institution or hospital.

Management of Exposures

If a health-care worker has a parenteral (e.g., needlestick or cut) or mucous membrane (e.g., splash to the eye or mouth) exposure to blood or other body fluids or has a cutaneous exposure involving large amounts of blood or prolonged contact with blood—especially when the exposed skin is chapped, abraded, or afflicted with dermatitis—the source patient should be informed of the incident and tested for serologic evidence of HIV infection after consent is obtained. Policies should be developed for testing source patients in situations in which consent cannot be obtained (e.g., an unconscious patient).

If the source patient has AIDS, is positive for HIV antibody, or refuses the test, the health-care worker should be counseled regarding the risk of infection and evaluated clinically and serologically for evidence of HIV infections as soon as possible after the exposure. The health-care worker should be advised to report and seek medical evaluation for any acute febrile illness that occurs within 12 weeks after the exposure. Such an illness—particularly one characterized by fever, rash, or lymphadenopathy—may be indicative of recent HIV infection. Seronegative health-care workers should be retested 6 weeks post-exposure and on a periodic basis thereafter (e.g., 12 weeks and 6 months after exposure) to determine whether transmission has occurred. During this follow-up period—especially the first 6–12 weeks after exposure, when most infected persons are expected to seroconvert—exposed health-care workers should follow U.S. Public Health Service (PHS) recommendations for preventing transmission of HIV (36,37).

No further follow-up of a health-care worker exposed to infection as described above is necessary if the source patient is seronegative unless the source patient is at high risk of HIV infection. In the latter case, a subsequent specimen (e.g., 12 weeks following exposure) may be obtained from the health-care worker for antibody testing. If the source patient cannot be identified, decisions regarding appropriate follow-up should be individualized. Serologic testing should be available to all health-care workers who are concerned that they may have been infected with HIV.

If a patient has a parenteral or mucous membrane exposure to blood or other body fluid of a health-care worker, the patient should be informed of the incident, and the same procedure outlined above for management of exposures should be followed for both the source health-care worker and the exposed patient.

REFERENCES

1. CDC. Acquired immunodeficiency syndrome (AIDS): precautions for clinical and laboratory staffs. *MMWR* 1982;31:577–80.

2. CDC. Acquired immunodeficiency syndrome (AIDS): precautions for health-care workers and allied professionals. *MMWR* 1983;32:450–1.

3. CDC. Recommendations for preventing transmission of infection with human T-lymphotropic virus type III/lymphadenopathy-associated virus in the workplace. *MMWR* 1985;34:681–6, 691–5.

4. CDC. Recommendations for preventing transmission of infection with human T-lymphotropic virus type III/lymphadenopathy-associated virus during invasive procedures. *MMWR* 1986;35:221–3.

5. CDC. Recommendations for preventing possible transmission of human T-lymphotropic virus type III/lymphadenopathy-associated virus from tears. *MMWR* 1985;34:533–4.

6. CDC. Recommendations for providing dialysis treatment to patients infected with human T-lymphotropic virus type III/lymphadenopathy-associated virus infection. *MMWR* 1986;35:376–8, 383.

7. Garner JS, Simmons BP. Guideline for isolation precautions in hospitals. *Infect Control* 1983;4 (suppl):245–325 .

8. CDC. Recommended infection control practices for dentistry. *MMWR* 1986;35:237–42.

9. McCray E, the Cooperative Needlestick Surveillance Group. Occupational risk of the acquired immunodeficieney syndrome among health care workers. *N Engl J Med* 1986;314:1127–32.

10. Henderson DK, Saah AJ, Zak BJ, et al. Risk of nosocomial infection with human T-cell lymphotropic virus type III/lymphadenopathy-associated virus in a large cohort of intensively exposed health are workers. *Ann Intern Med* 1986;104:644–7.

11. Gerberding JL, Bryant-LeBlanc CE, Nelson K, et al. Risk of transmitting the human immunodeficiency virus, cytomegalovirus, and hepatitis B virus to health care workers exposed to patients with AIDS and AIDS-related conditions. *J Infect Dis* 1987;156:1–8.

12. McEvoy M, Porter K, Mortimer P, Simmons N, Shanson D. Prospective study of clinical, laboratory, and ancillary staff with accidental exposures to blood or other body fluids from patients infected with HIV. *Br Med J* 1987;294:1595–7.

13. Anonymous. Needlestick transmission of HTLV-III from a patient infected in Africa. *Lancet* 1984;2:1376–7.

14. Oksenhendler E, Harzic M, Le Roux JM, Rabian C, Clauvel JP. HIV infection with seroconversion after a superficial needlestick injury to the finger. *N Engl J Med* 1986;315:582.

15. Neisson-Vernant C, Arfi S, Mathez D, Leibowitch J, Monplaisir N. Needlestick HIV seroconversion in a nurse. *Lancet* 1986;2:814.

16. Grint P, McEvoy M. Two associated cases of the acquired immune deficiency syndrome (AIDS). *PHLS Commun Dis Rep* 1985;42:4.

17. CDC. Apparent transmission of human T-lymphotropic virus type

III/lymphadenopathy-associated virus from a child to a mother providing health care. *MMWR* 1986,35:76–9.

18. CDC. Update: human immunodeficiency virus infections in health-care workers exposed to blood of infected patients. *MMWR* 1987;36:285–9.

19. Kline RS, Phelan J, Friedland GH, et al. Low occupational risk for HIV infection for dental professionals [Abstract]. In: *Abstracts from the III International Conference on AIDS,* June 1-5 1985, Washington, DC:155.

20. Baker JL, Kelen GD, Sivertson KT, Quinn TC. Unsuspected human immunodeficiency virus in critically ill emergency patients. *JAMA* 1987;257:2609–11.

21. Favero MS. Dialysis-associated diseases and their control. In: Bennett JV, Brachman PS, eds. *Hospital infections.* Boston: Little, Brown, 1985:267–84.

22. Richardson JH, Barkley WE, eds. *Biosafety in microbiological and biomedical laboratories, 1984.* Washington, DC: U.S. Department of Health and Human Services, Public Health Service. HHS publication no. (CDC)84-8395.

23. CDC. Human T-lymphotropic virus type III/lymphadenopathy-associated virus: agent summary statement. *MMWR* 1986;35:540–2, 547–9.

24. Environmental Protection Agency. *EPA guide for infectious waste management.* Washington, DC: U.S. Environmental Protection Agency, May 1986 publication no. EPA/530-SW-86-014.

25. Favero MS. Sterilization, disinfection, and antisepsis in the hospital. In: *Manual of clinical microbiology.* 4th ed. Washington, DC: American Society for Microbiology, 1985;129–37.

26. Garner JS, Favero MS. *Guideline for handwashing and hospital environmental control, 1985.* Atlanta: Public Health Service, Centers for Disease Control, 1985. HHS publication no. 991117.

27. Spire B, Montagnier L, Barre-Sinoussi F, Chermann JC. Inactivation of lymphadenopathy associated virus by chemical disinfectants. *Lancet* 1984;2:899–901.

28. Martin LS, McDougall JS, Loskoski SL. Disinfection and inactivation of the human T lymphotropic virus type III/lymphadenopathy-associated virus. *J Infect Dis* 1985;152:400–3.

29. McDougal JS, Martin LS, Cort SP, et al. Thermal inactivation of the acquired immunodeficiency syndrome virus-III/lymphadenopathy-associated virus, with special reference to antihemophilic factor. *J Clin Invest* 1985;76:875–7.

30. Spire B, Barre-Sinoussi F, Dormont D, Montagnier L, Chermann JC. Inactivation of lymphadenopathy-associated virus by heat, gamma rays, and ultraviolet light. *Lancet* 1985;1:188–9.

31. Resnik L, Veren K, Salahuddin SZ, Tondreau S, Markham PD. Stability and inactivation of HTLV-III/LAV under clinical and laboratory environments. *JAMA* 1986;255:1887–91.

32. CDC. Public Health Service (PHS) guidelines for counseling and antibody testing to prevent HIV infection and AIDS. *MMWR* 1987;3:509–15.
33. Kane MA, Lethu LA. Transmission of HBV from dental personnel to patients. *J Am Dent Assoc* 1985;110:634–6.
34. Lettau LA, Smith JD, Williams D, et al. Transmission of hepatitis B with resultant restriction of surgical practice. *JAMA* 1986;255:934–7.
35. Williams WW. Guideline for infection control in hospital personnel. *Infect Control* 1983;4(suppl):326–9.
36. CDC. Prevention of acquired immune deficiency syndrome (AIDS): report of inter-agency recommendations. *MMWR* 1983;32:101–3.
37. CDC. Provisional Public Health Service inter-agency recommendations for screening donated blood and plasma for antibody to the virus causing acquired immunodeficiency syndrome. *MMWR* 1985;34:1–5.

Index